Introduction to
Renal Therapeutics

Introduction to Renal Therapeutics

Edited by

Caroline Ashley

MSc, BPharm (Hons), MRPharmS
Lead Specialist Pharmacist, Renal Services
Royal Free Hospital
Royal Free Hampstead NHS Trust
London, UK

Clare Morlidge

BPharm (Hons), DipClinPharm, MRPharmS
Cardiothoracic Directorate Pharmacist
Lister Hospital
East and North Hertfordshire NHS Trust
Hertfordshire, UK

On behalf of the UK Renal Pharmacy Group

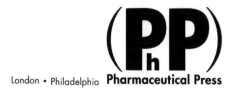

London • Philadelphia **Pharmaceutical Press**

Published by Pharmaceutical Press

1 Lambeth High Street, London SE1 7JN, UK

University City Science Center, Suite 5E, 3624 Market Street,
Philadelphia, USA, PA 19104

© Pharmaceutical Press 2008

(**PP**) is a trade mark of Pharmaceutical Press

Pharmaceutical Press is the publishing division of the Royal
Pharmaceutical Society of Great Britain

First published 2008

Typeset by Photoprint Torquay, Devon, United Kingdom
Printed and bound by CPI Group (UK) Ltd, Croydon, CT0 4YY

ISBN 978 0 85369 688 9

A catalogue record for this book is available from the British Library.

Contents

Preface

Welcome to the first edition of the *Introduction to Renal Therapeutics*. In 1995, the UK Renal Pharmacy Group recognised that there was a lack of readily accessible information for pharmacists, either with an interest in renal medicine, or newly appointed as specialist practitioners in the renal field. As a result, members of the RPG wrote and produced the *Beginner's Guide to Renal Pharmacy*. It was designed to be a comprehensive introductory guide to the causes, effects and management of renal failure, and as such, a copy has since been given to each new member of the RPG. In addition, the *Beginner's Guide* has become required reading for some post-graduate pharmacy courses.

The *Beginner's Guide* has now been updated and expanded to become the *Introduction to Renal Therapeutics*. This guide has been written by practising renal pharmacists and other healthcare professionals who work in renal units. The mix of authors and the depth of their 'hands on' experience has been used to provide a text that directs the reader to the important factors in renal therapies. It highlights points that may not be readily accessible in any other single text, but still bears in mind the practitioner new to renal pharmacy.

This book is not meant to be exclusive to pharmacists working in renal units, but should be used by all those who wish to familiarise themselves with the issues concerning drug therapy for the renally impaired. The aim of this book is to help pharmacy students, pharmacists and other healthcare workers to understand and promote the safe and effective use of drug therapies in renal failure.

The case studies and questions have been kept separate from the answers in order to encourage readers to formulate their own answers before reading the author's. The answers section illustrates how the questions should be approached and what factors need to be taken into consideration when formulating a response. The answers are based on clinical opinion at the time of writing, but they also represent, to some degree, the opinions of the authors themselves. As time passes and new drugs and new information become available, some readers may disagree with the decisions arrived at by the authors, which is entirely appropriate.

We would like to take this opportunity to thank all those pharmacists, dieticians and nurses who have contributed chapters for this book. Writing these chapters requires an enormous amount of time and effort, and everyone has given unstintingly of both. We hope that this book will be of use to all those pharmacists who aspire to become a specialist renal pharmacist, as well as those who just wish to improve their renal knowledge.

Caroline Ashley
Clare Morlidge
July 2007

About the editors

Clare Morlidge BPharm (Hons), DipClinPharm, MRPharmS graduated from Bradford University, and undertook the clinical pharmacy diploma whilst working as a basic grade pharmacist in Worcester Hospital. Clare moved to Walsgrave Hospital, Coventry where she worked as a renal pharmacist for a number of years. During this time Clare wrote articles in the *Pharmaceutical Journal, Nephrology Dialysis and Transplantation* and *British Journal of Renal Medicine*. She was also involved in writing the renal unit's *Help I've got Renal Failure* book, Dr Andy Stein's *Kidney Dialysis and Transplantation*, and was on the editorial board for the Renal Pharmacy Group's *Renal Drug Handbook* 2004 edition.

Clare currently works at the Lister Hospital in Stevenage as a senior cardiothoracic pharmacist.

Caroline A Ashley MSc, BPharm (Hons), MRPharmS has worked as a hospital pharmacist for 20 years, and is currently the lead specialist pharmacist for renal services at the Royal Free Hospital in London. She is the Chair of the UK Renal Pharmacy Group, has served on the Council of the British Renal Society, and was involved with the development of the Renal National Service Framework.

Caroline studied pharmacy at the School of Pharmacy, University of London, and later gained an MSc in Clinical Pharmacology from the University of East London. Her interest in renal medicine began during her time as a basic grade pharmacist at Guy's Hospital, and she has been specialist renal pharmacist at the Royal Free since 1991. She is co-editor of the *Renal Drug Handbook* and has written numerous articles for various pharmacy journals, including the *Pharmaceutical Journal* and *Hospital Pharmacist*. In addition, she has contributed chapters to several books, including *Drugs in Use*, and the forthcoming edition of the *Oxford Textbook of Medicine*. She has recently been invited to join the editorial board of the *British Journal of Renal Medicine*.

Contributors

Caroline Ashley MSc, BPharm (Hons), MRPharmS
Lead Specialist Pharmacist, Renal Services, Royal Free Hospital Hampstead NHS Trust, London

Stephen Ashmore MPhil, BPharm, MRPharmS
Clinical Pharmacy Team Leader, Acute Medicine/ Renal Medicine, Leeds General Infirmary, Leeds Teaching Hospitals NHS Trust

Robert Bradley MSc, BPharm, MRPharmS
Lead Pharmacist for Nephrology and Renal Transplantation, University Hospital of Wales, Cardiff & Vale NHS Trust

Aileen Currie BSc (Hons), MRPharmS
Renal Pharmacist, Crosshouse Hospital, Kilmarnock

John Dade BPharm, MPharm, MRPharmS
Clinical Pharmacist – Critical Care, St James's University Hospital, Leeds Teaching Hospitals NHS Trust

Andrea Devaney BPharm, DipClinPharm, MRPharmS
Renal Pharmacy Team Manager, Oxford Transplant Centre, Oxford Radcliffe Hospitals NHS Trust

James Dunleavy BSc, MSc, MRPharmS
Senior Clinical Pharmacist – Renal Services, Monklands Hospital, Airdrie, Lanarkshire

Roger Fernandes MSc, BPharm, MRPharmS
Deputy Chief Pharmacist, Mayday University Hospital, Croydon

Diane Green BSc (Hons), SRD
Dietetic Manager, Hope Hospital, Salford PCT

Elizabeth Lamerton BSc, DipClinPharm, MRPharmS
Senior Clinical Pharmacist, Renal Medicine, Salford Royal NHS Foundation Trust

Mark Lee BSc (Hons), MRPharmS
Advanced Level Pharmacist, Renal Transplant, Leeds Teaching Hospitals NHS Trust

Anne Millsop BSc (Hons), DipClinPharm, Cert Clin Pharm Teach, MRPharmS
Renal Pharmacist, Oxford Transplant Centre, Oxford Radcliffe Hospitals NHS Trust

Clare Morlidge BPharm (Hons), DipClinPharm, MRPharmS
Cardiothoracic Pharmacist, Lister Hospital, Stevenage

Emma Murphy RN, DipNurStudies
Clinical Nurse Specialist – Renal Palliative Care – Modernisation Initiative, Guy's and St Thomas' NHS Foundation Trust, London

Fliss Murtagh EM, MRCGP, MSc
Clinical Research Training Fellow, Dept of Palliative Care, Policy & Rehabilitation, King's College London

Mrudula Patel MSc, BPharm, DipClinPharm Pract, MRPharmS
Renal Directorate Pharmacist, Churchill Hospital, Oxford

Susan Patey BSc (Pharmacy), MRPharmS
Lead Pharmacist, Nephrology, Great Ormond
Street Hospital for Children NHS Trust London

Jane Pearson BSc (Hons), DipClinPharm, MRPharmS
Senior Pharmacist Renal Medicine, Royal
Infirmary of Edinburgh

John Sexton, MSc, BPharm (Hons), MCPP, MRPharmS
Principal Pharmacist Lecturer-Practitioner, Royal
Liverpool and Broadgreen University Hospitals
NHS Trust & Liverpool John Moores University

Zoe Thain BSc, DipClinPharm, MRPharmS
Senior Pharmacist, Renal Services, Lancashire
Teaching Hospitals NHS Trust

Marc Vincent BPharm, DipClinPharm, MRPharmS
Lead Pharmacist Renal Services, Manchester
Royal Infirmary

Hayley Wells MSc, BPharm, MRPharmS
Senior Clinical Pharmacist, Renal Services, Guy's
and St. Thomas' NHS Foundation Trust, London

Abbreviations

ACE	angiotensin-converting enzyme
ACR	albumin:creatinine ratio
ACT	activated clotting time
ADH	antidiuretic hormone
ADPKD	autosomal dominant polycystic disease
AERD	aspirin-exacerbated respiratory disease
AGE	advanced glycation end-products
AIN	acute interstitial nephritis
AMR	antibody-mediated rejection
ANA	antinuclear antibodies
ANCA	antineutrophil cytoplasmic antibodies
APA	anti-phospholipid antibodies
APC	antigen-presenting cells
APD	automated peritoneal dialysis
APTT	activated partial thromboplastin time
ARF	acute renal failure
AT-II	angiotensin II
ATG	antithymocyte globulin
ATN	acute tubular necrosis
ATP	adenosine triphosphate
AUC	area under the curve
BP	blood pressure
BSA	body surface area
BUN	blood urea nitrogen
CAN	chronic allograft nephropathy
CAPD	continuous ambulatory peritoneal dialysis
CAVH/CAVHF	continuous arterio-venous haemofiltration
CAVHD	continuous arterio-venous haemodialysis
CAVHDF	continuous arterio-venous haemodiafiltration
CCPD	continuous cycling peritoneal dialysis
CHD	coronary heart disease
CKD	chronic kidney disease
CMV	cytomegalovirus
CNI	calcineurin inhibitor
CNS	central nervous system
COX	cyclo-oxygenase
CrCl	creatinine clearance

CRF	chronic renal failure
CRP	C-reactive protein
CRRT	continuous renal replacement therapy
CSS	Churg–Strauss syndrome
CT	computed tomography
CVP	central venous pressure
CVS	cerebrovascular system
CVVH/CVVHF	continuous veno-venous haemofiltration
CVVHDF	continuous veno-venous haemodiafiltration
DGF	delayed graft function
DIC	disseminated intravascular coagulation
DNA	deoxyribonucleic acid
DSA	donor specific antibodies
DTPA	diethylenetriamine penta-acetic acid
DVT	deep vein thrombosis
EABV	effective arteriolar blood volume
EBCT	electron beam computed tomography
EBPG	European Best Practice guidelines
EBV	Epstein-Barr virus
ECG	electrocardiogram
ECHO	echocardiogram
EDTA	ethylenediamine tetra-acetic acid
eGFR	estimated glomerular filtration rate
EHIC	European Health Insurance Card
ESA	erythropoiesis-stimulating agent
ESR	erythrocyte sedimentation rate
ESRD	end stage renal disease
ESRF	end stage renal failure
GBM	glomerular basement membrane
GFR	glomerular filtration rate
GI	gastrointestinal
GLP-1	glucagon-like peptide 1
H3G	hydromorphone-3-glucuronide
HD	intermittent haemodialysis
HDU	high dependency unit
HES	hydroxyethyl starch
HIT	heparin-induced thrombocytopenia
HIV	human immunodeficiency virus
HLA	human leukocyte antigens
HMG-CoA	3-hydroxy-3-methylglutaryl coenzyme A
HPT	hyperparathyroidism
HRT	hormone replacement therapy
HSP	Henoch–Schönlein purpura
HUS	haemolytic uraemic syndrome
IBW	ideal body weight
ICU	intensive care unit
IDDM	insulin-dependent diabetes mellitus
IDH	ischaemic heart disease
IDPN	intradialytic parenteral nutrition
IL-2	interleukin-2

IM	intramuscular
INR	international normalised ratio
IP	intraperitoneally
iu	international units
IV	intravenous
IVP	intravenous pyelogram
IVU	intravenous excretory urogram
KCTT	kaolin cephalin clotting time
LFT	liver function test
LMWH	low molecular weight heparin
LVF	left ventricular failure
LVH	left ventricular hypertrophy
M3G	morphine-3-glucuronide
M6G	morphine-6-glucuronide
MAM	monoacetylmorphine
MDRD	modified diet in renal disease
MHC	major histocompatibility complex
MHRA	Medicines and Healthcare Products Regulatory Agency
MI	myocardial infarction
MMF	mycophenolate mofetil
MPA	mycophenolic acid OR microscopic angitis
MPO	myeloperoxidase
M/R	modified release
MRI	magnetic resonance imaging
MRSA	methicillin-resistant *Staphylococcus aureus*
MTOR	mammalian target of rapamycin
mw	molecular weight
NICE	National Institute for Health and Clinical Excellence
NIDDM	non-insulin-dependent diabetes mellitus
NKF-K/DOQU	National Kidney Federation Dialysis Outcomes Quality Initiative
NMDA	*N*-methyl-D-aspartate
NNH	number needed to harm
NNT	number needed to treat
NSAID	non-steroidal anti-inflammatory drug
OD	once daily
OHA	oral hypoglycaemic agent
OTC	over the counter (medicine)
PCA	patient-controlled analgesia
PCP	*Pneumocystis carinii* pneumonia (now *Pneumocystis jiroveci*)
PCR	protein-creatinine ratio
PD	peritoneal dialysis
PDF	peritoneal dialysis fluid
PE	pulmonary embolism
PET	peritoneal equilibrium test
PKD	polycystic kidney disease
PR3	proteinase-3
PRA	panel reactive antibodies
PRCA	pure red cell aplasia
PTH	parathyroid hormone
PTFE	polytetrafluoroethylene

PTLD   post-transplant lymphoproliferative disease
RAS   renal artery stenosis
RBC   red blood cells
RNA   ribonucleic acid
RNI   recommended nutrient intake
ROD   renal osteodystrophy
RPGN   rapidly progressive glomerulonephritis
RRT   renal replacement therapy
SC   subcutaneous
SCUF   slow continuous ultrafiltration
SIRS   systemic inflammatory response syndrome
SLE   systemic lupus erythematosus
SPC   summary of product characteristics
SPF   sun protection factor
SSRI   selective serotonin reuptake inhibitor
SUN   serum urea nitrogen
t1/2   elimination half life
TB   tuberculosis
TCA   tricyclic antidepressant
TDM   therapeutic drug monitoring
Th-cell   T-helper lymphocyte
TIBC   total iron binding capacity
TTT   total therapy time (for APD and CCPD)
TTV   total therapy volume (for APD and CCPD)
TZD   thiazolidinediones (glitazones)
U&Es   urea and electrolytes
UKM   urea kinetic modelling
URR   urea reduction ratio
US   ultrasound
USS   ultrasound scan
UTI   urinary tract infection
VLPD   very low-protein diet
WCC   white cell count
WG   Wegener's granulomatosis

1

What are the functions of the kidney?

Caroline Ashley

The main functions of the kidneys may be summarised as follows:

- Regulation of the water and electrolyte content of the body by filtration, secretion and reabsorption
- Retention of substances vital to the body such as protein and glucose
- Maintenance of acid/base balance
- Excretion of waste products, water soluble toxic substances and drugs
- Endocrine functions – the kidney activates both erythropoietin and vitamin D. It also produces renin (in the afferent arteriole), which affects various aspects of water and electrolyte homeostasis.

The functional anatomy of the kidney

In a normal human adult, each kidney is about 10 cm long, 5.5 cm in width and about 3 cm thick, weighing 150 g. Together, kidneys weigh about 0.5% of a person's total body weight. The kidneys are 'bean-shaped' organs, and have a concave side facing inwards (medially).

There are three major anatomical demarcations in the kidney: the cortex, the medulla, and the renal pelvis. The cortex receives most of the blood flow, and is mostly concerned with reabsorbing filtered material. The medulla is a highly metabolically active area, which serves to concentrate the urine. The pelvis collects urine for excretion (Figure 1.1).

Terms

- **Renal capsule**: the membranous covering of the kidney
- **Cortex**: the outer layer over the internal medulla. It contains blood vessels, glomeruli (which are the kidneys' 'filters') and tubules, and is supported by a fibrous matrix
- **Hilus**: the opening in the middle of the concave medial border for nerves and blood vessels to pass into the renal sinus
- **Renal column**: the structures which support the cortex. They consist of lines of blood vessels and tubules, and a fibrous material
- **Renal sinus**: the cavity that houses the renal pyramids
- **Calyces**: (singular calyx) the recesses in the internal medulla which hold the pyramids. They are used to subdivide the sections of the kidney
- **Papillae**: (singular papilla) the small conical projections along the wall of the renal sinus. They have openings through which urine passes into the calyces
- **Renal pyramids**: the conical segments within the internal medulla. They contain the secreting apparatus and tubules, and are also called malpighian pyramids
- **Renal artery**: two renal arteries come from the aorta, each connecting to a kidney. The artery divides into five branches, each of which leads to a ball of capillaries. The arteries supply unfiltered blood to the kidneys. The left kidney receives about 60% of the renal bloodflow
- **Renal vein**: the filtered blood returns to the systemic circulation through the renal veins which join into the inferior vena cava

1

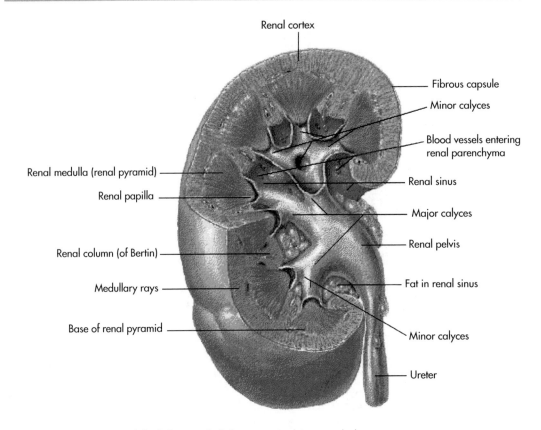

Figure 1.1   The anatomy of the kidney. Right kidney sectioned in several planes.

- **Renal pelvis:** basically just a funnel, the renal pelvis accepts the urine and channels it out of the hilus into the ureter
- **Ureter:** a narrow tube 40 cm long and 4 mm in diameter, passing from the renal pelvis out of the hilus and down to the bladder. The ureter carries urine from the kidneys to the bladder by means of peristalsis
- **Renal lobe:** each pyramid together with the associated overlying cortex forms a renal lobe.

The nephron

The functional unit of the kidney is the nephron (Figure 1.2). Each kidney consists of about one million nephrons. There are five parts of the nephron:

1 The glomerulus, which is the blood kidney interface, plasma is filtered from capillaries into the Bowman's capsule.

2 The proximal convoluted tubule, which reabsorbs most of the filtered load, including nutrients and electrolytes.

3 The loop of Henle, which, depending on its length, concentrates urine by increasing the osmolality of surrounding tissue and filtrate.

4 The distal convoluted tubule, which reabsorbs water and sodium depending on needs.

5 The collecting system, which collects urine for excretion. There are two types of nephrons, those localised to the cortex, and those extending into the medulla. The latter are characterised by long loops of Henle, and are more metabolically active.

The nephron makes urine by

- Simple filtration – the blood is filtered of its small molecules and ions
- Reabsorption – the required amounts of useful materials are reclaimed by selective and passive reabsorption

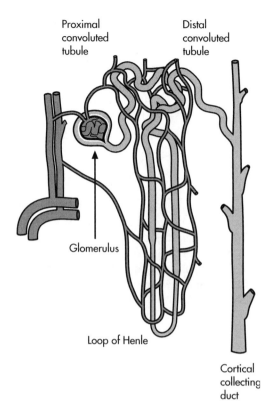

Proximal convoluted tubule

Distal convoluted tubule

Glomerulus

Loop of Henle

Cortical collecting duct

Figure 1.2 The nephron – the functional unit of the kidney.

- Excretion – surplus or waste molecules and ions are left to flow out as urine.

In 24 hours the human kidneys reclaim

- ~1300 g of NaCl
- ~400 g $NaHCO_3$
- ~180 g glucose
- almost all of the 180 L of water that entered the tubules.

The glomerulus

Renal blood flow is 25% of cardiac output (1200 mL/min). Approximately 99% of the blood flow goes to the cortex and 1% to the medulla. Renal plasma flow is about 660 mL/min, and 120 mL/min is filtered out of the blood and into the nephron. Ultimately approximately 1.2 mL of this fluid is excreted as urine (1% of filtered load). The rate at which fluid is filtered by the glomerulus is called the glomerular filtration rate (GFR). The major determinants of GFR are:

1 Renal blood flow and renal perfusion pressure
2 The hydrostatic pressure difference between the tubule and the capillaries
3 The surface area available for ultrafiltration.

Filtration takes place through the semipermeable walls of the glomerular capillaries, which are almost impermeable to proteins and large molecules. The filtrate is thus virtually free of protein and has no cellular elements. The glomerular filtrate is formed by squeezing fluid through the glomerular capillary bed. The driving hydrostatic pressure (head of pressure) is controlled by the afferent and efferent arterioles, and provided by arterial pressure (Figure 1.3). About 20% of renal plasma flow is filtered each minute (120 mL/min).

In order to keep the renal blood flow and GFR relatively constant, the hydrostatic pressure in the glomerulus has to be kept fairly constant. When there is a change in arterial blood pressure, there is constriction or dilatation of the afferent and efferent arterioles, the muscular walled vessels leading to and from

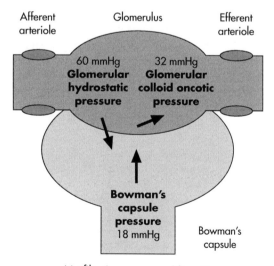

Afferent arteriole   Glomerulus   Efferent arteriole

60 mmHg
Glomerular hydrostatic pressure

32 mmHg
Glomerular colloid oncotic pressure

Bowman's capsule pressure
18 mmHg

Bowman's capsule

Net filtration pressure = 10 mmHg

Figure 1.3 Glomerular filtration.

each glomerulus. This process is called auto-regulation.

Proximal tubule (Figure 1.4)

The function of the renal tubule is to reabsorb selectively about 99% of the glomerular filtrate. The proximal tubule reabsorbs 60% of all solutes, which includes 100% of glucose and amino acids, 90% of bicarbonate and 80–90% of inorganic phosphate, vitamins and water.

Reabsorption is by either active or passive transport. Active transport requires energy to move solute against an electrochemical or a concentration gradient. It is the main determinant of oxygen consumption by the kidney. Passive transport is where reabsorption occurs down an electrochemical, pressure or concentration gradient.

Most of the solute reabsorption is active, with water being freely permeable and therefore moving by osmosis. When the active reabsorbtion of solute from the tubule occurs, there is a fall in concentration and hence osmotic activity within the tubule. Water then moves because of osmotic forces to the area outside the tubule, where the concentration of solutes is higher.

Loop of Henle

The loop of Henle is the part of the tubule which dips or 'loops' from the cortex into the medulla (descending limb) and then returns to the cortex (ascending limb). It is this part of the tubule where urine is concentrated if necessary. This is possible because of the high concentration of solute in the substance or interstitium of the medulla. This high medullary interstitial

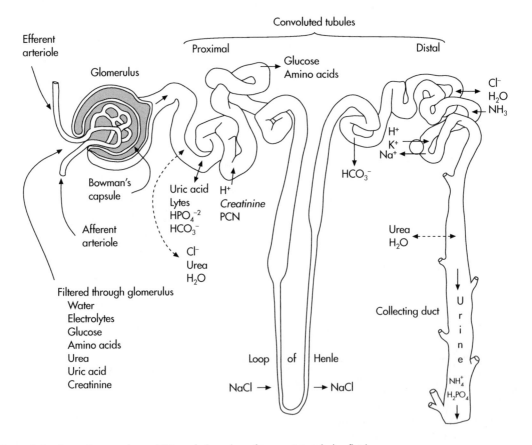

Figure 1.4   Sites of removal or addition of electrolytes from or into tubular fluid.

concentration of solutes is maintained by the counter-current multiplier system which gives the kidney the ability to concentrate urine. The loop of Henle is the counter-current multiplier and the vasa recta is the counter-current exchanger. The system works as follows:

- The descending loop of Henle is relatively impermeable to solutes but permeable to water so that water moves out by osmosis, and the fluid in the tubule becomes hypertonic.
- The thin section of the ascending loop of Henle is virtually impermeable to water but permeable to solutes, especially sodium and chloride ions. Thus sodium and chloride ions move out down the concentration gradient and the fluid within the tubule becomes first isotonic then hypotonic as more ions leave. Urea, which was absorbed into the medullary interstitium from the collecting duct, diffuses into the ascending limb. This keeps the urea within the interstitium of the medulla where it also has a role in concentrating urine.
- The thick section of the ascending loop and early distal tubule are virtually impermeable to water. Sodium and chloride ions, however, are actively transported out of the tubule, making the tubular fluid very hypotonic. A sodium–potassium–chloride ($1Na^+:1K^+:2Cl^-$) pump actively extracts these electrolytes from the tubular fluid in the thick ascending limb.

Distal tubule and collecting ducts

The final concentration of urine depends upon the amount of antidiuretic hormone (ADH) secreted by the posterior lobe of the pituitary. If ADH is present, the distal tubule and collecting ducts become permeable to water. As the collecting duct passes through the medulla with a high solute concentration in the interstitium, the water moves out of the lumen of the duct and concentrated urine is formed. In the absence of ADH the tubule is minimally permeable to water so a large quantity of dilute urine is formed.

There is a close link between the hypothalamus of the brain and the posterior pituitary.

Cells within the hypothalamus called osmo-receptors are sensitive to changes in osmotic pressure of the blood. If there is low water intake, there is a rise in the osmotic pressure of the blood; after excess intake of water, the osmotic pressure of the blood falls. Nerve impulses from the hypothalamus stimulate the posterior pituitary to produce ADH when the osmotic pressure of the blood rises. As a result water loss in the kidney is reduced because ADH is secreted, and water is reabsorbed in the collecting duct.

The result of this 'counter-current multiplier' system is threefold:

1 The high concentration of sodium and chloride (and urea) in the medullary interstitium makes this part of the kidney hyperosmolar.
2 Fluid delivered to the distal convoluted tubule is hypotonic. So, as this fluid passes down through this tubule and the collecting duct, it is exposed to very high osmolar pressures in the surrounding tissues. If the patient is dehydrated, the pituitary gland produces ADH, which makes the collecting ducts permeable to water, and water is rapidly reabsorbed along the concentration gradient. If not, a dilute urine is excreted.
3 Extracellular fluid volume depends on the amount of sodium in the body, so it is essential that the kidney is capable of conserving sodium. If the extracellular volume drops, a complex series of neurohormonal interactions lead to the release of aldosterone, which makes the collecting ducts permeable to sodium, which is absorbed.

Other functions of the kidneys

Acid/base balance

The lungs and kidneys work together to produce a normal extracellular fluid and arterial pH of 7.35–7.45 (34–46 nmol/L H^+ concentration). Carbon dioxide (CO_2), when dissolved in the blood is an acid, and is excreted by the lungs. The kidney excretes fixed acid and performs three functions to achieve this:

1 The majority of the filtered bicarbonate is reabsorbed (90% in the proximal tubule). The H^+, released as the tubular secretion of acid, forms carbonic acid with the bicarbonate (HCO_3^-).

$$H^+ + HCO_3^- \Leftrightarrow H_2CO_3 \Leftrightarrow H_2O + CO_2$$

The enzyme carbonic anhydrase, found in the proximal tubular cells, catalyses the reaction to carbon dioxide (CO_2) and water (H_2O). The CO_2 diffuses into the cell where it again forms carbonic acid in the presence of carbonic anhydrase. The carbonic acid ionises to H^+ and HCO_3^-. The H^+ is then pumped out of the cell back to the lumen of the tubule by the Na^+/H^+ pump and the sodium is returned to the plasma by the Na^+/K^+ pump. Water is absorbed passively.

2 Other buffers include inorganic phosphate (HPO_4^-), urate and creatinine ions which are excreted in urine as acid when combined with H^+ ions secreted in the distal nephron.

3 Ammonia is produced enzymatically from glutamine and other amino acids, and is secreted in the tubules. Ammonia (NH_3) combines with secreted H^+ ions to form a non-diffusible ammonium ion (NH_4^+) which is excreted in the urine. Ammonia production is increased by a severe metabolic acidosis to as much as 700 mmol/day.

Hormones and the kidney

Renin

Renin is a vital component of the renin–angiotensin system, and increases the production of angiotensin II which is released when there is a fall in intravascular volume (e.g. haemorrhage or dehydration). This leads to:

- Constriction of the efferent arteriole to maintain GFR, by increasing the filtration pressure in the glomerulus
- Release of aldosterone from the adrenal cortex
- Increased release of ADH from the posterior pituitary
- Thirst

- Inotropic myocardial stimulation and systemic arterial constriction.

The opposite occurs when fluid overload occurs.

Aldosterone

Aldosterone promotes sodium ion and water reabsorption in the distal tubule and collecting duct where Na^+ is exchanged for potassium (K^+) and hydrogen ions by a specific cellular pump. Aldosterone is also released when there is a decrease in serum sodium ion concentration. This can occur, for example, when there are large losses of gastric juice. Gastric juice contains significant concentrations of sodium, chloride, hydrogen and potassium ions. Therefore it is impossible to correct the resulting alkalosis and hypokalaemia without first replacing the sodium ions using sodium chloride 0.9% solutions.

Atrial natruretic peptide

Atrial natruretic peptide (ANP) is released when atrial pressure is increased (e.g. in heart failure or fluid overload). It promotes loss of sodium and chloride ions and water, chiefly by increasing GFR.

Antidiuretic hormone

Antidiuretic hormone (ADH) – also known as vasopressin – increases the water permeability of the distal tubule and collecting duct, thus increasing the concentration of urine. In contrast, when secretion of ADH is inhibited, it allows dilute urine to be formed. This occurs mainly when plasma sodium concentration falls, such as following drinking large quantities of water. This fall is detected by the osmoreceptors in the hypothalamus.

Erythropoietin

Decreased oxygen delivery to the kidney stimulates the release of renal erythropoietic factor which acts on a liver globulin to produce erythropoietin. Erythropoietin acts as a mitosis-stimulating factor and differentiation hormone to specifically stimulate the formation of erythrocytes from its committed progenitors in the bone marrow.

Vitamin D

The kidneys produce the active form of vitamin D, namely calcitriol (1,25-dihydroxychole-calciferol).

Other hormones

The following hormones are degraded or excreted by the kidneys:

- Parathyroid hormone
- Growth hormone
- Secretin
- Cholecystokinin
- Glucagon
- Gastrin
- Insulin.

Any of these hormones may increase in circulation in the patient with renal dysfunction if the kidney is unable to excrete or degrade the hormone.

Excretory functions

As cells perform their various metabolic processes, protein and nucleic acids, both of which contain nitrogen, are broken down. Other metabolic by-products include water and carbon dioxide. Chemical groups such as nitrogen, sulfur and phosphorus must be stripped from the large molecules to which they were formerly attached, as part of the process to prepare them for energy conversion. This continuous production of metabolic wastes establishes a steep concentration gradient across the plasma membrane, causing wastes to diffuse out of cells and into the extracellular fluid.

Some of the nitrogen is used to manufacture new nitrogen-containing molecules, but most of it cannot be used for this purpose and must be disposed of by the body. Typically, the first nitrogen-containing molecule that forms is ammonia (NH_3), which is very water-soluble, forming NH_4OH, a strong base, which must be excreted before it raises the pH of the body fluids. The two most common substances used to get rid of excess nitrogen are urea and uric acid. Ammonia is converted to urea, which is water-soluble and excreted in a water-based solution. While the major portion of human nitrogenous waste is in the form of urea, humans typically excrete some uric acid too.

In a similar fashion, the kidneys are also responsible for the excretion of many water-soluble drugs.

Conclusion

In general, humans can live normally with just one kidney, as they have more functioning renal tissue than is needed for survival. Only when the amount of functioning kidney tissue is greatly diminished will chronic renal failure develop. If the glomerular filtration rate has fallen very low (end stage renal failure), or if the renal dysfunction leads to severe symptoms, then renal replacement therapy is indicated, either as dialysis or renal transplantation. As can be seen from the diverse functions of the kidneys, renal failure generates a complex group of symptoms, which are discussed in the chapters of this book.

2

Laboratory tests and investigations

Elizabeth Lamerton

Most patients admitted to hospital undergo a series of standard or routine blood tests performed on admission and/or during their stay. Some of these tests relate to renal function. Such tests can be used to detect and diagnose kidney disease, kidney damage and kidney function and to monitor response to treatment.

Renal patients will have a wide range of tests and investigations on top of the standard tests. It is important to consider each test not in isolation but in the context of other results for each individual patient. In this chapter routine tests for adult patients will be discussed. Paediatric patients may have additional tests and investigations; these are discussed in more detail in Chapter 13.[1-3]

In this chapter we will cover:

- Common biochemistry tests
- Common haematological tests
- Urine tests
- Renal biopsy
- Immunological tests
- Radiological investigations
- Classification or staging of chronic kidney disease
- Measurement and estimation of kidney function.

Standard tests and investigations for the general adult patient population

Each laboratory has a specific reference range for blood test results. When identifying high or low values for your patients, it is essential that you refer to the local laboratory range. The reference range assumes that 95% of the population's values will be within the 2.5–97.5 percentile. Reference ranges do not generally take individual characteristics such as age, sex, weight or disease state into consideration.

A list of common biochemical tests used in the biochemistry laboratory to analyse blood samples quantitively for a variety of electrolytes is shown in Table 2.1.

Creatinine

Creatinine is produced continuously in muscle and is a function of muscle mass. The production is usually constant although the rate of production declines with age and in low muscle mass or cachectic states. Creatinine is eliminated from the body by the kidneys, predominantly through glomerular filtration, with an additional 30% eliminated by active tubular secretion. The plasma concentration of creatinine is therefore linked both to body muscle mass and the ability of the kidney to excrete the creatinine effectively. As a crude indicator, at steady state, a doubling of serum creatinine may indicate a 50% reduction in glomerular filtration rate.[1-3]

Creatinine clearance is routinely used as a measure of kidney function.

Urea

Urea is produced when protein or amino acids are broken down in the liver. Protein is sourced from both the diet and from body tissues. Like creatinine, urea is normally cleared by

Table 2.1   Common biochemical tests

Test	Sample	Approximate reference range for general population
Creatinine	Plasma	50–120 µmol/L
Urea	Plasma	3.0–6.5 mmol/L
Potassium	Plasma	3.5–5.0 mmol/L
Sodium	Plasma	135–145 mmol/L
Calcium	Serum	2.20–2.55 mmol/L
Phosphate	Serum	0.8–1.6 mmol/L
Magnesium	Serum	0.8–1.0 mmol/L
Albumin	Serum	40 g/L
Bicarbonate	Plasma	20–30 mmol/L
Glucose	Serum	Fasting 3.3–6.7 mmol/L
		Non-fasting <10 mmol/L
Ferritin		24–300 µg/L males
		15–300 µg/L females
Total iron-binding capacity		45–70 µmol/L
Serum iron		12–30 mmol/L

glomerular filtration and is reabsorbed in the kidney tubules. It is a weakly alkaline substance and osmotic diuretic.

The urea concentration may be increased following consumption of a high protein diet, states of increased catabolism due to tissue damage, sepsis or starvation and by increased absorption of amino acids, which may occur following large gastric haemorrhage where blood is digested.

When the glomerular filtration rate is reduced, this is often reflected more rapidly in serum urea levels than in the serum creatinine concentrations.[1]

Factors that affect urea are listed in Table 2.2.

Potassium

The total amount of potassium in the adult body is approximately 3000 mmol, most of which (98%) is found within the cells. Although they represent a small proportion of total body potassium, it is the extracellular potassium ions that have the physiological effects on membrane potential and therefore nerve and muscle function. Changes in extracellular potassium can have an immediate effect irrespective of the intracellular potassium concentration, with both hypokalaemia and hyperkalaemia having potentially fatal consequences. The intracellular potassium acts as a reservoir for the extracellular potassium.

Normal potassium intake is 60–100 mmol/day and comes from the diet via the intestines, the kidneys (glomeruli and tubular cells) and through cell membranes.

Within the kidney, potassium handling occurs through glomerular filtration, tubular reabsorption and tubular secretion.

Potassium undergoes glomerular filtration at

Table 2.2   Factors affecting serum urea concentration

Factor	Effect
Fluid status	
Oedema (excess fluid)	↓ urea
Dehydration	↑ urea
Low protein intake from the diet	↓ urea
Concurrent infection	↑ urea
Gastric blood loss	↑ urea
Liver function	↓ liver function ↓ urea
Pregnancy	↓ urea
Burns	↓ urea
Chronic nutritional status	Cachectic = ↓ urea

Table 2.3 Symptoms of hypokalaemia and hyperkalaemia

	Potassium (mmol/L)	Symptoms
Hypokalaemia	3.0–3.5	Malaise, muscle fatigue, cramps
	2.5–3.0	ECG changes, more prominent malaise, muscle fatigue and cramps
	<2.5	ECG changes, paralysis of legs or trunk can lead to respiratory arrest
Hyperkalaemia	>6.5	ECG changes, then ventricular fibrillation and cardiac arrest

the same rate as plasma and approximately 60–80% is reabsorbed by the proximal tubular cells through passive transport. Damage to the renal tubular cells may impair this function and result in hypokalaemia. Potassium is secreted in the distal tubules and collecting ducts in exchange for sodium. Hydrogen ions may compete in this exchange.

Some potassium moves into the filtrate in the thin descending limb of the loop of Henle; however, this is counterbalanced by movement of potassium into the medullary collecting ducts. Reabsorption of potassium also occurs in the thick ascending limb of the Loop of Henle. Approximately 30% of the filtered potassium will be reabsorbed here and is linked to sodium reabsorption.

Approximately 10% of filtered potassium reaches the distal tubule, with 95% of this being reabsorbed. The high luminal sodium concentration, and low luminal chloride concentration stimulates the potassium-chloride co-transporter to secrete potassium. In the cortical collecting duct, potassium is both secreted and reabsorbed, and this is the main site of potassium secretion in the kidney. As the plasma potassium concentration rises, so does the rate of excretion of potassium via the kidneys.

A rise in the potassium level of the extracellular fluid of the adrenal cortex will result in the release of aldosterone. In the cortical collecting duct, aldosterone promotes the synthesis of Na^+/K^+ ATPases and their subsequent insertion into the basolateral membrane. This effect on the cell creates an electrical potential favouring the movement of potassium from the cell to the urine. Apical sodium and potassium channel activity is also stimulated by aldosterone release, resulting in an increase in both sodium reabsorption and potassium secretion. In addition to hyperkalaemia, aldosterone release can also be stimulated by volume depletion and low plasma sodium osmolality.[2,3]

Management of hyper- and hypokalaemia in the renal dialysis patient

The usual range for random serum potassium concentrations is 3.5–5.3 mmol/L. Patients with kidney disease are generally less able to excrete potassium and most patients will have potassium concentrations in the upper limits of the 'normal range'. The symptoms of hypokalaemia and hyperkalaemia are summarised in Table 2.3.

The following checklist of questions should be used when dealing with the patient with kidney disease:

- Is the potassium result a true value and is it reliable? Could the blood sampling method have affected the result? Could the blood have haemolysed in the sample container?
- Is this a pre- or immediately post-dialysis reading? Pre-dialysis readings are usually high and immediate post-dialysis samples are low until the patient re-equilibrates (up to 4 hours post dialysis).
- Is the patient due to have imminent haemodialysis or peritoneal dialysis? High potassium: If the potassium level is not life threatening and haemodialysis is planned within 12 hours no action may be required. Low potassium: Advise the dialysis team and consider amending the dialysis prescription to a higher potassium dialysate.
- Is there a previous value? Is this acute or

chronic? Does the patient often have a high or low serum potassium?

- What are the patient's other electrolyte values? Remember always to check magnesium in patients with low potassium.
- Is there a drug cause (e.g. ACE inhibitor, angiotensin receptor blocker, NSAIDs, potassium supplements, amiloride, spironolactone)? Can the drug be stopped safely? Will this be enough action?

Immediately following haemodialysis a patient's serum potassium levels will be temporarily lower and levels measured at this time will not accurately reflect the actual potassium level. If necessary potassium should be checked at least 4 hours after haemodialysis.

- Serum potassium >3.0 mmol/L and <3.5 mmol/L: Ask the patient if they have a potassium-restricted diet. If the answer is yes, temporarily remove the restriction!
- Serum potassium <3.0 mmol/L but >2.5 mmol/L: Oral potassium supplements may be indicated. Recheck potassium concentration daily.
- Serum potassium <2.5 mmol/L: Intravenous potassium 40 mmol in 500 mL 0.9 NaCl or 5% glucose over 12 hours or, for fluid-restricted patients, IV KCl 40 mmol in 100 mL via central line, over 6 hours. Note potassium may also be added to peritoneal dialysis fluid. Recheck potassium level 4 hours after the end of the infusion and repeat if necessary.

For hyperkalaemia K^+ >5.3 mmol/L, remember that dialysis is the only reliable method of removing potassium from the body in dialysis-dependent patients. Consider planning dialysis at an early stage! Remember to stop any causative medicines or fluids.

If ECG changes are present (bradycardia, absent P-waves, broad QRS complexes and tall T-waves) or if K^+ >7.0, urgent action is required. Give IV calcium gluconate to stabilise cardiac muscle and reduce the risk of arrhythmia: 2.2 mmol = 10 mL of calcium gluconate 10% by slow IV bolus injection into a large vein. Calcium gluconate is highly irritant and causes severe damage when extravasated. The effect of

giving IV calcium will be seen in 1–5 minutes and the duration of action is 1 hour. Repeat if necessary after 1 hour.

For all patients with hyperkalaemia, give therapy to drive potassium into the cells: 10 units of soluble insulin in 50 mL of 50% glucose by IV infusion over 30 minutes. Increasing the availability of insulin drives the potassium into the cells by enhancing the Na^+/K^+-ATPase pump in skeletal muscle. Expect a drop in serum potassium of 0.5–1.5 mmol/L and monitor closely for hypoglycaemia. The effect begins in 15 minutes, peaks at 60 minutes and lasts for 4–6 hours. An additional dose may be given. If necessary prescribe additional emergency therapy to drive potassium into the cells: Salbutamol nebulised 5 mg every 2–3 hours. Take caution with this therapy, as sympathetic activity will be increased causing tachycardia, arrhythmias and fine tremors.

In addition, sodium bicarbonate may be given, either 1000 mg three times a day orally or 500 mL 1.26–1.4% IV (via central or peripheral line) over 6 hours. Raising the systemic pH results in hydrogen ion release from the cells and moves potassium into the cells. There is also a direct effect independent of pH. Effects begin within 30–60 minutes and last for 6–8 hours. It should be noted that this strategy can cause salt and water overload – exercise caution in fluid restricted patients. NEVER give bicarbonate and calcium together through the same line as precipitation will occur.

A longer-term strategy is to remove potassium from the body: Calcium polystyrene sulfonate (Calcium Resonium) 15 g four times a day orally or 30 g rectally. This is an ion exchange resin that exchanges calcium for potassium in the gut. This is more useful in chronic hyperkalaemia than acute hyperkalaemia as effects begin in 2–24 hours and last for 24–48 hours after stopping. Therapy must only be given for 48 hours. It can cause severe constipation, therefore always prescribe laxatives concomitantly and monitor. If the patient has a high serum calcium level, consider using sodium polystyrene resonium (Resonium-A) instead.

Sodium

Sodium is found in the extracellular fluid. There are approximately 3000 mmol of osmotically active sodium in the human body. Normal sodium intake is approximately 60–150 mmol per day. Net daily losses of sodium are 100 mmol of sodium in urine and 15 mmol in faeces and less than 30 mmol of sodium in sweat.

Renal blood flow and aldosterone control sodium balance. Aldosterone exerts its action by controlling loss of sodium from the distal renal tubule and the colon in exchange for potassium and hydrogen ions.[3]

Calcium

The total amount of calcium in the body depends upon the dietary intake of calcium and the calcium lost. The average adult will ingest 25 mmol of calcium and absorb 6–12 mmol. Calcium is lost from the body in faeces following formation of insoluble complexes with phosphate or fatty acids in the intestine. Urinary loss of calcium is a function of a combination of glomerular filtration and tubular function.

Calcium is present in the plasma as both free ionised calcium, which is the physiologically active form, and as protein-bound calcium.[2] The amount of calcium present in the body that is not bound to albumin and that is therefore physiologically active is known as corrected calcium.

Some laboratories measure total plasma calcium concentrations. To calculate the concentration of physiologically active calcium, the following formula may be used to correct for the percentage of calcium that is bound to albumin:[3]

If the serum albumin level is <40 mmol/L:

> Corrected calcium = [total concentration of calcium, mmol/L] + 0.02 (40 – [albumin concentration, g/L]) mmol/L

If the serum albumin level is >45 mmol/L:

> Corrected calcium = [total concentration

of calcium, mmol/L] – 0.02 ([albumin concentration, g/L] – 45) mmol/L

Haematological tests and investigations

Some common haematological laboratory tests and reference ranges are listed in Table 2.4.[3]

- Red blood cell count: Erythropoiesis is the production of red blood cells in the bone marrow and is stimulated by a hormone produced in the kidney called erythropoietin. Further discussion about erythropoeitin and red blood cell production can be found in Chapter 5 on renal anaemia.
- Haemoglobin: The higher concentration of red blood cells found in men compared with women is responsible for the higher haemaglobin concentration in men.
- Platelets: Another function of the bone marrow is the production of platelets. Once released into the circulation, platelets have a relatively short lifespan of 8–12 days.
- White cell count: White blood cells or leukocytes contain nuclei. There are two main types – granular and agranular. The granular leukocytes may be identified by staining and are subdivided into eosinophils, basophils and neutrophils. Agranular leukocytes comprise T-lymphocytes, B-lymphocytes and monocytes.

Table 2.4 Haematological blood tests

Test	Reference range
Haemoglobin	13.5–18.0 g/dL (males)
	12.0–16.0 g/dL (females)
White blood cell count (WCC)	$3.5–11.0 \times 10^9$/L
Red blood cell count (RBC)	$4.5–6.5 \times 10^{12}$/L (males)
	$4.4–6.0 \times 10^{12}$/L (females)
Platelets	$150–400 \times 10^9$/L
Prothrombin time (Pt)	Measured in seconds
Activated prothrombin time (APTT)	28–34 seconds

Urine tests

Urine is relatively easy to investigate in a variety of ways and has the advantage usually of providing a non-invasive test and investigation. Urine can be easily tested using urinalysis dipsticks to detect:

- Protein
- Microscopic haematuria (traces of blood)
- Sugar
- Infection.

This test is easy to do and convenient and thus is commonly perfomed at home, in the GP surgery, outpatient clinic or at the bedside.

Blood and protein should not routinely be present in urine although this is relatively common in people with kidney disease. Protein or albumin in the urine detected on dipstick tests may indicate bladder infection or indeed kidney disease and is suggestive of glomerulonephritis or vasculitis. Microalbuminuria is diagnosed if the albumin:creatinine ratio is greater than or equal to 2.5 mg/mmol in men or 3.5 mg/mmol in women.

Twenty-four-hour urine collection

Most patients with kidney disease provide a 24-hour urine collection for analysis where possible. The volume of urine collected over a 24-hour period provides a useful indication of renal function. The collection can be both quantitively and qualitatively analysed for:

- The actual volume of urine produced in a strict 24-hour time period
- Urinary creatinine clearance
- Urinary protein
- Calcium
- Oxalate
- Uric acid.

When giving a patient instructions on how to take a 24-hour urine, it is important to make sure they understand that they should go to the toilet as usual first thing on the morning of the collection, then collect the urine for the whole of the day and first thing the next morning. That completes the 24-hour collection.

Volume of urine produced in 24 hours.

A patient with normal kidney function should produce 2–5 L of urine in 24 hours, depending on the patient's hydration status. For example, a dehydrated patient will produce significantly less urine. Oliguric patients produce <500 mL in 24 hours; anuric patients produce <200 mL in 24 hours; and polyuric patients produce >5000 mL in 24 hours.

The 24-hour urine collection can also be qualitatively analysed for protein concentration, cortisol, osmolality, phosphate, potassium and sodium.

Urine microscopy

Samples of urine can be examined under the microscope to detect red blood cells, white blood cells, crystals and bacteria. The identification of red cell casts in the urine is diagnostic of glomerulonephritis.

Urinary protein.

Protein excretion of less than 150 mg per day is considered to be normal. Approximately 30 mg of this amount will be albumin. Persistent protein loss of more than 150 mg per day suggests renal or systemic disease.

Microalbuminuria is the presence of albumin in the urine at quantities above the normal range of 30 mg/L but below the amount (approximately 300 mg/L) detected by dipstick. As proteinuria increases, the albumin forms a relatively larger fraction of the total protein loss. Proteinuria is best measured on an early morning spot urine sample to enable calculation of the protein-creatinine ratio (PCR). Relating the urine protein loss to creatinine enables a correction for variations in urine concentration, and is an important prognostic factor in the management of kidney disease. In many cases, single samples may be used in place of a 24-hour urine collection.

Unexpected abnormal results should be repeated at least three times. Proteinuria greater than 3.0 g in 24 hours is considered to be in the nephrotic range.

Renal biopsy

Renal biopsy may be performed to diagnose the cause of the kidney disease. Native kidney biopsies are usually carried out in the radiology department under radiological guidance to ensure accuracy.

Prior to the biopsy, anticoagulant and antiplatelet therapy must be discontinued to reduce the risk of post biopsy bleeding. Local policies should be followed, but common recommendations include:

* Stop aspirin or clopidogrel for 7 days
* Avoid NSAIDs for at least 24 hours before and after biopsy
* Stop coumarin anticoagulant therapy for at least 2–5 days and replace with heparin if continuous anticoagulation is required
* Continue antihypertensive medication and ensure blood pressure is adequately controlled.

In some units, prophylactic desmopresssin (DDAVP) is given to control uraemic bleeding, which is often abnormal when urea is greater than 18 mmol/L. This is an unlicensed indication for desmopressin (see Table 2.5). Factor VIII concentrations will be increased two- to fourfold within 1 hour of administration and doses can be repeated every 4 hours if necessary

Immunological tests

The presence of autoimmune antibodies in blood or urine detects immunological disease. These diseases are discussed in detail in Chapter 14. Selected blood tests may indicate specific disease or diagnoses.

Routine tests

Routine tests include:

* Antineutrophil cytoplasmic antibodies (ANCA) to look for systemic vasculitis such as Wegener's granulomatosis or microscopic polyangiitis. Those patients with Wegener's granulomatosis exhibit c-ANCA reactivity again proteinase 3 (PR3), while those with microscopic polyangitiis have p-ANCA reactivity against myeloperoxidase (MPO).
* Antiglobular basement membrane antibodies (anti-GBM) as markers of Goodpastures's disease
* Double-strand DNA (anti-dsDNA) as a marker of systemic lupus erythematosus (SLE).
* Complement factors – C3 and C4 to look for systemic lupus erythematosus, infective endocarditis, cryoglobulinaemia
* Myeloperoxidase (MPO) is positive in 80% of cases of pauci-immune crescentic glomerular nephritis and systemic vasculitis
* Immunoglobulins – IgG, IgA
* Bence Jones proteins, light chains, heavy chains and kappa bands, which can indicate amyloid or myeloma.

Serum and urine electrophoresis

Serum protein electrophoresis is used as a screening tool to detect monoclonal proteins (M-proteins), which can be classified into six general regions, namely albumin, $\alpha 1$, $\alpha 2$, $\beta 1$ $\beta 2$ and γ immunoglobulins.

Albuminuria is usually associated with renal disease. Microalbuminuria is defined as protein loss between 3 and 300 mg in 24 hours and is often seen in patients with diabetes or hypertension.

Table 2.5 Unlicensed use of desmopressin in renal biopsy

Agent	Dose	Onset of action	Peak effect	Duration
IV desmopressin	0.3–0.4 µg/kg in 50 mL of 0.9% NaCl over 20 min	Less than 60 min	1–4 h	4–8 h

Bence Jones proteins are lights chains excreted in the urine in patients with myeloma. Bence Jones proteins are not detected using dipstick urinalysis.

Radiological tests

Renal imaging is an essential investigation in renal medicine. Imaging tests are used to investigate the size and location of kidneys and look for structural damage or blockages. This is especially useful to detect hydronephrosis suggestive of obstruction – a potentially reversible cause of acute renal failure.

Imaging techniques include ultrasound, computed tomography (CT), isotope scans and intravenous pyelograms (IVP). X-ray procedures include intravenous urograms, mictuating cystograms, magnetic resonance imaging (MRI) and renal angiograms. Isotope scans such as chromium-labelled ethylenediamine tetra-acetic acid (^{Cr} – EDTA) can assess both overall and individual kidney function within a given person, and are currently the most accurate way of assessing renal function.

X-ray and ultrasound

The easiest and often first radiological tests are a plain radiograph of the kidneys, ureter and bladder to look for renal calculi, accompanied by a renal and bladder ultrasound.

A healthy adult with normal kidneys would be expected to have two kidneys, measuring approximately 12 cm in length and of equal size. Small kidneys may indicate either a congenital abnormality or long-term (chronic) damage. Large kidneys may indicate the presence of cysts. This can be seen in patients with polycystic kidney disease.

Renal angiogram

Renal angiograms are performed to visualise the renal artery to confirm a diagnosis of renal artery stenosis and, if possible, the cause of the stenosis. The renal angiogram is a means of investigating the anatomy of the renal vascular bed.

Renal angiograms carry an associated risk of acute renal failure caused by the use of X-ray contrast media. This is termed contrast nephropathy and will be discussed in Chapter 3.

Intravenous excretory urogram

The intravenous excretory urogram (IVU) is a radiological test that uses radiocontrast media to produce a series of radiological images. This test will identify renal perfusion, structural abnormalities and the adequacy of lower urinary tract voiding. It is generally performed in children or adolescents to ascertain perfusion abnormalities, especially reflux nephropathy, where urine returns to the kidney and can cause scarring of the nephrons and chronic kidney damage.

Describing and measuring renal function

The concentration of serum creatinine, as discussed earlier, is determined not only by the rate of renal excretion of creatinine but also by the rate of production, which is in turn dependent upon muscle mass. Thus serum creatinine may be above the upper limit of normal in patients with normal kidney function but higher than average muscle mass, often observed in young men, and similarly the serum creatinine may remain within the reference range despite marked kidney disease in patients with low muscle mass, such as slight elderly women. This variation is illustrated in Table 2.6.

Traditionally biochemistry laboratories have reported serum creatinine as a measure of kidney function. However, this method is not ideal as it is insufficiently sensitive to detect moderate chronic kidney disease, and serum creatinine concentrations can be affected by other factors as discussed above. Assessing the degree of renal impairment usually involves a measurement of glomerular filtration rate (GFR) (see Chapter 10 for more detail). GFR is considered to be the best

Table 2.6 Patients with serum creatinine of 130 µmol/L – calculated GFR varies with age, gender, body weight and race

Patient	Gender	Age	Weight (kg)	Race	Creatinine (µmol/L)	GFR (mL/min/1.73 m²)
1	Male	25	80	Black	130	100
2	Male	75	80	White	130	48
3	Female	25	50	White	130	45
4	Female	75	50	White	130	25

measure of overall kidney function and forms the basis of the five-stage classification of chronic kidney disease, which determines management and referral strategies for patients in whom chronic kidney disease has been identified.

Kidney disease is usually identified and described in terms of acute renal failure (ARF) or chronic kidney disease (CKD). As described earlier, many tests and investigations are used to identify kidney disease and to subsequently describe the stage of kidney disease. Internationally, chronic kidney disease is routinely classified according to the American National Kidney Foundation K/DOQI clinical practice guidelines.[4] In the UK the definition and classification shown in Table 2.7 has been adopted by most groups, for example the UK Renal Association, the UK Royal Colleges of Physicians and GPs, the British Geriatric Society, the Association of Clinical Biochemists and the National Service Framework 2005 for renal medicine.[5]

Measuring glomerular fitration rate

Glomerular filtration rate (GFR) can be either measured or estimated. An accurate GFR may be measured by injecting a small amount of

Table 2.7 Stages of chronic kidney disease

NFK-K/DOQI Guidelines stage of kidney disease	Comment:	GFR or eGFR using validated calculations (mL/min/1.73 m²)
	Patient is at risk of kidney damage	>90 but with risk factors for kidney disease
1	Some evidence of kidney damage[b] with normal or increased GFR	>90
2	Kidney damage evident[b] with some reduction in GFR	eGFR>60 but <89
3 Chronic kidney disease (CKD)[a]	Moderate reduction in GFR	30-60
4	Severe reduction in GFR	15-30
5	Kidney failure or renal replacement therapy (e.g. dialysis therapy)	<15

[a]Chronic kidney disease is defined as either kidney damage or GFR <60 mL/min/1.73 m² for >3 months.

[b]Kidney damage is defined as pathological abnormalities or markers of damage, including abnormalities in blood or urine tests or imaging studies for example patients with diabetes mellitis, microalbuminuria and normal GFR, patients with cysts in polycystic kidney disease.

radioactive substance and monitoring the rate of travel through the kidney, for example inulin clearance. This test is rarely done in routine clinical practice and is reserved for use in clinical trial settings where a more accurate measure of GFR may be necessary.

As methods of directly measuring creatinine clearance are cumbersome, the use of a formula to estimate renal function from serum creatinine is a practical way to assess kidney function.[4] A number of methods are available. The two equations most commonly used in practice are the Cockcroft and Gault equation and the Modified Diet in Renal Disease (MDRD) equation. Both equations have been validated.[6,7]

Cockroft and Gault equation

Creatinine clearance (CrCl) = (140 – age in years) $\times$ weight in kg/serum creatinine in µmol/L

multiplied by 1.04 females or 1.23 for males, where creatinine clearance is expressed in mL/min.

Modified Diet in Renal Disease equation

eGFR = 170 $\times$ $(P_{cr})^{-0.999}$ $\times$ $(age)^{-0.176}$ $\times$ (0.762 if female) $\times$ (1.180 if African American) $\times$ $[SUN]^{-0.170}$ $\times$ $[Alb]^{+0.318}$

where estimated GFR (eGFR) is expressed in mL/min/1.73 m^2, Pcr is plasma creatinine concentration in mg/dL, age is in years, SUN is serum urea nitrogen concentration in mg/dL and Alb is serum albumin concentration in g/dL. The equation was developed in patients with chronic kidney disease; they were predominantly white and did not have diabetic kidney disease or a kidney transplant. The equation has been validated for African Americans but no other ethnic groups.

The term CrCl from Cockcroft and Gault used to be interchangeable with the term GFR. More recently, with the advent of MDRD to calculate eGFR the waters have been muddied. The eGFR gives the individual's renal capacity if their body surface area was 1.73 m^2, whereas CrCl is what the kidneys are actually doing. It is important to know which calculation has been used to determine GFR and to be aware that eGFR often gives a lower number. In recommending drug dosing it is usually the CrCl that has been used not the eGFR in the summary of product characteristics.

Estimated GFR values are increasingly being reported directly from clinical biochemistry laboratories in place of serum creatinine.

Limitations of the Modified Diet in Renal Disease equation in calculating eGFR

The MDRD formula for estimating GFR should not be used in all situations. This is particularly important in situations where the creatinine production rate is increased or decreased, the volume of distribution is altered, or the creatinine excretion rate is modified.[6,7]

MDRD has not so far been validated in the following patient groups or clinical scenarios:

- Children
- Acute renal failure
- Pregnancy
- Oedematous states
- Muscle-wasting disease states
- Amputees
- Malnourished patients
- Asian patients
- Kidney transplants
- People with diabetes.

References

1. Davison AM, Cameron JS, Grunfeld JP *et al. Oxford Textbook of Nephrology*, 2nd edn. Oxford: Oxford Medical Publications, Oxford University Press, 1998.
2. Mayne Philip D, ed. *Clinical Chemistry in Diagnosis and Treatment*, 6th edn. London: Edward Arnold, 1994.
3. Trauls Scott L. *Basic Skills in Interpreting Lab Data*, 2nd edn. Bethesda, MD: American Society of Health Systems Pharmacists, 1996.
4. National Kidney Foundation. *KDOQI Clinical Practice Guidelines for Chronic Kidney Disease: Executive Summary*. New York: National Kidney Foundation, 2002.

5. Department of Health. *The National Service Framework for Renal Services. Part Two: Chronic Kidney Disease, Acute Renal Failure and End of Life Care.* London: Department of Health, February 2005.

6. Kuan Y, Hossain M, Surman J *et al.* GFR prediction using the MDRD and Cockroft and Gault equations in patients with end-stage renal disease. *Nephrol Dial Transplant* 2005; 20: 2394–2401

7. Froissart M, Rossert J, Jacquot C *et al.* Predictive performance of the Modification of Diet in Renal Disease and Cockroft-Gault equations for estimating renal function. *J Am Soc Nephrol* 2005; 16: 763–773.

3

Acute renal failure

Caroline Ashley

Acute renal failure (ARF) is defined as the rapid cessation of renal excretory function within a time frame of hours or days, accompanied by a rise in serum urea and creatinine, and accumulation of nitrogenous waste products in a patient whose renal function was previously normal. It is usually, but not always, accompanied by a fall in urine output. The condition is potentially reversible, and in routine clinical practice, measurement of serum creatinine is used to follow the changes in glomerular filtration rate (GFR).

Definition

There are various working definitions of ARF, including:

- an increase in serum creatinine of >50 µmol/L
- an increase in serum creatinine of >50% from baseline
- a reduction in calculated creatinine clearance of >50%
- the need for dialysis.

Confusingly, the patient may be anuric (<50 mL urine/24 hours), oliguric (<400 mL urine/24 hours), pass normal volumes of urine or may even be polyuric. The urine produced may be of poor quality, however, with very few waste products. The diagnosis of ARF is made on plasma biochemistry, with an elevated serum creatinine, urea and possibly potassium. Oliguria is usually indicative of failure of both glomerular and tubular function. In contrast to chronic renal failure, there is no early loss of endocrine function.

Caution is required when interpreting measurements of serum creatinine in ARF for several reasons:

- Creatinine production depends on muscle mass, and though normally constant for an individual, it can increase in patients with acute muscle injury.
- Because of the reciprocal relationship between creatinine concentration and GFR, small changes in GFR close to the normal range have much less effect on serum creatinine than small changes when GFR is already significantly reduced.
- Changes in serum creatinine concentration lag behind changes in GFR. The serum creatinine may continue to increase for several days after a marked reduction in the GFR, even if the GFR has subsequently started to improve.

Incidence

The incidence of ARF is difficult to state precisely because it depends on the parameters by which it is defined. The incidence of severe ARF (serum creatinine >500 µmol/L) in the general population is estimated to be approximately 70–140 per million of the population,[1] and around half of these will require dialysis. Less severe ARF (serum creatinine ≤177 µmol/L or an increase of 50% above baseline) occurs in about 210/million/year. One hospital survey revealed some degree of renal impairment in around 5% of all admissions.[2] In intensive care units (ICU), however, the figure is much higher, with at least 15% of admissions having renal impairment, of which the cause is sepsis in approximately 50% of cases. The financial implications of renal impairment are considerable: the cost of a survivor who had renal failure leaving ICU is 70 times that of a patient without renal impairment.[2]

Clinical features

Since ARF involves the acute retention of nitrogenous waste products, salt, water, potassium and acid, the physical signs and symptoms encountered include:

- nausea and vomiting
- peripheral oedema
- breathlessness
- pulmonary oedema
- itching
- pleural effusion
- weakness
- pericarditis
- depression of consciousness
- oliguria
- convulsions.

An episode of ARF usually lasts between 7 and 21 days providing the primary insult is corrected in a reasonable time.

Irreversible ARF usually occurs either in patients with pre-existing renal disease or in those who experience repeated ischaemic or nephrotoxic insults.

The mortality rate for ARF is variable. Patients with non-oliguric ARF have a relatively low mortality (10–40%), possibly because they have less severe underlying disease or perhaps because they have been treated more promptly or aggressively. A particularly high mortality rate (80–90%) is found in older patients and in those with serious complications such as pre-existing cardiovascular or respiratory disease, severe burns, hepatorenal syndrome, sepsis and multi-organ failure.

Causes

Conventionally, the causes of ARF are classified by renal anatomy into pre-renal, renal and post-renal causes. This approach is somewhat over-simplified, since many cases of ARF have a mixture of pre, post and renal components. Take, for example, a traumatic injury causing rhabdomyolysis and ARF. The injury and associated muscle swelling causes a fall in effective arteriolar blood volume (EABV) and hence pre-renal impairment. The myoglobin released from the muscle causes renal vasoconstriction (also pre-renal), tubular injury (renal) and tubular obstruction (post renal).[3] Nevertheless, since there is no alternative classification in clinical use and it is a useful way of considering the kidney, the causes of ARF will be described under these headings.

Pre-renal failure

Pre-renal ARF is caused by inadequate perfusion of essentially normal kidneys, in which the EABV is reduced. It is a normal physiological response to hypotension or hypovolaemia, resulting in intense renal conservation of sodium and water at the expense of a decreased GFR. Renal function usually returns to normal rapidly once the underlying cause is corrected.

The kidneys are adept at regulating their blood supply over a variety of perfusion pressures, and such autoregulation is highly effective in healthy individuals. This means that quite severe perturbations of blood pressure or interference with the usual adaptive responses of the kidney are required to cause renal dysfunction in the normal kidney. The operative word here is normal, since in disease states, for example hypertension, this autoregulation may be disordered or reset, leading to renal dysfunction at blood pressures that would ordinarily be quite adequate to maintain renal perfusion.

Table 3.1 lists some of the causes of ARF.

The traditional signs of sodium and water depletion include tachycardia, hypotension, postural hypotension, reduced skin turgor, reduced ocular tension (sunken eyes), collapsed

Table 3.1 Some of the causes of acute renal failure

Hypovolaemia	Trauma, burns, surgery, pancreatitis, haemorrhage, gastrointestinal losses, exudative dermatitis, liver failure, nephrotic syndrome, hepatorenal syndrome
Loss of peripheral resistance in which the vascular bed is dilated thereby reducing the circulating volume	Sepsis, endotoxaemia, shock, general anaesthesia, overuse of antihypertensives, anaphylactic shock, surgery
Decreased cardiac output	Cardiogenic shock, heart failure, pulmonary embolism, myocardial infarction, cardiac arrhythmias, post-cardiac surgery
Renovascular obstruction	Atherosclerosis, thrombosis, embolism, dissecting aneurysm
Altered renal autoregulation	NSAIDs, ACE inhibitors, ciclosporin, tacrolimus

peripheral veins and cold extremities. One of the physiological responses is a reduction in renal perfusion, which in turn may lead to intrinsic renal damage with a consequent acute deterioration in renal function. This state may be caused by a significant haemorrhage, or by septicaemia, in which the vascular bed is dilated thereby reducing the effective circulating volume. It may also be caused by excessive sodium and water loss from the skin, urinary tract or gastrointestinal tract. Excessive loss through the skin by sweating occurs in hot climates and is rare in the UK, but it also occurs after extensive burns. Gastrointestinal losses are associated with vomiting or diarrhoea. Urinary tract losses often result from excessive diuretic therapy but may also occur with the osmotic diuresis caused by hyperglycaemia and glycosuria in a diabetic patient.

Infection causes a large proportion of ARF by causing the systemic inflammatory response syndrome (SIRS). SIRS can be precipitated by a variety of organisms (including bacteria, viruses and fungi) and can lead to multi-organ failure which has a mortality in excess of 60%.[4] The mediators of multi-organ failure include haemodynamic changes (principally systemic hypotension and altered tissue bed perfusion), complement activation and cytokine release.

Acute tubular necrosis

Acute tubular necrosis (ATN) comes from the insults that cause pre-renal ARF, but in circumstances lasting long enough to cause ischaemic injury to renal tubules. This leads to a prolonged reduction in GFR that sometimes persists for weeks after correction of the initiating insult. However, the condition is potentially recoverable, provided the initial insult to the kidneys is removed, and renal perfusion is maintained.

Intrinsic renal failure

Intrinsic renal failure is caused by any factor that causes damage either to the kidney itself or the surrounding vasculature. Table 3.2 lists the numerous mechanisms that can lead to intrinsic ARF.

Renal causes of ARF can be be subdivided into four categories; vascular, glomerular, tubular and interstitial.

Vascular

Blockage of renal blood vessels caused by atheroembolic disease or foreign material leading to an inflammatory reaction which obliterates the lumen (e.g. cholesterol emboli) can cause ARF. Occasionally, endothelial damage causes intimal proliferation and luminal obliteration (e.g. in scleroderma renal crisis or accelerated phase hypertension).

The vasculitides cause inflammation and necrosis in the vessel wall upstream of, or in, the glomerular tuft (after all the glomerulus is merely a modified blood vessel). The size of the vessel involved determines the symptoms and

Table 3.2   Mechanisms that can lead to intrinsic acute renal failure

Acute tubular necrosis	General surgery Cardiac surgery Vascular surgery (e.g. repair of abdominal aortic aneurysm, involving cross-clamping of the aorta) Obstetric complications Sepsis Acute heart failure Burns
Nephrotoxicity	Including aminoglycosides and amphotericin
Intravascular coagulation	Including hypertension, pre-eclampsia, eclampsia, haemolytic–uraemic syndrome (HUS), thrombotic thrombocytopenic purpura (TTP), scleroderma, disseminated intravascular coagulation (DIC), sepsis
Acute tubular necrosis	Post-ischaemia Nephrotoxins (drugs, contrast media, organic solvents, herbal medicines, snake venom, mushrooms, heavy metals) Myoglobinaemia Hypercalcaemia
Contrast nephropathy	A specific form of nephrotoxicity characterised by renal vasoconstriction and avid sodium retention
Impaired renal perfusion + drug-induced impairment of autoregulation	ACE inhibitors, NSAIDs, plus atherosclerotic renal vascular disease or hypovolaemia
Hepatorenal syndrome	Reversible intense renal vasoconstriction and sodium retention complicating cirrhosis
Poisoning	Including paracetamol, often after recovery from liver damage
Rhabdomyolysis	Following crush injury, drug overdose, status epilepticus
Atheroembolism (cholesterol embolism)	Spontaneous or a complication of angiography, angioplasty or thrombolysis
Raised intra-abdominal pressure (abdominal compartment syndrome)	Caused by intra-abdominal pressure >25 mmHg (e.g. post-operative abdominal exploration, tense ascites)
Renal embolism	Endocarditis, cardiac thrombus
Infiltration	Including leukaemias, lymphoma, multiple myeloma
Urate nephropathy	Complication of chemotherapy for acute leukaemia or lymphoma
Myeloma	Cast nephropathy, light-chain deposition disease, amyloidosis, sepsis and hypercalcaemia can all cause renal damage
Hypercalcaemia	Sarcoidosis, myeloma
Intravenous immunoglobulin	Probably results from osmotic damage to proximal tubular cells caused by sucrose in some IV immunoglobulin preparations
Renal parenchymal disease	Rapidly progressive glomerulonephritis (systemic vasculitis, Goodpasture's syndrome, systemic lupus erythematosus, Wegener's granulomatosus) Acute interstitial nephritis Haemolytic uraemic syndrome Cryoglobulinaemia

→

Table 3.2   (continued)

Renal parenchymal disease (continued)	Acute allergic tubulo-interstitial nephritis (penicillins, NSAIDs, recreational drugs) Bacterial endocarditis Infections (Legionnaires' disease) Granulomas (tuberculosis) Crystals (hyperuricaemia, hypercalcaemia)
Malignant hypertension	Untreated primary ('essential') hypertension or a complication of chronic glomerulonephritis, or scleroderma renal crisis
Renal vein thrombosis	Complication of malignancy or pre-existing nephritic syndrome
Acute pyelonephritis	Seldom causes acute renal failure, although may be more likely to do so in the elderly and in those taking NSAIDs Infection in patients with diabetes and partial obstruction (e.g. from papillary necrosis) may cause pyelonephritis and acute renal failure

signs and also provides a way of classifying these diseases.

Microangiopathic haemolytic processes are processes in which endothelial damage is the prime mover, leading to activation of coagulation, red cell destruction, tubular obliteration and downstream necrosis. The classical examples include pre-eclampsia and the haemolytic uraemic syndrome.

Glomerular

The glomuruli may be affected by various usually immune-mediated insults classified by their histological appearance (the glomerulonephritides). These can present either as the nephrotic syndrome (proteinuria >3 g/24 hours, oedema, hypoalbuminaemia) with or without renal dysfunction, or as a nephritic illness with nephrotic features and/or hypertension and haematuria, often accompanied by renal dysfunction. Drugs are sometimes responsible for inducing glomerular disease.

Tubular

Tubular function may be compromised by numerous insults. Tubular cells have adapted to exist in an ischaemic environment normally, but any insult which reduces further the already critical supply of metabolites can cause renal dysfunction by causing acute tubular necrosis. Tubular damage usually results in a reduction in urine output, although the reasons for this have not been completely elucidated. Certainly when tubular cells are damaged they slough off the tubular basement membrane into the tubular lumen causing some degree of tubular obstruction. In addition, glomerular filtrate is not constrained within the tubular lumen and leaks back into the capillaries without change in composition. Finally, and probably most importantly, renal blood flow is reduced in ATN and blood is diverted towards the medulla away from the cortex, bypassing the glomeruli. Renal vasoconstriction is caused by, among other things, tubuloglomerular feedback from increased sodium chloride delivery to the macula densa, sympathetic stimulation, angiotensin II, endothelin and thromboxanes.

Metabolic derangements may also lead to renal dysfunction, the most common cause of which is probably hypercalcaemia, which can cause ARF. Another metabolic problem that can lead to ARF is hypothyroidism.

Interstitial

The interstitium is that part of the kidney that is not vascular, glomerular or tubular. As the kidney relies on its tightly coordinated structure to function, any disruption to this highly interdependent architecture can result in renal failure. An interstitial infiltration with inflammatory cells including eosinophils is a characteristic of many drug-associated cases of ARF.

Acute bacterial pyelonephritis can lead to infiltration with inflammatory cells and interstitial scarring and some viral infections are associated with marked interstitial oedema that can cause ARF. Autoimmune diseases (e.g. systemic lupus erythematosus or mixed connective tissue diseases) cause an interstitial infiltrate that may be irreversible. Very occasionally, the kidney is infiltrated with cells from lymphoma or leukaemia causing interstitial expansion and ARF. One unusual cause of renal failure is that of the compressed or 'Page kidney'. In this situation compression of the renal parenchyma by a haematoma (e.g. following a renal biopsy or trauma) can cause acute renal dysfunction.[5]

Analgesic nephropathy is a special form of renal disease in which there is often renal papillary necrosis and a history of analgesic administration. It is now much less common in the UK where many of the strongly associated drugs have been withdrawn (e.g. phenacetin).[6]

Drug-induced acute renal disease

Drug-induced renal failure is well recognised, but the frequency with which it occurs with particular drugs is unknown. It is, however, important to be aware of the types of drug that can induce renal failure because there may be a specific antidote or, if suspected and acted on early, the failure may be reversible.

Despite a large blood supply, the kidneys are always in a state of incipient hypoxia because of their high metabolic activity, and any condition that causes the kidney to be underperfused may be associated with an acute deterioration in renal function. However, such a deterioration may also be produced by nephrotoxic agents, including drugs.

- **Non-steroidal anti-inflammatory drugs (NSAIDs)** in particular are associated with renal damage, and even a short course of an NSAID (such as diclofenac) has been associated with ARF, especially in older patients. The main cause of NSAID-induced renal damage is inhibition of prostaglandin synthesis in the kidney, particularly prostaglandins E2, D2 and I2 (prostacyclin). These prostaglandins are all potent vasodilators and consequently produce an increase in blood flow to the glomerulus and the medulla. The maintenance of blood pressure in a variety of clinical conditions, such as volume depletion, biventricular cardiac failure or hepatic cirrhosis with ascites, may rely on the release of vasoconstrictor substances such as angiotensin II. In these states, inhibition of prostaglandin synthesis may cause unopposed renal arteriolar vasoconstriction, which again leads to renal hypoperfusion. NSAIDs impair the ability of the renovasculature to adapt to a fall in perfusion pressure or to an increase in vasoconstrictor balance.

- **Angiotensin-converting enzyme (ACE) inhibitors** may also produce a reduction in renal function by preventing the angiotensin II-mediated vasoconstriction of the efferent glomerular arteriole, which contributes to the high-pressure gradient across the glomerulus. This problem is important only in patients with renal vascular disease, particularly those with bilateral renal artery stenoses, causing renal perfusion to fall. In order to maintain the pressure gradient across the glomerulus, the efferent arteriolar resistance must rise. This is predominantly accomplished by angiotensin-induced efferent vasoconstriction, as is shown in Figure 3.1. If ACE inhibitors are administered, this system is rendered inoperable and there is no longer any way of maintaining an effective filtration pressure. This leads to a fall in GRF and the development of ARF.

- **Contrast media**, especially the ionic variety (iodinated) used for radiological scans, are also known nephrotoxins, especially in patients with already compromised renal function. There are thought to be two mechanisms of action behind this toxicity. The contrast media cause vasospasm which in turn leads to tubular ischaemia and reduced oxygen tension. In addition, oxidative stress causes an increased formation of free radicals within the tubules, leading to further damage.

- **Iatrogenic factors**, including fluid and electrolyte imbalance and drug nephrotoxicity, can be identified in over 50% of cases of ARF and also play a large role in many cases

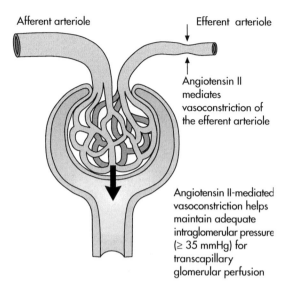

Afferent arteriole

Efferent arteriole

Angiotensin II mediates vasoconstriction of the efferent arteriole

Angiotensin II-mediated vasoconstriction helps maintain adequate intraglomerular pressure (≥ 35 mmHg) for transcapillary glomerular perfusion

Figure 3.1 The role of angiotensin II in maintaining adequate intraglomular pressure.

Table 3.3 Common causes of obstructive nephropathy	
Bladder outflow	Benign prostatic hypertrophy or prostatic carcinoma Infiltrative bladder cancer causing bilateral vesico-ureteric obstruction Neurogenic bladder
Ureteric obstruction	Bilateral stone disease Crystal deposition (urate, sulfonamides, aciclovir, cisplatin) Pelvic tumours Papillary necrosis Retroperitoneal fibrosis (with or without abdominal aortic aneurysm) Radiation fibrosis Urethral strictures

of community-acquired ARF. Other causes of drug-induced renal failure are discussed in Chapter 11. It has been estimated that up to 20% of individuals over the age of 65 are prescribed diuretics, with a lesser number receiving an NSAID; consequently, there is a large population of elderly patients susceptible to renal damage in the event of any insult to the kidney. ARF that requires dialysis is fortunately rare, with only 50–70 patients per million of the population affected annually, but less severe degrees of impairment may occur in up to 5% of hospital inpatients.

Post-renal failure (obstruction)

Post-renal failure or obstructive nephropathy involves obstruction of urinary outflow, leading to increased pressure within the renal collecting systems and resulting in reduced GFR, reduced tubular reabsorption of sodium and water, and acquired renal tubular acidosis, phosphaturia and other abnormalities of tubular function. These abnormalities may persist even after relief of the cause of the obstruction. Table 3.3 lists the most common causes of obstructive nephropathy.

Symptoms/signs

The initial cause of the ARF is important in determining the symptoms and signs of the presentation. There may be none until late on, when signs of fluid overload, oedema and hypertension and hyperkalemia might be presenting features.

Hyperkalaemia may cause cardiac arrest without warning. Not all patients have the same susceptibility to the cardiac effects of hyperkalaemia, but the risk of cardiac arrest can be judged by electrocardiogram (ECG). Pulmonary oedema is the most serious complication of salt and water overload in ARF, often arising from inappropriate administration of intravenous fluids to oliguric patients. In severe cases, patients are restless and confused, with sweating, cyanosis, tachypnoea, tachycardia and widespread wheeze or crepitations in the chest. Further investigation will show arterial hypoxaemia and widespread interstitial shadowing on chest X-ray.

Distinguishing acute from chronic renal impairment

One question that must be asked is whether the renal failure is really acute. Raised serum creatinine in an acutely unwell patient can be caused by acute (ARF), acute-on-chronic, or chronic (CRF) renal failure. These presentations have different prognoses and may require fundamentally different management. Points to help distinguish between them include:

- Comparing any previous measurements of serum creatinine with the patient's current biochemistry. Pre-existing chronic renal impairment can be excluded if a relatively recent previous measurement of renal function was normal.
- A history of several months' vague ill-health, nocturia or pruritus, and findings of skin pigmentation, anaemia, long-standing hypertension or neuropathy suggest a more chronic disease.
- Renal ultrasonography to determine size and echogenicity of the kidneys. It is noteworthy that renal size is normal in most patients with ARF.
- Anaemia is a major feature of CRF, but it may occur early in the course of many diseases that cause ARF.
- Bone disease – evidence of long-standing renal bone disease (e.g. radiological evidence of hyperparathyroidism, greatly elevated parathyroid hormone (PTH) levels) is diagnostic of CRF, but hypocalcaemia and hyperphosphataemia may occur in both ARF and CRF.

Management

Regardless of the cause, the same general treatment principles apply to all patients who develop ARF. These include removing nephrotoxic insults (e,g. drugs): in some instances the nephrotoxins may need to be removed by dialysis or adsorption (e.g. after aspirin overdose) or specific antidotes may be needed in addition to dialysis (e.g. N-acetylcysteine in paracetamol overdose). In the case of obstructive ARF, the cause of the obstruction should be removed if possible.

Fluids

In pre-renal failure, urine output and renal function should improve when intravascular volume is restored, thus improving renal perfusion. The fluid infused should be blood, colloid or sodium chloride, and should mimic the nature of the fluid lost as closely as possible. Aggressive, early fluid resuscitation is the intervention most likely to have a positive effect on the course of pre-renal ARF and ARF caused by ATN. It must be guided by regular clinical assessment of the patient's circulating volume, aided by measurements of central venous pressure (CVP) or even pulmonary capillary wedge pressure.

Sodium chloride 0.9% is an appropriate choice of intravenous fluid, as it replaces both water and sodium ions in a concentration approximately equal to plasma. Conversely, should water depletion with hypernatraemia occur, isotonic solutions that are either free of, or low in, sodium are available (e.g. dextrose 5% or sodium chloride 0.18% with dextrose 4%). Patients should be observed continuously and the infusion stopped ideally when features of volume depletion have been resolved but before volume overload has been induced.

Fluid balance

Strict fluid balance charts are often ordered in patients with ARF. It is useful to know the fluid input and output, but these charts are notoriously inaccurate. Over-reliance on them also carries the danger that fluid replacement will be adjusted according to the recent output rather than the clinical state of the patient. Positive fluid balance is a necessary part of the resuscitation process for patients with effective or true hypovolaemia.

However, in extremely overloaded patients, it may be necessary to restrict fluid intake to the urine volume passed in the previous 24 hours + other losses, for example, insensible losses of 500 mL/day. This fluid allowance may be increased if the patient exhibits signs of hyperventilation, sweating, fever, wound or drain losses.

Possibly the most common cause of ARF is the peripheral vasodilation that occurs in septic shock. In such cases it would be appropriate to infuse a colloid as well as sodium chloride as this would help to restore the circulating volume. It is important to remember, however, that not all shocked patients are hypovolaemic and some, notably those in cardiogenic shock, could be adversely affected by a fluid challenge.

Urine output

Another reason for measuring urine output is to assess renal function. Anuria and severe oliguria are diagnostic of severe ARF, but otherwise urine volume is of little help. For example, a GFR of 100 mL/min (6000 mL/h) normally gives a urine flow rate of about 60 mL/h because of reabsorption of 99% of the filtrate delivered to the renal tubules. However, a GFR of 1 mL/min combined with complete failure of tubular reabsorption (resulting from tubular damage, as in ATN, or from high doses of drugs that inhibit tubular reabsorption (e.g. dopamine, furosemide) would also give a urine output of 60 mL/h. Changes in urine flow are therefore a very poor guide to changes in GFR, and must be interpreted along with all other available clinical information. Urethral catheters are often placed to enable accurate measurement of urine flow rate. However, they are the single most important source of hospital-acquired Gram-negative sepsis, so should not be placed without good reason, and should be removed as soon as possible.

Fluid challenges

These are often given in the hope that they will stimulate diuresis. It is both illogical and dangerous to give further fluid to a patient who has already been fully resuscitated. If the patient remains oliguric, the extra fluid load may cause life-threatening pulmonary oedema. The only rational use of a 500 mL fluid bolus is when given in combination with CVP measurements; administration of a fluid bolus to a hypovolaemic patient causes only a transient increase in CVP, whereas a more sustained rise is seen in patients approaching euvolaemia.

Dopamine, loop diuretics and mannitol

In ATN, volume repletion does not restore renal function, and urine output usually remains low (<30 mL/h). There is no evidence that any treatment improves renal function or accelerates renal recovery. Dopamine has been used at low doses (~2 ng/kg per min) for many years as a reno-protective agent, in the belief that it causes vasodilatation of the renal vascular bed, restores renal blood flow and thereby improves GFR. While its use has been controversial, a multi-centre randomised double-blinded placebo-controlled trial has shown no benefit to using low-dose dopamine infusion in patients with renal dysfunction with the systemic inflammatory response syndrome.[7] The weight of evidence has swung firmly against the use of low-dose dopamine and its routine use in incipient or established ARF should be discontinued.

The use of a loop diuretic infusion in patients with non-oliguric ARF has been popular. The theory is that the most metabolically active cells in the nephron are the first to suffer tubular necrosis in renal underperfusion. Loop diuretics reduce the activity of the $Na^+/K^+/2Cl^-$ pump, which is highly metabolically active, thus releasing some metabolic energy towards essential subcellular pathways favouring survival in a critical incipient tubular cell death. They are also purported to flush out tubular casts. Many units give a trial of furosemide (e.g. 500 mg IV over 8 hours, or 1 g over 24 hours, if a small dose has produced no effect). Treatment is then continued according to response, although if the urine output in a euvolaemic patient does not respond to a large dose of furosemide, further therapy should be discontinued in order to prevent further damage to the tubules.[8]

Mannitol has been used to promote an osmotic diuresis and has been advocated by some in cases of incipient ARF and contrast media-induced nephrotoxicity. However it has not been shown to offer any reno-protective effects in any field of ARF and may cause significant renal impairment itself by causing an osmotic nephrosis and increase tubular workload by increasing solute delivery.[9]

Loop diuretics and dopamine can both increase urine output by reducing tubular reabsorption of filtrate, which give the false impression that GFR has improved. The ability to mount a diuresis in response to either drug is probably an indication that the patient may have a better prognosis overall. Unless the patient is significantly volume overloaded, the diuresis caused by these drugs can exacerbate ATN by causing further hypovolaemia. Administration of diuretics to patients with a low CVP or to those at risk of hypovolaemia is similarly clinically unjustified.

Choice of resuscitation fluid

Adequate intravascular volume replacement is essential in the management of ARF. However, controversy continues over the optimal fluid for correction of hypovolaemia.

Crystalloids

Crystalloids (e.g. 0.9% sodium chloride, 5% glucose, Hartmann's solution) are cheap and safe, but rapidly distribute between the vascular space and the extracellular space, resulting in oedema, pleural effusions and ascites if used in large volumes, particularly in the presence of increased endothelial permeability (as in systemic inflammatory response syndrome). In cases where the patient has symptomatic metabolic acidosis, 1.26% sodium bicarbonate solution may be infused instead of 0.9% sodium chloride. The two solutions are both isotonic with blood, but the bicarbonate will help correct the acidosis.

Colloids

Colloids (e.g. human albumin, dextrans, hydroxyethyl starch (HES), modified gelatins) are used in the hope that they will remain in the vascular space for longer and hence restore microcirculatory flow more efficiently. This theory holds true for cases of simple hypo-

volaemia. However, when plasma protein levels may be increased as a result of haemoconcentration, crystalloids will probably be more effective. In sicker patients with sepsis, endothelial permeability to macromolecules is often increased, with the danger that these molecules will leave the circulation, elevate interstitial oncotic pressure and exacerbate the accumulation of fluid in the extracellular space.

In the UK, the available colloid solutions include gelatin preparations, dextran solutions and HES solutions. None of the available preparations are free of potentially serious side-effects. In particular, dextrans can cause anaphylactoid reactions and HES solutions may disrupt coagulation mechanisms and cause renal impairment. In a trial comparing gelatin with HES 200/0.62 in critically ill patients there was twice the incidence of ARF in the HES-treated group. However, more recent trials comparing gelatin solution with the low-molecular-weight, low-substitution HES 130/0.4 solution have shown a vastly improved safety profile with regard to renal function and coagulation with the new HES.[10,11]

A Cochrane meta-analysis comparing synthetic colloids with crystalloids concluded that there was no proven clinical benefit for the use of colloids in resuscitation. However, they continue to be widely used in clinical practice on the basis of their theoretical advantages.

Renal replacement therapy

Many patients with mild-to-moderate ARF can be managed on general medical or surgical wards, but those with multiple organ failure should be managed on an ICU. Patients with ARF requiring renal replacement therapy (RRT) (i.e. those with rapidly increasing serum creatinine, oliguria, especially those with impending or established pulmonary oedema, hyperkalaemia and severe metabolic acidosis) should be managed on either a renal ward or an ICU.

There is currently little evidence to guide decisions on when to instigate RRT in ARF. The options for RRT are usually continuous arterio-venous or veno-venous haemofiltration (CAVH/CVVH), continuous arterio-venous or veno-venous haemodiafiltration (CAVHDF/CVVHDF) and intermittent haemodialysis.

Additional points

There are several other practical points to be considered in the management of patients with ARF, some of which are especially relevant to pharmacists. These include:

- Amendment of drug doses: prescriptions should be closely scrutinised and, where necessary, the doses of drugs must be altered so that they are appropriate for the patient's level of renal function. Since the level of renal function may be in a state of flux in someone with ARF, it is important to continue to monitor renal function and re-adjust doses as necessary.
- In order to allow the already damaged kidneys to recover, it is also vital to avoid any further nephrotoxic insults wherever possible, for example, the use of NSAIDs and aminoglycosides. If they must be used, ensure that the dose is appropriate, and minimise the length of treatment. Try to use an alternative, non-nephrotoxic agent wherever possible.
- Maintain adequate nutritional therapy: a good rough guide is a protein intake of 0.6 g/kg per day, increasing to 1 g/kg if the patient being dialysed. Calorie intake should be 50–100% above the patient's resting energy expenditure (25 kcal/kg per day). Consult a specialist renal dietician where possible.
- Monitor the patient's biochemical parameters closely, including daily weight, fluid balance, U + Es (especially potassium, calcium and phosphate), a full blood count, and liver function tests. Treat any serious anomalies appropriately.
- Treat hyperkalaemia if the serum potassium is >6 mmol/L (see also Chapter 2). Severe hyperkalaemia with changes in the ECG should be treated as an emergency. Dialysis will correct hyperkalaemia, but it may not be possible to initiate this measure immediately.

A salbutamol nebuliser will lower serum potassium levels transiently by stimulating uptake into cells. Intravenous calcium (10% calcium gluconate, 10 mL over 60 seconds) is given to 'stabilise' the cardiac membranes, but does not alter the serum potassium level. Rapidly acting insulin 10 units (with 50% glucose, 50 mL) given IV over 5–10 minutes, stimulates the Na^+/K^+-ATPase in muscle and liver, driving potassium into cells and reducing the serum concentration by 1–2 mmol/L over 30–60 minutes. This does, however, render the potassium 'unavailable' to a dialysis procedure and should therefore be avoided if imminent dialysis is contemplated. Cation exchange resins (e.g. calcium polystyrene sulfonate (Calcium Resonium) 15 g) orally or rectally 6-hourly may be given to absorb potassium into the gut lumen. They require 4 hours to take effect, and lead to severe constipation if taken without laxatives, but may be a useful 'stopgap' measure.

- Patients with ARF are very prone to developing stress ulceration, so a proton pump inhibitor, H_2 blocker or sucralfate should be prescribed as per local protocol.

Outcome

Acute renal failure is a life-threatening condition. In a series of more than 1000 patients requiring dialysis, mortality was 40%.[12] Outcome depends directly on pathogenesis. If due to obstruction which is successfully relieved, or ATN where haemodynamic parameters return to normal quickly, then recovery approaches 100%. However if due to glomerulonephritis, prognosis depends on severity of damage and may be irrecoverable if too many glomeruli are involved. In such cases, the patient will need to remain on dialysis permanently.

Conclusion

Acute renal failure is common in hospitalised patients and is most often due to ATN. It is associated with a significant mortality and morbidity and is expensive to treat. Drugs play an important role in the pathogenesis of ARF. The pharmacist can play an important role in identifying possible pathogens, ensuring that the patient does not receive any further nephrotoxic compounds during the recovery phase, and advising on appropriate dose adjustments for drugs given to the patient while undergoing RRT.

 CASE STUDY

Mr VC is a 65-year-old man (68 kg, 175 cm) who presents to casualty with nausea, vomiting and profound diarrhoea. Two weeks ago he presented to his GP with a painful right metatarsal pharyngeal joint (due to gout), for which his GP prescribed colchicine 500 µg 4-hourly for 2 days. Unfortunately, the patient became violently sick after four doses and discontinued this medication and went back to the GP who then prescribed:

- Indometacin 50 mg three times a day
- Ranitidine 150 mg twice daily.

The gout pain is now resolving.
    On admission, Mr VC was pale, lethargic and breathless.

Past medical history:

- Hypertension 1 year
- Type 2 diabetes 5 years.

Medication:

- Bendroflumethiazide 5 mg every morning (for the last six months – increased from 2.5 mg)
- Ramipril 2.5 mg every morning (started six months ago)
- Gliclazide 40 mg twice daily.

Biochemistry:

- Sodium 137 mmol/L (135–150 mmol/L)
- Potassium 6.9 mmol/L (3.5–5.2 mmol/L)
- Urea 28.5 mmol/L (3.2–6.6 mmol/L)
- Creatinine 386 µmol/L (60–110 µmol/L)
- Bicarbonate 18 mmol/L (22–31 mmol/L)
- Phosphate 1.7 mmol/L (0.9–1.5 mmol/L)
- Corrected calcium 2.6 mmol/L (2.2–2.5 mmol/L)
- pH 7.26 (7.36–7.44)
- Glucose 10.8 mmol/L
- 24-hour urine output 600 mL.

Mr VC is admitted to hospital under the diabetic team.

$\rightarrow$

CASE STUDY (continued)

Q1. **What patient and pharmaceutical factors may have precipitated acute renal failure in this patient?**

Q2. **What are the main pharmaceutical problems and how might they be managed?**
Mr VC is treated for his hyperkalaemia, put on a sliding scale insulin infusion, and rehydrated with 4 L of sodium chloride 0.9%, until he has a central venous pressure (CVP) of 12.

After 2 days, his serum creatinine has fallen to 168 µmol/L. However, a further 2 days later, it is noted that he is again failing to pass urine, although he appears to have a palpable bladder, and his serum creatinine has again risen to 272 µmol/L. This suggests urinary retention, so the decision is made to insert a urinary catheter.

Following insertion of the catheter, Mr. VC passed 2 L of urine in the next 24 hours, but then spiked a temperature of 38.5°C and became hypotensive. A diagnosis of urinary sepsis was made, and because it was the weekend, and with no other laboratory data available, the new senior house officer (SHO) prescribed gentamicin 475 mg IV daily.

Q3. **Comment on the appropriateness of the prescribed antibiotic therapy. What advice would you provide regarding this?**
Mr VC is given the gentamicin dose of 475 mg IV on the Sunday. On Monday morning, the pharmacist notes that both the drug and the dose are inappropriate for Mr VC, given his degree of renal impairment. The drug is discontinued on the drug chart, but a gentamicin level is taken anyway, and is reported back as 8.6 mg/L, so it is calculated it will take Mr VC several more days to clear that one dose. The prescription is changed to co-amoxiclav IV 600 mg three times a day.

His serum creatinine is monitored, and over the course of the next few days, the serial levels are 272, 284, 290, 237, 188, 135 µmol/L. He is switched to oral co-amoxiclav, and his renal function continues to fall.

Mr VC is discharged from hospital on day 10, with a serum creatinine of 112 µmol/L.

References

1. Feest TG, Round A, Hamad S. Incidence of severe acute renal failure in adults: Results of a community based study. *BMJ* 1993; 306, 481–483.
2. Hou SH, Bushinksy DA, Wish JG *et al.* Hospital-acquired renal insufficiency: a prospective study. *Am J Med* 1983; 74: 243.
3. Holt S, Moore K. Pathogenesis of renal failure in rhabdomyolysis: the role of myoglobin. *Exp Nephrol* 2000; 8: 72–76.
4. Bone RC. Sepsis and SIRS. Nephrol Dial Transplant 1994; 9 (Suppl 14); 99–103.
5. Kingdon E, Brunton C, Holt S *et al.* The re-appearing kidney: an unusual complication of renal biopsy. *Nephrol Dial Transplant* 1999; 14: 1758–1760.
6. DeBroe M, Elseviers M. Analgesic nephropathy. *N Engl J Med* 1998; 228: 446.
7. Australian and New Zealand Intensive Care Society Clinical Trials Group. Low dose dopamine in patients with early renal dysfunction: a placebo controlled randomised trial. *Lancet* 2000; 356: 2139–2143.
8. Ho KM, Sheridan DJ. Meta-analysis of frusemide to prevent or treat acute renal failure. *BMJ* 2006; 333: 420.

9. Visweswaran P, Massin EK, Dubose TD. Mannitol-induced acute renal failure. *J Am Soc Nephrol* 1997; 8: 1028–1033.

10. Langeron O, Doelberg M, Ang ET *et al*. Voluven, a lower substituted hydroxyethyl starch (HES 130/0.4) causes fewer effects on coagulation in major orthopaedic surgery than HES 200/05. *Anesth Analg* 2001; 92: 855–862.

11. Boldt J, Brenner T, Lehmann A *et al*. Influence of two different volume replacement regimens on renal function in elderly patients undergoing cardiac surgery: comparison of a new starch preparation with gelatin. *Intensive Care Med* 2003; 29: 763–769.

12. Liano F, Pascual J. Epidemiology of acute renal failure: a prospective, multicenter, community-based study. *Kidney Int* 1996; 50: 811–818.

Further reading

Armitage AJ, Tomson C. Acute renal failure. *Medicine* 2003; 31: 43–48.

Dodds LJ. *Drugs in Use*, 3rd edn. London: Pharmaceutical Press, 2004.

Kumar P, Clark M. *Clinical Medicine*, 4th edn. Edinburgh: WB Saunders, 1998.

Walker R, Edwards C. *Clinical Pharmacy and Therapeutics*, 2nd edn. Edinburgh: Churchill Livingstone, 1998.

4

Chronic renal failure

Roger Fernandes

This chapter provides a general overview on the incidence, causes, consequence and treatments of chronic renal failure. The consequences of chronic renal failure, in particular anaemia and renal bone disease, are covered elsewhere in the book and only general principles will be covered here. The first part of this chapter looks at the causes and symptoms experienced in chronic renal failure with a brief discussion on the treatment options available for symptom control. The second part discusses drug handling in chronic renal failure. The case study at the end highlights some important learning points which should be attempted on completion of the chapter.

Definition

In health, the kidney performs a phenomenal workload: it is perfused with 20% of the heart's output every minute, every day 180 litres of fluid and 1.6 kg of sodium chloride are filtered out of and then reabsorbed into the circulation, yet minute changes in dietary salt and fluid intake are perfectly adjusted for. It primarily regulates serum electrolyte levels for sodium, potassium, chloride, calcium, magnesium and phosphate amongst others. It stimulates red cell production from the bone marrow by means of erthropoietin and promotes skeletal maintenance by the conversion of vitamin D to 25-hydroxycholecalciferol. It is primarily responsible for the excretion of water-soluble waste products of metabolism. Figure 4.1 shows the glomerulus, the part of the kidney responsible for filtering plasma from capillaries into the Bowman's capsule.

The term chronic renal failure (CRF) describes a worsening, progressive and irreversible loss of a patient's kidney function. Unlike acute renal failure, where a complete recovery of renal function is possible, in CRF the kidneys are permanently damaged, potentially leading to dialysis or transplantation.[1]

Clinical features

Chronic renal failure is categorised by severity into grades 1 to 5 (Table 4.1). The severity can be determined by blood tests. This process begins when the glomerular filtration rate (GFR) falls below normal, less than 90 mL/min per 1.73 m^2.

During progression from acute renal failure (ARF) to CRF the regulatory capacity of the kidneys attempts to compensate for renal damage by increasing filtration through the remaining working nephrons. If the renal function falls below about 30 mL/min per 1.73 m^2, this process causes further damage to the kidney and generalised wasting. This is often manifested in shrinking of kidney size and scarring within all parts of the kidney. Patients may often not present with any symptoms until over 80% of normal kidney function is lost, indicating the abundant capacity of the organ.[1] A proportion of all CRF patients will progress to end stage renal failure (ESRF) necessitating renal replacement therapy in the form of continuous ambulatory peritoneal dialysis (CAPD), haemodialysis and/or kidney transplantation (see Chapter 8).

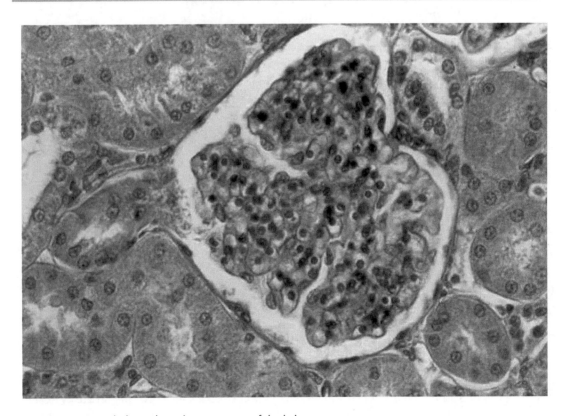

Figure 4.1   A normal glomerulus – the sieving unit of the kidney.

Table 4.1   Stages of chronic kidney disease (Renal Association)

Stage	GFR (mL/min per 1.73 m^2)	Description	Actions
1	90+	Normal kidney function but urine findings or structural abnormalities or genetic trait point to kidney disease	Observation, control of blood pressure
2	60–89	Mildly reduced kidney function, and other findings (as for stage 1) point to kidney disease	Observation, control of blood pressure and risk factors
3	30–59	Moderately reduced kidney function	Observation, control of blood pressure and risk factors
4	15–29	Severely reduced kidney function	Planning for end stage renal failure
5	<15	Very severe, or end stage kidney failure	Treatment choices

Incidence

Data taken from 22 819 patients from the databases of UK general practitioners in East Kent, West Surrey and Salford showed an estimated prevalence of stages 3–5 chronic kidney disease of 5.1% in the general population.[2]

Causes

There are three main ways in which kidney damage can occur: pre-renal, post-renal and renal CRF.[3] With pre-renal causes, conditions like hypovolaemia, as in major bleeds, or poor cardiac function or stenosis of the renal arteries can cause continuous hypoperfusion which may ultimately lead to kidney ischaemia and necrosis, resulting in CRF. In post-renal CRF, a disruption of urine flow from the kidneys by bladder obstruction, ureteric stones, retroperitoneal fibrosis, etc. increases pressure within the kidneys, eventually damaging nephrons and resulting in CRF. The most common causes of irreversible damage occur primarily within the kidney (renal CRF) and include diabetic nephropathy, hypertensive nephrosclerosis, vasculitis (including lupus and Wegener's granulomatosis), interstitial nephritis, and polycystic kidney disease.[1] Table 4.2 shows data from the 2004 UK Renal Registry.

Diagnosis is founded on a detailed medical history, physical examination and a considerable array of immunological and other serological tests. Precise diagnosis is important for identifying and treating potentially reversible causes. It can also assist nephrologists with assessing prognosis and planning for replacement therapy. Kidney biopsies are sometime inconclusive as late in the disease diffuse scarring may obscure the primary cause. In these cases or where a biopsy was not performed the diagnosis may be given as unknown.

Glomerulonephritis is a term used to describe a variety of disorders which affect the glomeruli. These allow protein and red blood cells that normally circulate only in the bloodstream to pass into the urine. This clinical picture is often accompanied by hypertension, oedema and impaired renal function. Clinical presentation ranges from an acute onset which can be corrected with treatment, to a chronic insidious onset that can progress to established CRF after many years.[4,5]

Polycystic kidney disease (PKD) refers to hereditary cystic diseases. Autosomal recessive polycystic disease is a rare form in children, autosomal dominant polycystic kidney disease (ADPKD) presents in adults and the genetic defect is present in about 0.1% of the white population and accounts for about 6% of patients presenting for dialysis in the UK. In ADPKD, if one parent is affected, approximately 50% of

Table 4.2 Percentage primary renal diagnosis by age and gender ratio in England and Wales (Renal Registry 2004)

Diagnosis	<65 years	>65 years	All	M:F
Aetiology unc./GN NP[a]	19.7	29.6	24.6	1.5
Glomerulonephritis	12.9	5.9	9.4	2.4
Pyelonephritis	7.8	7.4	7.6	1.4
Diabetes	20.9	14.9	17.9	1.6
Renal vascular disease	2.4	13.2	7.7	1.6
Hypertension	4.7	5.6	5.1	2.3
Polycystic kidney	9.4	2.7	6.1	1.3
Other	15.7	13.4	14.6	1.4
Not sent	6.6	7.3	6.9	2.4
No. of patients	1992	1942	3934	

[a] GN NP, glomerulonephritis not proven.

their children will develop the disease at some stage of life.[1] In PKD, the kidneys consist of a compact mass of cysts equally distributed through the cortex and medulla causing considerable enlargement of kidney size. Cysts increase in size and eventually rupture, causing infection, scar tissue formation and hence an overall reduction in functioning nephrons and renal function.

Symptoms and consequences

The symptoms experienced by patients are usually a direct sign of uraemia which tends to occur as the GFR falls to below 30 mL/min per 1.73 m[2].[6] The symptoms and signs include fatigue, electrolyte disturbances, hypertension, pruritis, 'restless leg' syndrome, anorexia, nausea and malnutrition as well as those of anaemia and of renal bone disease.[4]

Hypertension

Hypertension occurs in approximately 80–90% of renal patients.[1] It can be the cause or result of a decreased renal function. The kidneys attempt to autoregulate the pressure of blood entering the glomerular capillaries. Through secretion of renin acting on the renin–angiotensin pathway, the hydrostatic blood pressure remains constant, thereby maintaining a favourable filtration rate. In renal failure, falling filtration rates are usually associated with sodium and fluid retention and consequent hypertension. Conversely, if a patient presents with hypertension, there is a risk of damage to the blood vessels in the kidney. The renal artery and other smaller vessels become stenosed, leading to impaired blood flow through the organ, which stimulates renin release. This aggravates the hypertensive state of the patient and accelerates deterioration of renal function.

Tight blood pressure control can often be difficult to obtain and may result in patients being on maximal doses of many antihypertensive agents simultaneously (e.g. a cocktail of a beta-blocker, alpha-blocker, calcium channel blocker, angiotensin-converting enzyme (ACE) inhibitor, angiotensin II inhibitor and a diuretic). Drugs should, however, be initiated at low doses and

increased gradually whilst monitoring the patient's blood pressure. The majority of ESRF patients die from cardiovascular disease. Both hypertension and chronic fluid overload can lead to left ventricular hypertrophy (LVH) and systolic and diastolic left ventricular dysfunction.[1,6] Left ventricular hypertrophy has been shown to be a strong determinant of mortality and morbidity in haemodialysis patients. Hypertension also appears to be the major risk factor for the development of atherosclerosis in these patients. Patients experience a higher blood pressure and also lose the normal diurnal variation.

Treatment aims to correct chronic volume overload by fluid removal and optimisation of the patient's 'dry weight'. Patients are 'prescribed' a maximum amount of fluid to be taken per day and dietetic advice is also generally offered on the restriction of sodium in the diet. Beta-blockers, calcium antagonists and angiotensin enzyme inhibitors all have evidence of specifically improving left ventricular hypertrophy in the general population.[4] See Chapter 7 for further information.

Anaemia

Anaemia is common in patients with kidney disease. Healthy kidneys produce erythropoietin which stimulates the bone marrow to produce red blood cells needed to carry oxygen to vital tissues and organs. In CRF, kidney production of erythropoietin falls, causing a reduction in the stimulation of red blood cells by the bone marrow. Other causes of anaemia in CRF are loss of blood from haemodialysis and low levels of iron and folic acid.[1] Correcting anaemia can reduce lethargy and also decrease left ventricular hypertrophy, thereby reducing morbidity and mortality.

Anaemia may begin to develop in the early stages of kidney disease, when there is still 20–50% normal kidney function. This partial loss of kidney function is often called chronic renal insufficiency. Anaemia tends to worsen as kidney disease progresses. Most patients with end-stage kidney failure have a degree of anaemia present and will be on some form of treatment.[4]

In patients who present with greater than 50% loss in renal function and with a low haematocrit level, anaemia is usually caused by a reduced erythropoietin level. The European Best Practice Guidelines 2004 recommend that a detailed investigation of anaemia in patients with CRF is performed when haemoglobin levels fall below 11.5 g/dL in adult women, 13.5 g/dL in adult men or 12 g/dL in men over 70 years old.[7] The investigation will routinely include tests for iron deficiency and blood loss in the stool to exclude causes other than CRF.

The mainstay of treatment is administration of a genetically engineered form of erythropoietin (Eprex, NeoRecormon, Aranesp, etc.).[7] The European Best Practice Guidelines 2004 recommend achieving a target haemoglobin of greater than 11 g/dL within four months of starting treatment.[7]

Basic erythropoietin supplementation is not sufficient without monitoring of ferritin and percentage hypochromic red blood cells. Ferritin levels provide an indication of the amount of iron stored in the body. The current European guidelines aim for a ferritin level no lower than 100 µg/L and a percentage hypochromic red blood cells lower than 5%.[1] If iron levels are too low, administration of erythropoietin will be of limited benefit in raising haemoglobin levels and intravenous iron supplementation may be warranted. Both 'absolute' iron deficiency, due to depletion of iron stores, and 'functional' iron deficiency, due to inadequate mobilisation of iron stores to support demand, can be treated with iron therapy.[7] Administration of oral iron is of some benefit in renal patients. Intravenous iron supplementation (Venofer and CosmoFer) has been shown to produce better outcomes and response.[7]

In addition to erythropoietin and iron, some patients may also need additional vitamin B_{12} and folic acid supplementation. See Chapter 5 for further information.

Renal bone disease

Patients with CRF will exhibit some abnormality of electrolytes, potentially causing a varied degree of renal bone disease.

The kidneys aid the homeostatic balance between calcium and phosphate in the body.

With deteriorating renal function, phosphate filtration reduces, resulting in high phosphate levels and hence contributing to a low plasma calcium level. Lack of active vitamin D (which is necessary for normal absorption and utilisation of calcium) results in reduced gut calcium absorption, which further reduces plasma calcium levels, resulting in a combined effect of hypocalcaemia, hyperphosphataemia and low vitamin D levels, all contributing to the increased stimulation of parathyroid hormone secretion.[6] This increases calcium release from the bones, leading to renal osteodystrophy and fractures.

As can be seen from Figure 4.2, a number of abnormalities of calcium and phosphate homeostasis occur. Phosphate retention is associated with reciprocal depression of serum calcium level.[6]

Reduced calcium absorption occurs as the diseased kidney fails to hydroxylate 25-hydroxycholecalciferol to the more active form 1,25-dihydroxycholecalciferol (Figure 4.3). The resulting hypocalcaemia stimulates the parathyroid glands to return the serum calcium level to normal. This results in hypersecretion of the parathyroid gland and eventually hyperparathyroidism.[6]

The resulting effects are:

- Osteodystrophy (due to hyperparathyroidism)
- Osteomalacia (due to lack of vitamin D)
- Ectopic calcification.

Management of renal bone disease includes administration of phosphate binders, such as calcium carbonate, aluminium hydroxide, sevelamer, magnesium carbonate, lanthanum and vitamin D analogues (e.g. calcitriol, alfacalcidol, paricalcitol), suppression of parathyroid hormone (PTH), parathyroidectomy, control of aluminium and transplantation, and will be discussed in Chapter 6.

Oedema

This can result from sodium and water retention, and fluid restriction is usually advised to the patient. Careful compliance with fluid restriction is vital, but often inadequate. An

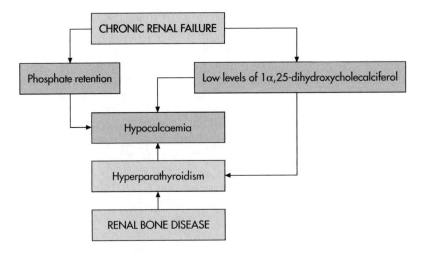

Figure 4.2 Abnormalities of calcium and phosphate homeostasis.

important consideration is the number of medicines that are prescribed to fluid-restricted patients as often a considerable amount of fluid is needed to take their tablets which forms part of their total daily allowance. Oedema can result in breathing difficulties if present in the lung and can also increase load on the heart. Diuretics can attempt to increase urine output, allowing patients to be able to drink more, but this also has corresponding effects on blood electrolyte levels.

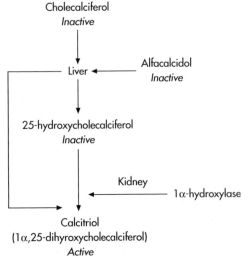

Figure 4.3 Flow diagram for hydroxylation of cholecalciferol to calcitriol.

Pruritis

Itching is a common uraemic symptom which can be distressing to the patient, often worse at night and quite difficult to treat. Treatment consists of control of phosphate and calcium levels, hydrating the skin with topical moisturisers and the use of sedating antihistamines and ondansetron.[5]

'Restless leg' syndrome

Patients with this condition describe creeping, crawling, prickling sensations in the lower limbs, which are often worse at night and relieved by moving the legs. It is well recognised in patients with iron deficiency.[9] Clonazepam, haloperidol, carbamazepine, pramipexole, ropinirole or baclofen are of benefit for some patients.[4,5]

Nausea

Nausea is common in patients with CRF due to the accumulation of urea and other toxins. Routine antiemetics such as metoclopromide, prochloperazine, etc. are effective, with dialysis being the best treatment.

Stress ulceration

Uraemic patients have an increased risk of gastrointestinal lesions and are therefore prescribed ranitidine or a proton pump inhibitor as prophylaxis.

Aspirin, statins

Patients with CRF have an increased risk of cardiovascular disease due to diabetes or being on haemodialysis. Therefore they are frequently prescribed low-dose aspirin and statins to reduce this risk. Statins should be initiated at a low dose and increased slowly.

Diet

Patients with chronic renal impairment need regular advice on their diet. This is partly because of their poor appetite due to uraemia and general feeling of being unwell and partly through the need to restrict certain foods which contain excess potassium and sodium. Hyperkalaemia can be life-threatening, and fruit, vegetables and foods generally containing water-soluble vitamins are on a restricted list so patients may require supplements.[3] Renal multivitamins are available and often used in patients who appear deficient in vital vitamins (see Chapter 19).

Influence of chronic renal disease on drug handling

Absorption

Drug absorption can be reduced in patients with chronic renal disease due to:[10]

- oedema of the gastrointestinal tract ('soggy gut syndrome'),
- alteration in gastrointestinal tract transit time,
- alterations in gastrointestinal pH,
- vomiting and or diarrhoea, and

- use of phosphate binders and ion exchange resins.

The uraemic state can also alter drug handling. This can be affected in three ways:

1 Reduced protein binding
2 Reduced tissue binding
3 Increased volume of distribution.

Metabolism

The main hepatic pathways of drug metabolism appear to be unaffected in renal impairment. The kidney has some metabolic activity and some of the kidney's enzymes are thought to have comparable activity to those in the liver.[1] This metabolic activity is reduced in CRF and therefore there is reduced hydroxylation of vitamin D. The kidney is also the main site of metabolism of insulin, so as a patient's renal function deteriorates they may require reduced doses of exogenous insulin.

Excretion

The failure of the excretory function of the kidneys may lead to the accumulation of drugs, with consequent toxicity. It is therefore important to decrease this risk by making appropriate alterations either in dose and/or frequency of dosing of drugs that are renally excreted or preferably ensuring an alternative drug is administered.[3]

Particular care should be taken with drugs possessing a narrow therapeutic index. Drugs which have an active metabolite that is excreted renally (e.g. morphine-6-glucuronide) should also be used with great care or preferably avoided in CRF.

Dose adjustments

When making dose adjustments, important questions to remember are:

- What proportion of the drug is normally cleared by the kidney?

- What proportion is normally cleared through other routes, such as metabolism?
- How toxic is the drug?

These points are discussed in more depth in Chapter 10.

Renal replacement therapies

The progression to end stage renal disease will result in patients receiving either a form of renal replacement therapy or palliative treatments. This is covered in detail in Chapter 8.

Conclusion

Chronic renal failure is a progressive illness which usually results from a primary renal disease or a renal complication of a multi-system disease. The resulting fall in GFR is progressive and treatment aims to delay progression to end stage renal disease as well as treat the symptoms experienced by the patient. Symptoms are multifactorial and involve a range of body systems, with which patients usually present in clinic. Drug therapy is often complex and the choice and dose is tailored to specific biochemical markers and patient compliance.

Preserving renal function and delaying progression to dialysis is the primary aim of management and all nephrotoxic agents and factors need to be minimised. Drug handling during CRF alters, and care must be taken in determining specific effects of drugs in the patient.

Monitoring is essential and continuous multidisciplinary input is needed to ensure patients receive the best treatment, care and advice possible.

Acknowledgement

I wish to acknowledge the help, review and additions made to this chapter by Dr Charles Soper, Consultant Nephrologist, Mayday University NHS Trust.

 CASE STUDY

A 72-year-old retired journalist presents with a three-week history of feeling unwell, tired, nauseated and unable to climb the stairs because his muscles are too weak. He is known to have chronic renal failure (usual creatinine 350 μmol/L), hypertension, ischaemic heart disease and peripheral vascular disease. He last saw his GP about a month ago for hypertension and had been started on irbesartan.

In A&E, he is pale, grey and weak. Blood pressure 140/80 with pedal oedema.

Medication:

- Calcium carbonate (Calcichew) 2 tabs three times daily
- Alfacalcidol 0.25 μg once daily
- Irbesartan 75 mg once daily
- Amlodipine 5 mg od
- Atorvastatin 10 mg at night
- Vitamin supplement (Ketovite) 1 tab once daily

→

CASE STUDY (continued)

- Ferrous sulfate 200 mg once daily
- Furosemide 500 mg once daily
- Epoetin beta (NeoRecormon) 2000 U SC three times a week.

Blood tests:

- Urea 49 mmol/L
- Creatinine 960 µmol/L
- Potassium 7.2 mmol/L
- Sodium 139 mmol/L
- Bicarbonate 17 mmol/L
- Corrected calcium 2.24 mmol/L
- Phosphate 2.3 mmol/L
- Haemoglobin 9.0 g/dL
- WBC 7.0×10^9/L
- Platelets 190×10^9/L
- % hypochromic red cells 6.0.

Q1. What are the metabolic abnormalities?

Q2. What has caused the abnormalities?

Q3. What is the life-threatening complication and how would you treat it?

Q4. What is the rest of his medication for and how much does it cost per year?

References

1. Goldsmith D. Management of renal impairment. *Medicine* 2003; 31: 52–56.
2. O'Donoghue D, Stevens P, Farmer C *et al.* Evaluating the prevalence of chronic kidney disease in the UK using GP computerised records. Renal Association 2004, Aberdeen, cited in the Renal Registry Report 2004.
3. Ashley C. Renal failure – how drugs can damage the kidney. *Hospital Pharmacist* 2004; 11: 48–53.
4. Morlidge C, Richards T. Managing chronic renal disease. *Pharm J* 2001; 266: 655–657.
5. Shaw L. *Chronic Renal Failure; The Beginner's Guide to Renal Pharmacy*. London: UK Renal Pharmacy Group, 2001.
6. El Nahas AM, Winearls CG. Chronic renal failure and its treatment. In: Weatherall DJ, Ledingham JGG, Warrell DA, eds. *Oxford Textbook of Medicine*, 3rd edn. Vol. 3. New York: Oxford University Press, 1996; 322–333.
7. Sexton J, Vincent M. Managing anaemia in renal failure. *Pharm J* 2004; 273: 603–605.
8. National Kidney Foundation. Clinical practice guidelines and clinical practice recommendations for anemia in chronic kidney disease. *Am J Kidney Dis* 2006; 47 (Suppl 3): S1–S145.
9. Kryger MH, Otake K, Foerster J. Low body stores of iron and restless legs syndrome: a correctable cause of insomnia in adolescents and teenagers. *Sleep Med* 2002; 3: 127–132.
10. *Renal Disease and Dysfunction*. Certificate in Applied Therapeutics, University of Brighton, 2006. http://www.londonpharmacy.nhs.uk/Clinical/Applied_Therapeutics_Modules.asp
11. Renal Association. *UK Renal Registry Report* 2004. http://www.renalreg.com/Front_Frame.htm

Further reading

Feest T. Epidemiology and causes of chronic renal failure. *Medicine* 2003; 31: 49–52.

Macdougall IC. How to get the best out of r-HuEPO. *Nephrol Dial Transplant* 1995; 10 (Suppl 2): 85–91.

Morlidge C, Richards T. Managing chronic renal disease. *Pharm J* 2001; 266: 655–657.

Renal Association. Adult Section 7: Anaemia in patients with chronic renal failure. *Treatment of Adults and Children with Renal Failure: Standards and Audit Measures*, 3rd edn. London: Royal College of Physicians: 2002. Available at www.renal.org/Standards/RenalStandards_2002b.pdf

5

Renal anaemia

John Sexton

Anaemia is a common feature of chronic kidney disease (CKD), which has a substantial impact on morbidity and mortality. This chapter reviews:

- The maintenance of serum haemoglobin in healthy individuals
- The reasons why patients with CKD become anaemic
- The consequences of anaemia in renal impairment, if left uncorrected
- The standards for initiation and treatment of anaemia in renal failure
- The management of renal anaemia by correcting causes, iron supplementation and use of erythropoiesis-stimulating agents (ESAs)
- Iron supplements and ESAs available on the UK market
- The management of patients who fail to respond to therapy.

Maintenance of serum haemoglobin in the healthy individual

The red blood cells (RBC) or erythrocytes are the most numerous cells in the blood, and carry an iron-containing protein called haemoglobin which is responsible for transporting oxygen in the circulation to the peripheral tissues that need it. The manufacture of erythrocytes, called erythropoiesis, of which typically 2 million are made every second, is controlled by the body in order to maintain serum haemoglobin in a tight range. The peritubular cells in the kidney are sensitive to falls in serum oxygenation, and they respond to hypoxia by increasing production of a hormone known as erythropoietin, a protein whose existence was first speculated about in 1897 though it was not actually purified until 1975. Once released, erythropoietin then acts on cells in the bone marrow to stimulate RBC production. During erythropoiesis, erythroid-progenitor cells incorporate haemoglobin and develop through immature RBCs called reticulocytes into mature erythrocytes, losing their nuclei in the process. The RBCs have a mean half-life of up to 12 weeks in the circulation, although this is reduced in uraemia, after which they are recycled.

It is worth commenting here that athletes seek to train at high altitude because, in addition to developing greater aerobic fitness, the altitude-related hypoxia they experience will result in increased erythropoietin production and a rise in serum haemoglobin that persists on return to lower altitudes.

The normal adult human body contains a typical 4 g of iron, though this can vary from 2 to 6 g, depending on sex, age and nutritional status. Very little of this iron is free in the circulation: free iron is toxic to many organ systems, but rather it is to be found in three main locations: in haemoglobin, in storage and in transport.

Iron in haemoglobin

The majority of the iron in the body at any time, about 3 g, is found in haemoglobin within the erythrocytes, performing its primary function as a carrier of oxygen from the lungs to the peripheral tissues.

Storage iron

There is considerable storage of iron, typically 1 g, especially in the liver and bone marrow, including that bound within a hollow protein called ferritin from which it can be released for use. This storage is hard to assess, but measurement of serum ferritin, which does not carry or contain significant iron, is considered to provide an indicator which reflects tissue ferritin and therefore total available iron stores in the body. Raised serum ferritin may indicate high levels of stored iron but can also be raised for other reasons such as inflammation or infection. In these situations, a consideration of the level of C-reactive protein (CRP) will enable differentiation of high ferritin levels. Low serum ferritin levels usually indicate insufficient iron stores in the body to supply erythropoiesis; this is known as **absolute iron deficiency**.

Transport iron

A small amount of iron, 4–5 mg at any time, is carried around the body bound to the protein transferrin. Transferrin carries the iron between the stores and the erythropoietic cells in the bone marrow where it is incorporated into new haemoglobin-containing RBCs and also between the reticulo-endothelial system, where RBCs are broken down and recycled, back into stores again. Normally about 20–50% of the transferrin is carrying iron at any time, leaving capacity to quickly mop up any iron entering the circulation. Transferrin saturation (TSAT, the ratio of serum iron to total iron-binding capacity), which can be assessed in the laboratory, provides a good indicator of iron availability for erythropoiesis. Like the forklift driver delivering parts to a factory production line, insufficient transferrin iron will limit erythropoiesis; this is known as **functional iron deficiency**.

Given the typical life of a RBC, about 1% of them are being turned over every day. To do this, every day, the bone marrow requires 30–40 mg of iron for erythropoiesis, and a similar amount is being recycled back into store again.

Much smaller amounts of iron are absorbed from the diet and excreted from the body each day. Normal iron losses in minor bleeds, menstruation and turnover of the gastrointestinal mucosa amount to 1–2 mg, and a similar amount therefore needs to be absorbed from the gut. The normal diet contains about 10–20 mg daily of iron, and so it will be seen that only 10% or so gets absorbed, though this can rise to about 20% during periods of iron demand. Haem iron from red meat is fairly predictably absorbed, but the absorption of other iron of non-haem origin such as in green vegetables is much more variable. It is impaired by tea, coffee and milk, consumption of which should be separated from mealtimes.

Absorption is also impaired by phosphate binders and antacids, and drugs which raise the pH of the gastrointestinal tract such as proton-pump inhibitors. Iron absorption can be promoted, however, by the consumption of fruit drinks containing ascorbic acid with meals.

Where iron absorption into the body falls below the loss of iron from the body for prolonged periods, absolute iron deficiency will eventually develop, followed by functional iron deficiency, and finally anaemia. This can occur in malnutrition, pregnancy, prolonged minor gastrointestinal bleeding, heavy menstruation and similar conditions. The iron cycle is shown in Figure 5.1.

Anaemia, a serum haemoglobin concentration which has been reduced to a level affecting tissue oxygenation, is most commonly associated with an inadequate iron intake or increased losses of blood, such as in menstruating women or following trauma. Blood transfusions may be administered to correct severe anaemia, but for most patients, supplementation with sufficient iron over time will suffice to restore serum haemoglobin over a period of weeks to months. More rarely in general practice, anaemia can present in the absence of an underlying iron deficiency, due to a failure of erythropoiesis for other reasons. This is seen in inflammatory conditions such as rheumatoid arthritis, a variety of vitamin deficiencies, some malignancies, or the failure of erythropoietin production in CKD.

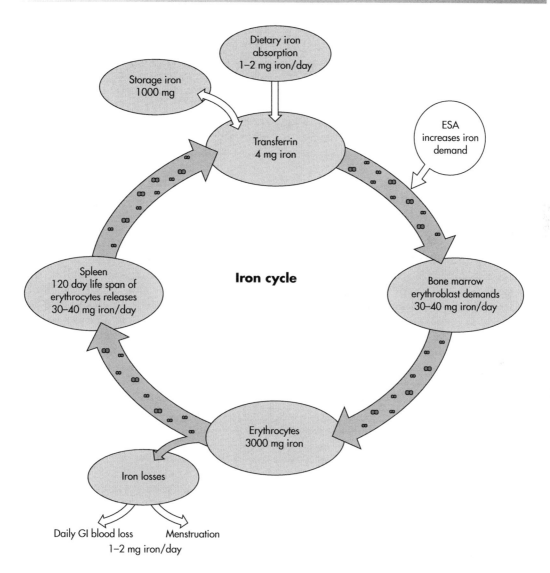

Figure 5.1   Iron turnover in the body.

The development and consequences of anaemia of chronic kidney disease

In addition to the reduced survival of RBCs in uraemia, the numerous reasons why patients with renal impairment might become anaemic can be divided into two main groups. The first set of reasons relates to the non-availability of sufficient iron for erythropoiesis: each 1 g/dL rise in serum haemoglobin requires 150 mg of iron delivered from its ferritin storage sites bound to transferrin. In absolute iron deficiency, or where the iron needs of erythropoiesis are increased, such as when erythropoietin analogues are administered, transferrin saturation may fall below that necessary to fuel RBC production, a situation previously referred to as functional iron deficiency. The second group of reasons relates to situations in which even if sufficient iron were available to supply the needs of erythropoiesis, this process would be retarded. That is to say, the bone marrow is unable to utilise adequate iron stores to make adequate numbers of functional RBCs. Of course, several or many of these reasons can also exist concurrently with absolute or functional iron deficiency. Failure of the renal peritubular cells to synthesise adequate erythropoietin is an important reason, but there are a variety of other factors that may impair erythropoiesis. These reasons are listed in Table 5.1.

In the light of the above, it should not be surprising that anaemia is a common problem in patients with renal disease, or would be if action were not taken to both prevent and treat it as it arises. There is some evidence that the processes that lead to anaemia are at work early in the course of CKD, although reported prevalence varies widely depending on the definition of anaemia, any treatments received, co-morbidities and the rapidity of onset of the renal disease.

Anaemia can manifest itself at any stage of CKD (see Chapter 4 for stages of CKD), but the prevalence of anaemia in the natural course of the disease begins to increase once the glomerular filtration rate has dropped below 60 mL/min, as the patients progress through stage 3 CKD. Untreated, most patients with stage 4 or 5 CKD would be expected to have some anaemia. Anaemia is more prevalent and severe in diabetic patients, and in those receiving haemodialysis, who have greater iron losses due to blood loss in extracorporeal circuits.

The anaemia developed by renal patients has serious effects on their morbidity and mortality. Patients will feel tired and there may be a deterioration in both physical and cognitive functioning, leading to an impairment of quality of life. However, it must be remembered that CKD has its major morbidity and mortality through cardiovascular ill-health, as blood pressure, lipids, electrolytes and other risk factors are often deranged. Anaemia is an independent risk factor for the development of left

Table 5.1 Common contributory factors to the development of anaemia in chronic kidney disease

Absolute or functional iron deficiency	
Dietary inadequacy	Anorexia due to nausea of uraemia
	Dietary restriction to reduce phosphate
Poor iron absorption	Absorption poor in uraemia
	Absorption affected by drinking tea with meals, calcium/aluminium phosphate binders, or proton-pump inhibitors
Increased blood losses	Stress ulceration (minor gastrointestinal losses) of chronic disease, possibly exacerbated by aspirin and NSAIDs
	Sampling losses for analysis
	Losses in haemodialysis circuit – EBPG says IV iron usually required in haemodialysis
Reduced erythropoiesis	
Inadequate erythropoietin	Reduced renal synthesis in CKD
	Missed doses of ESAs – hypertensive when dose was due or poor compliance in self-administration
Impaired erythropoiesis in presence of adequate erythropoietin and iron	Inflammation or infection
	Uraemia – inadequate dialysis
	Raised aluminium or parathyroid hormone
	ACE inhibitors, immunosuppressant drugs
	Infection/inflammatory conditions
	Vitamin B_{12}/folate deficiency

NSAIDs, non-steroidal anti-inflammatory drugs; EBPG, European Best Practice Guidelines; CKD, chronic kidney disease; ESA, erythropoiesis-stimulating agent; ACE, angiotensin-converting enzyme.

ventricular hypertrophy. In one study over 12 months, a fall in haemoglobin of 0.5 g/dL carried three times the risks of a rise in systolic blood pressure of 5 mmHg.[1] Anaemia also is associated with a rise in left ventricular dilatation, heart failure and death. Once coronary heart disease is established, either as a result of anaemia or hypertension, diabetes mellitus, dyslipidaemia, uraemia or some other cause, the effects of anaemia continue to impair outcomes. By reducing blood oxygen levels in a similar manner to cigarette smoking, the existence of anaemia will not only mean that the heart will have to work harder to supply the peripheral oxygen demands of the body, but also that the blood reaching it through the coronary arteries will contain less oxygen. Anginal attacks will therefore be more likely, and it has been shown that the outcomes after myocardial infarction are worse in the presence of anaemia.

There is a clear consensus from pooling the trial data of ESAs that the correction of anaemia 'provides important clinical and quality-of-life benefits whilst substantially reducing hospitalisations and transfusions'.[1] The avoidance of transfusions in populations who may be the future recipients of renal transplants is especially important to avoid pre-sensitisation to foreign antigens which might increase the chances of graft rejection. Unfortunately, the longer term benefits of anaemia correction are less clear-cut, especially in the area of cardiovascular morbidity and mortality, and what information exists is conflicting. Older pharmacists will remember a similar situation that formerly existed with antihypertensive medication. Every antihypertensive on the market, to obtain a product licence, has been through a clinical trials process that shows that it is effective in lowering blood pressure with an acceptable adverse event profile. Until recently, however, few had been tested in trials powered to show that they produced the intended outcomes of a reduction in cardiovascular morbidity and mortality.[1–3]

So it is with anaemia correction in CKD. It should not be surprising that in a group of patients with so many cardiovascular risk factors the correction of just one of these fails to make much impact on overall mortality. In addition, since until very recently most ESA use had been in patients with severe CKD, and especially those requiring dialysis, outcome measures from early prevention and correction of developing anaemia whilst patients are still reasonably healthy are scarce. Several large trials are currently in progress to try to quantify the cardiovascular benefits of anaemia correction in more representative cohorts of patients, especially in such early disease. One other possible benefit of anaemia correction might be on the progression of the CKD itself.

In short, more work is needed to quantify:

1 the overall (especially cardiovascular) risks and benefits of prevention and correction of renal anaemia, and
2 the most appropriate target haemoglobin once treatment is initiated that will optimise the benefits against risk and costs of anaemia correction.

Assessing the anaemia of chronic kidney disease

The most detailed guidelines on the management of renal anaemia are those produced by the joint working group of the European Renal Association and the European Dialysis and Transplant Association in 2004, and known as the Revised European Best Practice Guidelines for the management of patients with chronic renal failure (EBPG).[2] The UK Renal Association expanded its own guidance in 2006 and published *Chronic Kidney Disease in Adults: UK Guidelines for Identification, Management and Referral*, which includes guidance on renal anaemia.[1] Finally, the UK National Institute for Health and Clinical Excellence (NICE) published minimum standards for the National Health Service in England and Wales in September 2006, the guidelines 'Anaemia management in people with chronic kidney disease' being available via the NICE website.[3] Similar guidance has been published for the United States by the National Kidney Foundation Dialysis Outcomes Quality Initiative (NKF K/DOQI). There are slight differences between the different guidelines in their definitions of anaemia, thresholds for treatment, target haemoglobin levels and other standards but since they all draw on the same evidence base a certain commonality is seen and that shared vision is more important than small differences in approach reflecting the different needs and views of their intended users.

Healthy adults have serum haemoglobin concentrations which usually fall in the range of 12–15 g/dL for women and 14–18 g/dL for men, though different laboratories cite different reference ranges. The EBPG state that the investigation of anaemia in CKD should begin when haemoglobin concentrations fall below:

- 11.5 g/dL in adult women
- 13.5 g/dL in adult men
- <12 g/dL in adult men over 70 years of age.[2]

These guidelines state that the actual degree of CKD is irrelevant. As was discussed earlier, anaemia is more common as CKD advances but anecdotal evidence suggests that most renal centres formerly felt a need to set arbitrary serum creatinine concentrations for either referral to anaemia clinics or the prescription of ESAs. In the absence of NICE guidance and funding streams, limits have often been set to direct treatment to patients for whom the cost-benefit base is clear, or for whom resources can be made available. In many UK centres, resources to treat patients other than those who have started dialysis have only become available in the last few years and the EBPG guidance merely highlights how artificial this practice was.

Both Renal Association and NICE guidance take a slightly different approach.[1,3] The Renal Association guidance in 2006 lists anaemia as something to be checked when CKD reaches stage 3 (creatinine clearance <60 mL/min) and recommends treatment with ESAs for those patients with a haemoglobin of <11 g/dL. (Older Renal Association standards had previously only set a target haemoglobin of >10 g/dL in 2002.[4]) This guidance no longer conflicts with the EBPG guidance, which itself recommends ESA therapy when haemoglobin falls to 11 g/dL and all other causes of anaemia have been excluded or corrected. The draft NICE guidance simply suggests that management of anaemia should be consid-

ered if the patient has CKD (stage not specified) and a haemoglobin of 11 g/dL or less.[3] Unlike the other guidance NICE has not restricted care to any particular degree of CKD, though reference is made to CKD stage 3 when considering the assessment of anaemia.

The assessment of renal anaemia is clearly documented in the EBPG but includes an assessment of:

- the nature and severity of the CKD
- the actual haemoglobin being currently achieved
- iron stores as reflected by serum ferritin (to exclude absolute iron deficiency)
- available iron as determined by transferrin saturation or % hypochromic RBCs (to exclude functional iron deficiency)
- other causes/contributing factors towards renal anaemia (see Table 5.1)
- other medical reasons why the patient might be anaemic.[2]

Once haemoglobin has fallen to 11 g/dL or below, and contributing factors have been dealt with as far as possible, then all the guidelines agree that therapy with ESAs and/or iron should be initiated, as appropriate.

Target haemoglobin levels once treatment is initiated

In a similar manner to their selection of patients for assessment, the EBPG stress that treatment availability and targets for haemoglobin to be achieved should apply to all patients, though this is not always the case in current UK practice. So, the EBPG consider equally:

- Non-dialysing patients with CKD in stages 1–5
- Patients with CKD stage 5 receiving haemodialysis or peritoneal dialysis
- Transplant patients with chronic renal insufficiency (undefined) and anaemia.[2]

The target in the EBPG is to raise haemoglobin and maintain it at above 11 g/dL, this target to be reached within four months after treatment initiation. The majority of patients should be able to achieve this, but the upper

Table 5.2 Targets for iron stores during therapy for renal anaemia

Target	EBPG 2004	EBPG 2004 population target	NICE 2006 Guidance
Serum ferritin (to avoid absolute iron deficiency)	>100 µg/L (and avoid >800 µg/L)	200–500 µg/L	100–500 µg/L (non-HD) 200–500 µg/L (HD)
Transferrin saturation (to avoid functional iron deficiency)	>20%	30–40%	>20% (unless ferritin >800 µg/L)
% Hypochromic RBCs (where available) – (better measure of functional iron deficiency)	<10%	<2.5%	<6% (unless ferritin >800 µg/L)

EBPG, European Best Practice Guidelines; NICE, National Institute for Health and Clinical Excellence; HD, haemodialysis; RBCs, red blood cells.

limit to be achieved is still unclear. The guidelines say that pre-dialysis haemoglobin levels of higher than 14 g/dL should be avoided in patients on haemodialysis, as the blood further concentrates during haemodialysis, and that until more is known, patients with diabetes or heart disease should be restricted to a maximum of 12 g/dL. If angina is a problem or if there is a hypoxia due to concurrent airways disease it may be necessary to aim higher. Some younger, fitter patients, especially those with families to raise or work to go to may feel better with haemoglobins towards 14 g/dL, but the evidence base is unclear and there is a law of diminishing returns in relation to ESA therapy – it takes increasingly high doses and therefore cost to raise haemoglobin above 12 g/dL. The Renal Association guidelines simply recommend maintaining haemoglobin in the range 11–12 g/dL and the NICE guidance a similar 10.5–12.5 g/dL, with therapeutic changes made and action taken if it falls outside the range 11–12 g/dL.[1,3]

Iron store targets

ESAs will not work effectively if functional iron stores are low, as once transferrin cannot deliver adequate iron to the bone marrow, initially the RBCs will become hypochromic and then erythropoiesis will cease. In addition, since functional iron stores are replenished from stored iron, absolute iron deficiency must also be avoided. Iron stores may be adequate initially, but will fall rapidly once erythropoiesis is stimulated with ESAs. The guidelines all give standards to ensure that functional and absolute iron deficiency does not impair treatment. Of course, if functional iron deficiency has been the cause of the renal anaemia rather than a deficiency in erythropoietin, simply replacing iron may be sufficient to generate a rise in serum haemoglobin. Oral iron supplements such as ferrous sulfate tablets may be sufficient for many patients to maintain iron stores. However, in haemodialysis patients where iron losses are higher, where initiation of ESAs is creating an increased demand for available iron, or where the patient is starting from a position of depleted stores, intravenous iron therapy may be required.

The targets for adequate iron stores for erythropoiesis are shown in Table 5.2. It will be seen that the EBPG gives population targets as well; these will be higher to make sure that the majority of patients in the population reach the minimum individual targets.

Iron and erythropoiesis-stimulating agents available for the correction of renal anaemia

Once a patient's haemoglobin has fallen below 11 g/dL, they will need treatment for their anaemia. Twenty years ago, the only treatments available were iron dextran infusions, and, once these were ineffective, blood transfusions. Many renal patients became transfusion-dependent to maintain haemoglobin. Apart from the infection risks and fluid load this carried, the success of future transplants is impaired if patients are repeatedly exposed to foreign antigens. In addition, each unit of blood contains up to 200 mg of iron. Over time, multiple transfusions in patients without major blood (and iron) losses leads to iron overload and the need to treat patients with chelating agents such as desferrioxamine. However, the increasing availability since the early 1990s of both synthetic recombinant human erythropoietin and safer intravenous iron preparations has revolutionised therapy to the extent that renal anaemia is now a manageable condition in most patients. The recombinant erythropoietins available in the UK are:

- Epoetin alfa (marketed in Europe as Eprex by Janssen-Cilag, now Ortho-Biotech)
- Epoetin beta (marketed in Europe as NeoRecormon by Boehringer Ingelheim, now part of Roche)
- Darbepoetin (marketed by Amgen as Aranesp).

Much work has been done to compare darbepoetin with epoetin, especially epoetin alfa, and a large body of work now exists comparing the two drugs in different situations. Most sources would conclude that the erythropoiesis stimulating agents epoetin and darbepoetin are broadly similar in terms of ability to achieve target haemoglobin levels, and adverse-event profiles. This should be remembered when considering the differences between products, some of which are listed below.[5]

Presentations

All ESAs are available in a selection of pre-filled syringes providing different strengths to enable either nurse or patient/carer administration. In addition, Roche market NeoRecormon as a multiple-use vial for ward or satellite unit use, and cartridges for use in a pen-type administration device. Amgen supply a smaller range of strengths of Aranesp in an automatic dis-

posable injector that may facilitate patient self-administration. Patients report more favourably on issues such as the 'sharpness' of the needle and ease of injection with particular products. ESAs are temperature-sensitive and need to be stored in a refrigerator and the room temperature period which the product is considered safe to use within varies between products.

Route of administration

For patients receiving haemodialysis, intravenous administration during dialysis would avoid the need to give the patient unnecessary injections. However, the shorter half-life of epoetin means that the product is less efficient when given intravenously compared with subcutaneous administration – dose increases of 25% or more have been required to maintain haemoglobin levels in some studies. This can add considerable cost across a population, and many units have traditionally had to administer epoetin subcutaneously even though vascular access is available during the haemodialysis session. One advantage of Aranesp is that this loss of efficiency is not seen, and thus intravenous administration is possible without incurring extra costs. For all other patients, subcutaneous administration is the only route practical. With the removal of the Eprex licence for subcutaneous administration in 2002, this product essentially was no longer an option for peritoneal dialysis or non-dialysing patients. The subcutaneous route was reinstated in late 2006, but the summary of product characteristics (SPC) now says that the intravenous route is preferable and should be used wherever possible.

Frequency of administration

Epoetin was originally administered three times a week, with some early studies suggesting that attempting to reduce this increased the required weekly dose and costs. NeoRecormon is now licensed for subcutaneous use in stable patients at once-weekly dosing, with a possible use as little as fortnightly. Aranesp, because of its longer half-life, can be initiated weekly and reduced to as little as once a month in stable, non-haemodialysis patients.

Iron preparations

Oral iron preparations such as ferrous sulfate are cheap, readily available, and do increase iron availability from the gastrointestinal tract. Where an absolute iron deficiency has not yet developed, or is not severe, oral iron may be sufficient to restore absolute and functional iron status. However, once iron deficiency has become established, or continuing losses are elevated, this may not be the case: the EBPG observe that most haemodialysing patients will require intravenous iron. Oral iron can, however, irritate the gastric mucosa and lead to nausea, constipation or diarrhoea. Unfortunately, whilst taking iron tablets with food reduces some of these side-effects, it also means that if the patient is taking phosphate binders, which are also taken with food, this will impair iron absorption.

In the UK, two main intravenous iron preparations are available. Although a preparation of intravenous iron dextran was used formerly, this product had a poor reputation for anaphylaxis and was replaced by an iron sucrose product. Iron sucrose, also referred to by other names such as iron saccharate, is supplied in ampoules containing 100 mg of ferric iron as Venofer by Syner-Med. Iron sucrose can be easily administered as a slow intravenous injection of up to 200 mg, or slowly infused in a small volume of 0.9% sodium chloride. On first use, a test dose of 25 mg over 15 minutes is required by the product licence, and whilst this is good practice it is not the case in some other countries or required in the EBPG. Several doses may be required to restore iron stores, followed by maintenance doses at intervals of weekly to monthly depending on the patient's iron losses.

More recently, a lower molecular weight iron dextran than that used previously has been licensed as CosmoFer by Vitaline. As with iron sucrose, iron dextran can administered by intravenous injection or infusion. One advantage of CosmoFer is that its product licence allows large infusions of up to 20 mg/kg, the so-called total dose infusion. In patients who are not receiving haemodialysis, this removes the need to have to repeatedly attend a clinic or hospital, although administration may take several hours. This practice was also formerly commonly practised with Venofer but the off-label (outside the product licence) nature of this method of administration has reduced its popularity. The SPCs for both iron preparations require administration to take place where facilities for cardiopulmonary resuscitation are available, and in the case of iron dextran, with a doctor in attendance.

Venofer remains the dominant product in the UK; many sources and the EBPG consider it to be safer, faster working, and the product of choice.[2] However, CosmoFer use is considerable and the licensed availability of total dose infusions offers advantages in some situations.

Initiating iron and erythropoiesis-stimulating agents therapy

Practice does vary between units, and the guidelines take slightly differing approaches. The major decisions to be made in a CKD patient whose haemoglobin has dropped below 11 g/dL are whether to start iron, ESAs or both. The forthcoming NICE guidance contains helpful algorithms when initiating ESAs and iron therapy.[3] In patients with functional iron deficiency (TSAT <20% or hypochromic cells >6%), then up to 1 g of ferric iron should be administered over a few weeks, unless serum ferritin is high, typically greater than 800 µg/L. ESAs can be initiated at the same time, or after a month to see if the iron replacement has had any effect on the serum haemoglobin. The SPCs for darbepoetin and epoetin can be consulted for precise initiating dose regimens, but epoetin is generally initiated twice weekly in the UK in non-dialysing populations, and three times a week otherwise. Darbepoetin is typically initiated weekly before reducing the frequency of administration. Checking blood pressure and haemoglobin fortnightly to monthly, haemoglobin is typically allowed to rise at about 1–2 g/L per month, increasing and reducing ESA dose to achieve this until the target haemoglobin is achieved.

It cannot be stressed too strongly that adequate iron stores are required if ESA therapy is to be efficient, and any other contributing factors to renal anaemia (Table 5.1) need the optimum control possible. ESAs are generally well tolerated, their major dose-limiting problems being cost and the effects on blood pressure.

Failure to respond to therapy

Some patients will fail to respond to ESA therapy, for a variety of reasons, mostly already included in Table 5.1 as a contributory cause of the renal anaemia in the first place. The most common reasons for inadequate response are considered to be either inadequate functional or absolute iron stores, or inflammatory disorders. However, in self-administering patients noncompliance must be excluded. Even in those patients who receive ESA therapy from their dialysis nurse or community nursing teams, patients may miss doses for a variety of reasons (hypertension, non-availability of the product at the required time, poor communication, etc.). There is a whole chapter in the EBPG on the response to a patient not responding to darbepoetin at >100 µg weekly or epoetin at >20 000 units weekly.[2] More worryingly is the failure to respond to ESAs due to the development of antibodies to ESAs. The most severe manifestation of this is known as pure red cell aplasia (PRCA), a severe anaemia where haemoglobin, RBCs and reticulocyte counts fall steadily in the presence of normal white cell and platelet counts. No ESA can be administered to a patient with PRCA, and lifelong transfusions will be required. PRCA can occur spontaneously but is most associated with subcutaneous epoetin therapy for more than four weeks.

A rise in the incidence of PRCA was noted since 1998, in particular with epoetin alfa (Eprex). As a result, the licence to administer Eprex subcutaneously for renal patients was revoked in most European countries. The cause of PRCA with Eprex is probably multifactoral

and seems to be related to a change in the formulation or manufacturing process. Interesting points are:

- The US epoetin alfa made by Amgen was not associated with the same rise in PRCA cases as Eprex
- Intravenous use is associated with a much lower incidence of PRCA
- Use of Eprex in cancer patients did not lead to a rise in PRCA, possibly because of the shorter durations of therapy that are typical in malignant disease, or possibly there is some other factor at play in CKD
- Ortho Biotech postulate a possible reaction between the stabiliser polysorbate 80 and the formerly uncoated rubber stoppers used until 2003.[6]

Ortho Biotech has now reformulated Eprex and had produced sufficient data to allow the recent reinstatement of the subcutaneous route, albeit with the proviso that the intravenous route is preferable. Pharmacists should remain vigilant for signs of PRCA in a patient receiving any ESA therapy.

Summary

In the last 10 years the incidence of renal anaemia has declined sharply, due to the development of ESAs and safer parenteral iron therapy. The challenge of the future is to develop systems that ensure funding streams are in place so that all patients requiring ESAs receive them, and that units purchase and use ESAs in the most efficient way. Newer ESAs are on the verge of licensing, and it seems likely that these will work their way into clinical practice. Uptake will be slower than previously, due to the increasing commitment of NHS Trusts to exclusive purchasing arrangements, and fears about the comparatively lower safety data of newer products, especially in the light of the PRCA experience. However, patients with CKD need no longer fear the debilitating effects of renal anaemia and the NHS has delivered effective correction of haemoglobin levels in the majority of patients with CKD.

CASE STUDY

Mrs AP is a 56-year-old woman with chronic kidney disease secondary to type 2 diabetes mellitus, which has been worsening over several years. She smokes 20 cigarettes a day, drinks 4 units weekly, is tired and breathless, and blood tests are performed.

Blood results:

- Potassium 5.2 mmol/L (3.5–5.5 mmol/L)
- Creatinine 281 μmol/L (<130 μmol/L)
- Phosphate 2.21 mmol/L (0.7–1.4 mmol/L)
- Calcium 2.05 mmol/L (2.2–2.6 mmol/L)
- HbA1c 9.2%
- Haemoglobin 10.1 g/dL (12–15 g/dL)
- Blood pressure 165/95 mmHg.

Medication:

- Atenolol 50 mg every morning
- Amlodipine 5 mg every morning
- Isosorbide mononitrate SR 60 mg every morning
- Glyceryl trinitrate (GTN) spray when required
- Sodium bicarbonate 1 g three time daily
- Aluminium hydroxide (Alu-Caps) 2 three times daily
- Sevelamer 2 three times daily
- Alfacalcidol 1μg twice weekly
- Co-codamol 30/500 four times daily
- Diclofenac 50 mg twice daily.

Q1. **The Senior House Officer (SHO) asks if Mrs AP could be started on ESA therapy. Give three reasons why you might advise against this at this point.**

Q2. **If ESA therapy is to be initiated, what are the choices in terms of initial dose and monitoring?**

Q3. **What factors might contribute to reduced efficiency of ESA therapy in Mrs AP?**

Q4. **What factors affect the choice of ESA for Mrs AP?**

References

1. Joint Specialty Committee on Renal Medicine of the Royal College of Physicians and the Renal Association, and the Royal College of General Practitioners. *Chronic Kidney Disease in Adults: UK Guidelines for Identification, Management and Referral.* London: Royal College of Physicians, 2006.
2. Locatelli F, Alijama P, Barany P *et al.* Revised European best practice guidelines for the manage-

ment of anaemia in patients with chronic renal failure. *Nephrol Dial Transplant* 2004; 19 (Suppl 2): 1–47.

3. NICE. Anaemia management in people with chronic kidney disease. NICE Guideline. London: National Institute for Health and Clinical Excellence (NICE), 2006.

4. Renal Association. Adult Section 7: Anaemia in patients with chronic renal failure. In: *Treatment of Adults and Children with Renal Failure: Standards and Audit Measures*, 3rd edn. London: Royal College of Physicians of London and the Renal Association, 2002.

5. Dreicher R, Horl WH. Differentiating factors between erythropoiesis-stimulating agents. *Drugs* 2004; 64: 499–509.

6. Locatelli F, Aljama P, Barany P *et al*. Erythropoiesis-stimulating agents and antibody-mediated pure red-cell aplasia: where are we now and where do we go from here? *Nephrol Dial Transplant* 2004; 19: 288–293.

6

Renal bone disease

Robert Bradley

Renal bone disease is one of the classic complications associated with chronic kidney disease (CKD). The normal physiological mechanisms regulating blood levels of phosphate, calcium, vitamin D and parathyroid hormone are disrupted and this has important implications for the structural integrity and long-term health of bone. It is now clear that the complex pathophysiology is not restricted to bone and that the increased risk of calcification, especially of the cardiovascular system, is extremely important and probably has a role in the high cardiovascular morbidity and mortality in this population of patients. Drug therapy with phosphate binders and vitamin D is the mainstay of treatment. Patient education is crucial, particularly for phosphate binders, which must be taken appropriately in relation to meals to demonstrate any benefit. Drug therapy can also exacerbate renal bone disease – hypercalcaemia or oversuppression of parathyroid hormone, for example, need to be avoided. Therapeutic targets for the various parameters of bone biochemistry are evolving, research into calcification processes is ongoing and new pharmacological agents have recently become available. All of this will, it is hoped, improve the management of this complicated and serious condition.

Pathophysiology

Renal bone disease (or renal osteodystrophy, ROD) is a breakdown in the homeostatic mechanisms that control bone biochemistry, triggered by a decline in renal function (the glomerular filtration rate, GFR). The relevant biochemical parameters are serum phosphate, serum calcium, calcium–phosphate product, vitamin D levels and parathyroid hormone (PTH) levels. Each is important but it is the complex interaction between them that can be used to describe why ROD occurs.

The kidneys play a vital role in controlling each of the above parameters so virtually all CKD patients, particularly those at stage 4 and 5 CKD, will at some point exhibit a set of blood results that include risk factors for ROD. See Chapter 4 for stages of CKD.

Phosphate is excreted by the renal tubules, so in the presence of a reduced GFR, urinary clearance is reduced, leading to a build-up in the blood (hyperphosphataemia). The normal range (e.g. 0.8–1.45 mmol/L) is frequently exceeded and values well in excess of 2 mmol/L are regularly seen, particularly in the later stages of CKD.

Vitamin D is crucial for good bone health because it promotes the gastrointestinal absorption of calcium, influences the renal tubular reabsorption of calcium and aids the mineralisation process in the bone. Vitamin D is present in the body because of the action of sunlight on the skin and through dietary absorption. This form of vitamin D is inactive (cholecalciferol) and requires enzymatic hydroxylations in the kidney and the liver to become the active form of vitamin D, calcitriol (1α,25-dihydroxycholecalciferol). The renal reaction occurs under the control of 1α-hydroxylase – as renal mass reduces and enzyme levels fall there is reduced capacity for this vital stage of the process and activated vitamin D levels fall (Figure 6.1).

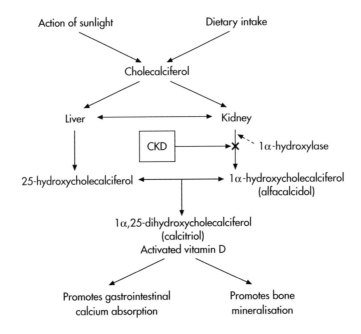

Figure 6.1   Vitamin D metabolism in chronic kidney disease.

Under conditions of normal calcium homeostasis, around half of the 1000 mg (25 mmol) of calcium that is generally ingested per day is absorbed from the gut. The vitamin D deficit and to a lesser extent the excess phosphate (via binding to free calcium in the blood) result in a fall in serum calcium below the normal range (e.g. 2.2–2.6 mmol/L) typically to just below 2 mmol/L. However, patients with CKD do not usually develop symptoms of hypocalcaemia.

Acute changes to phosphate, calcium and vitamin D as outlined above are unlikely to be a problem for a CKD patient but left uncorrected as CKD progresses they will increase the risk of developing ROD, especially as the parathyroid glands begin to respond to the abnormalities in bone biochemistry.

In early CKD when the GFR may be well above 25 mL/min small rises in phosphate are seen as filtration becomes defective. Renal activation of vitamin D also declines and the combination of these two changes will reduce calcium levels. As GFR continues to fall below 25 mL/min these abnormalities of bone mineral homeostasis become more pronounced. However, the fact that this process starts early in

CKD means that drug therapy should commence in CKD stage 4 and even stage 3 if indicated by blood results, rather than delaying until stage 5 when the consequences of ROD may already be established and drug management is more difficult.

The parathyroids are a set of four small glands situated, as their name suggests, in close proximity to the thyroid gland. They secrete parathyroid hormone (PTH), which is fundamentally important for the maintenance of normal bone turnover, and regulation of bone biochemistry. PTH secretion rises above the basal level in response to hypocalcaemia, vitamin D deficiency and/or hyperphosphataemia.

PTH has a variety of mechanisms to restore normality, for example:

- Decrease urinary clearance of calcium
- Increase urinary clearance of phosphate
- Increase synthesis of vitamin D
- Increase bone turnover to mobilise calcium from bone to serum.

Under normal physiological conditions the actions of PTH will correct the bone biochemistry and through negative feedback PTH secre-

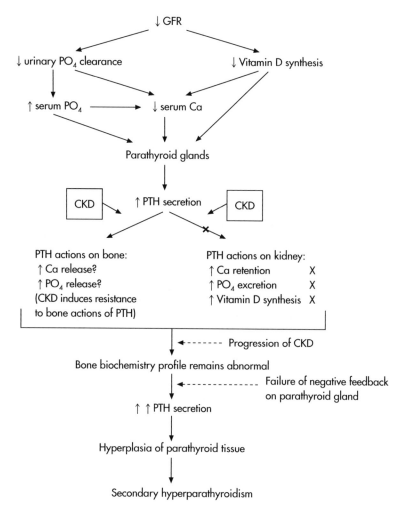

Figure 6.2   Secondary hyperparathyroidism in chronic kidney disease.

tion then falls back to basal levels. In CKD the first three actions listed above will be impaired because they rely on functioning renal tubules. However the extensive reserve capacity of the kidney means that as long as GFR is above 25 mL/min the response induced by PTH can be near to normal. The main focus is then to increase serum calcium by the non-renal actions of PTH on bone. This is unlikely to be sufficient to correct the calcium and meanwhile phosphate retention continues and vitamin D synthesis falls as GFR continues to drop. The negative feedback system now fails, the parathyroid glands continue to respond to these

stimuli and PTH secretion rises well above the normal range (0.9–5.4 pmol/L). At a cellular level within the parathyroid tissue hyperplasia will eventually occur and parathyroid glands will enlarge. The high PTH secretion will continue to increase bone turnover, causing bone damage and release of phosphate from the bone, exacerbating the hyperphosphataemia.

The response of the glands to bone biochemistry is now pathological and secondary hyperparathyroidism (HPT) is present (Figure 6.2). This complication is present to some degree in the majority of stage 5 CKD patients on regular dialysis therapy.

Complications for the skeleton and progression of renal bone disease

The complex bone biochemistry abnormalities that initiate renal bone disease result in equally complex changes to the skeleton, especially relating to rate of bone turnover (Figure 6.3).

Vitamin D deficiency may be associated with low bone turnover. Osteoblasts (bone formation cells) and osteoclasts (bone resorption cells) need vitamin D to function effectively. Without it, bone mineralisation is defective and osteoid (immature bone that has not yet undergone calcification) accumulates in the bone. This is known as osteomalacia and is associated with significant damage to the structural integrity of bone. There are other forms of low bone turnover states, some of which are related to treatment options in ROD, and will be described later.

Elevated PTH levels are associated with high bone turnover. There is increased remodelling of bone with greater activity of osteoclasts relative to osteoblasts. This weakens the bone architecture and induces fibrotic changes in the bone.

This is referred to as osteitis fibrosa and is the most common and important form of ROD.

Osteopenia is a condition of bone that occurs when bone resorption exceeds bone formation from whatever the cause. On radiographs this appears as increased radiolucency or 'poverty of bone'. Osteopenia can be associated with osteitis fibrosa and also with hypogonadism. For a variety of reasons, gonadal steroid hormone levels are low in both men and women with more advanced stages of CKD.

It is important to note that the pathogenesis of bone disease in CKD is a series of complicated processes and multifactorial in origin. Many patients will have mixed ROD, exhibiting bone damage secondary to both low and high turnover. The specific type of bone disease that a patient has can only be confirmed on bone biopsy. In practice this is a painful, invasive intervention that is rarely carried out. Drug therapy is based on the relative degree of abnormality of the bone biochemistry profile and on general principles to promote good bone health. A raised bone specific alkaline phosphatase level, indicative of bone damage, is often seen, particularly in the presence of osteitis fibrosa.

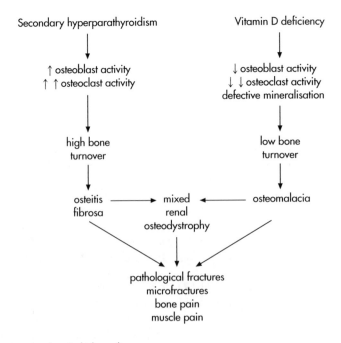

Figure 6.3   Bone diseases in chronic kidney disease.

The clinical consequences of all the effects of CKD and HPT on bone are to increase the risk of pathological fractures (e.g. vertebral fractures), bone pain, muscle pain, microfractures and even skeletal deformities.[1,2]

In spite of pharmacological intervention, bone biochemistry abnormalities may persist and the secondary HPT progresses as the parathyroid glands continue to be overworked. This results in:

- Further increases in PTH levels (can reach 8–10 times the normal range or more)
- Increased hyperplasia of parathyroid glands
- Reduced vitamin D receptors on the surface of the glands
- Reduced sensitivity of parathyroid tissue to the suppressive effects of calcium.

Over time, the parathyroid glands become less responsive while they continue to secrete more and more PTH. Bone turnover accelerates, worsening the osteitis fibrosa. More calcium and phosphate move from the bone to the serum under the influence of PTH, exacerbating hyperphosphataemia and increasing calcium levels. With advanced HPT the parathyroid gland has greatly reduced sensitivity to calcium levels because there are fewer calcium-sensing receptors on the surface of the gland. The set point at which calcium effects PTH secretion is raised. So as the PTH remains high, the serum calcium will eventually rise above the normal range. This stage of ROD is tertiary HPT and the glands are acting autonomously.

Clearly, pharmacological management now becomes increasingly difficult, the parathyroid glands become increasingly resistant to the action of drugs and surgical options (i.e. parathyroidectomy) may need to be considered.

Extraskeletal complications

It is becoming increasingly apparent that there are other consequences of the bone biochemical changes that are extremely important for CKD patients.

Other potential complications include:

- Pruritis
- Red, sore eyes

- Exacerbation of anaemia
- Soft tissue calcification
- Peripheral vascular calcification
- Cardiovascular calcification.

Hyperphosphataemia is primarily responsible for pruritis and red, sore eyes. Itching is a common problem for CKD patients and is related to their uraemic state. It is one of the most troublesome and distressing symptoms and management of high phosphate can contribute to symptom relief.

Hyperparathyroidism may cause bone marrow fibrosis which can contribute to the suboptimal haemoglobin of renal anaemia and be a factor in poor response to therapy with erythropoiesis-stimulating agents (ESAs).

Soft tissue, peripheral vascular and cardiovascular calcification are particularly important and are the focus of much research at present.[3] Calcium and phosphate remain soluble in the blood under normal physiological conditions and there are various factors that maintain the status quo. If serum levels of calcium, phosphate or both rise, there is a risk that the concentrations can reach a level where precipitation occurs, resulting in extraskeletal calcification. It is clear that CKD patients have potential risk factors for calcification, for example:

- Hyperphosphataemia
- Hypercalcaemia in the presence of severe HPT
- Hypercalcaemia related to drug therapy for ROD (e.g. vitamin D and calcium-based phosphate binders, to be described later)
- High calcium–phosphate product
- Vitamin D deficiency leading to poor calcium utilisation.

It also explains why the calcium–phosphate product is an important parameter to monitor in CKD patients; it is calculated simply by multiplying the serum concentration of calcium by that of phosphate and measured in $mmol^2/L^2$ (Figure 6.4).

Soft tissue calcification involving the peripheral arteries can develop into a rare but severe condition called calciphylaxis or calcific uraemic arteriolopathy. This is characterised by tissue and skin ischaemia leading to severe

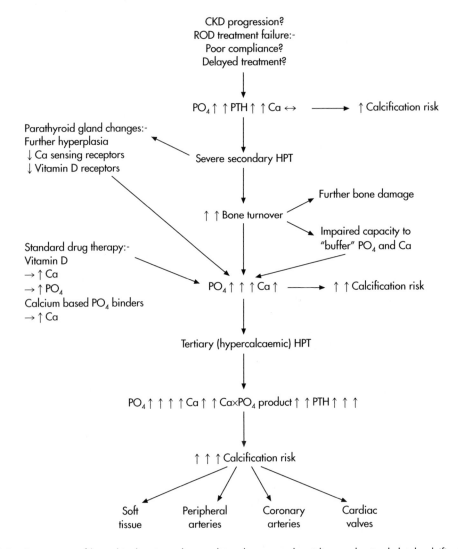

Figure 6.4 Progression of bone biochemistry abnormalities, hyperparathyroidism and extraskeletal calcification risk in chronic kidney disease.

necrosis. It is an extremely painful complication with a very high mortality rate, usually because of sepsis related to the necrotic skin lesions.

Metastatic calcification (of which calciphylaxis is an extreme form) can also occur in the lungs, cornea, conjunctivae, muscle, kidney and stomach. Simple but painful skin or periarticular deposition of calcium may be visible in CKD patients.

Calcification in the cardiovascular system (e.g. myocardium, coronary arteries, aorta and cardiac valves) is an extremely important issue for patients with CKD. It is well established that, in the end stage renal disease (ESRD) population, the most common cause of death is of cardiovascular origin. For example, the cardiovascular mortality of dialysis patients is on average 30 times that of the general population.[4] This figure is even higher when data are restricted to younger patients. Nearly half of all deaths in dialysis patients can be attributed to cardiovascular disease.[5] Disturbances to bone mineral homeostasis are increasingly being implicated in the high mortality rates.

The exact role of calcification in the high cardiovascular morbidity and mortality in CKD patients is yet to be fully determined. One hypothesis is that vascular smooth muscle cells are triggered by certain factors to undergo a change in phenotype to become bone-forming (osteoblast type) cells. It will be crucial to establish the precise nature of the pathology of vascular calcification and whether drug therapy for ROD can prevent or reverse cardiovascular calcification. The roles of other classical cardiovascular risks such as atherosclerosis related to dyslipidaemia, chronic inflammation, hypertension and diabetes need to be elucidated to complete the calcification jigsaw in CKD patients.

A consequence of arterial calcification is that vessels such as the aorta and coronary arteries become stiff. Left ventricular hypertrophy, reduced coronary artery blood flow during the diastolic phase and higher systolic blood pressure are all potential complications of greater arterial stiffness and reduced vascular compliance. Valvular calcification of the aortic or mitral valves can also occur and may contribute to heart failure.

Epidemiological studies provide data on the roles of abnormal phosphate, calcium and PTH values as risk factors for mortality in patients with ESRD.[6] Retrospective data in patients on haemodialysis have indicated a twofold mortality rise with serum phosphate above 2.26 mmol/L.[7] A similar retrospective study demonstrated a 27% higher mortality risk, adjusted for age and co-morbidities, in patients on haemodialysis with a phosphate over 2.10 mmol/L.[8] Even at lower phosphate levels than this the risk is still high and unfortunately, due to the difficulties in managing phosphate, around 50% of dialysis patients worldwide are estimated to have serum phosphate levels above 1.8 mmol/L.[9]

Hyperparathyroidism may have additional unfavourable effects on the cardiovascular system, such as myocardial interstitial fibrosis and thickening of arteriolar walls. Following on from this it is vital to elucidate if and to what extent modification of the risk factors related to ROD affect cardiovascular outcomes.

Treatment with phosphate binders

Managing hyperphosphataemia can be extremely difficult in CKD patients. Many of the pharmacological therapies used are poorly tolerated, and efficacy is totally reliant on the patient taking the prescribed agent at specific times. Phosphate binder drugs act to reduce the absorption of dietary phosphate so they must be taken either with or just before meals and so are plagued by concordance problems. All binders form a complex with phosphate in the gut which is not absorbed systemically and will be cleared from the body via the faecal route. By reducing the gastrointestinal absorption the blood levels are not continually topped up, allowing them to fall gradually.

Taking phosphate binders inappropriately, for example between meals, will have little effect on phosphate. This can lead to doses of binders being increased to address the elevated phosphate when a simple piece of patient education would address the problem while maintaining the same dose. For this reason renal healthcare professionals, including pharmacists, have an important role to play in talking to patients with CKD about the benefits of phosphate binders and how to take them correctly. Also, although phosphate binders are generally prescribed as a three times a day dosage, patients should be encouraged to adjust their doses according to their diet. For example, only two doses are required if the patient has only two meals a day and additional, smaller doses of binders should be taken with snacks.

The present range of available phosphate binders fall into three categories: calcium-based, aluminium-based and calcium/aluminium-free agents.

Calcium-based phosphate binders

- Calcium carbonate (e.g. Calcichew, 500 mg elemental calcium per tablet, chew 5–10 minutes before meals)
- Calcium acetate (e.g. Phosex, 250 mg elemental calcium per tablet, swallow whole with meals).

This group are the most widely prescribed, and will be first-line agents for most patients as they are cheap and relatively efficacious. Calcium binds to phosphate in the gut and the resulting complex is not absorbed. Some of the calcium that remains unbound will be absorbed, which is desirable in hypocalcaemic patients but limits or contraindicates their use in patients with more severe forms of HPT. The starting dose is one or two tablets at mealtimes. It is important that patients understand when to take them as doses being taken between meals act as a calcium supplement, with maximum absorption. Concordance issues include gastrointestinal disturbances such as nausea and poor palatability, since the chewable formulations have a chalky texture. There is conflicting evidence concerning the relative merits of Calcichew and Phosex on a milligram for milligram of elemental calcium basis with regard to effectiveness of binding gut phosphate and incidence of hypercalcaemia. The efficacy of calcium salts as phosphate binders is influenced by gut pH levels, so could be modified by acid suppression therapy, although this appears to be less of a problem with Phosex.

Aluminium-based phosphate binders

• Aluminium hydroxide (e.g. Alu-Cap capsules, 475 mg capsules, swallow whole with meals).

These agents are the most potent phosphate binders currently available.[10] Concerns over toxicity of absorbed aluminium, especially dementia, led to a reduction in their use. However the elevated serum aluminium levels seen in patients on haemodialysis were more likely to be related to absorption of the metal from the water used in the haemodialysis process. Water purification requirements are now more stringent and most aluminium is removed before it reaches the haemodialysis machine. Current evidence that phosphate should be controlled more aggressively to improve patient outcomes has led many renal units to increase prescribing of Alu-Cap capsules once more. However there are other significant adverse reactions linked to aluminium. It is

toxic to the bone marrow (so may worsen renal anaemia) and to bone cells, causing greatly reduced bone turnover (adynamic bone disease). A direct link between aluminium-based binders and these complications is not clear. Although serum aluminium levels can be monitored, their clinical usefulness is debated and there is no threshold level for aluminium-induced diseases.[11] The starting dose of these agents is one capsule with each meal and the main indication is as a second- or third-line agent or as an add-on therapy when a single agent has not adequately reduced phosphate levels. To minimise toxicity, aluminium-based binders are used only on a short-term basis. As with all phosphate binders, gastrointestinal intolerance, in this case constipation, is a problem.

Calcium/aluminium-free phosphate binders

• Sevelamer hydrochloride (Renagel, 800 mg tablets, swallow whole with meals).

Sevelamer is the newest phosphate binder available and is a completely new class of drug. It is a hydrogel of poly(allyamine hydrochloride), a polymer molecule with partially protonated amine groups which bind to intestinal phosphate. Its advantages are that, being free of calcium, it is safer to prescribe for patients who are hypercalcaemic or in those with evidence of calcification. Sevelamer has been shown to have a lower incidence of hypercalcaemia than calcium-based binders.[12] It is also aluminium-free so is a viable option when aluminium toxicity is a concern. Unbound sevelamer is not absorbed from the gut so it has no systemic side-effects but still has gastrointestinal side-effects such as nausea. It is probably the least effective of the current range of drugs, which can cause a problem with high tablet burden. There is some concern about risk of exacerbating metabolic acidosis in patients with CKD.[13] Cost is also an issue because sevelamer is much more expensive than traditional therapies. It is important to be able to justify its prescription on sound clinical grounds so that sevelamer can be utilised in a cost-effective manner.

An interesting effect of sevelamer is an action to bind bile acids in the gut, leading to a reduction in serum LDL (low-density lipoprotein) cholesterol by up to 20%. This may have benefits in terms of reducing cardiovascular risk factors in patients with CKD.[14]

The starting dose of sevelamer is one or two tablets with meals although doses of up to five tablets with each meal may be required. It is generally prescribed as a second- or third-line agent, or as an additional therapy in combination with calcium- or aluminium-based binders.

There are novel phosphate binders in clinical development or new to the market (e.g. lanthanum carbonate (Fosrenal)) but any di- or trivalent cation will bind phosphate. Iron- and magnesium-based compounds, for example, have been used as phosphate binders. Phosphate binders are chronic therapies producing gradual changes in the bone biochemistry so dose adjustments are usually not made more frequently than every two to four weeks during initial phase of treatment and then every four to eight weeks thereafter. Crucially, reduction in phosphate levels can provide a directly associated suppression of PTH secretion and, of less significance, an increase in free calcium levels in the serum. Gastrointestinal intolerance and issues around concordance and patient education are the most problematic issues with all of the phosphate binders.

Combination therapy with different phosphate binders may sometimes be seen in clinical practice. This could be indicated in cases of recalcitrant hyperphosphataemia, but in situations like this the combination is often intended to be short term to gain better control of phosphate. It is important to review such patients regularly to avoid polypharmacy and increasing the complexity of the drug regimen unnecessarily. Long-term therapy with two or more binders in high doses is rarely indicated – an elevated phosphate despite such intense therapy can suggest either a problem with concordance or the presence of severe bone disease. At the extremes of bone turnover states (adynamic or severe hyperparathyroid) the bone loses much of its ability to buffer bone minerals so reduction in the absorption of dietary phosphate may have less impact on serum levels.

Non-pharmacological management of hyperphosphataemia revolves around dietary modification. The issue of reducing phosphate intake in the diet is controversial. Many foods contain phosphate; dairy products and protein-rich foods such as meat are especially rich and would be restricted in a low-phosphate diet. However, nutrition in general can be a major problem for renal patients and a low-phosphate diet is protein and calorie poor. For this reason many nephrologists and dieticians advocate a nutritious diet with sufficient protein rather than phosphate restriction. It is then the role of phosphate binders to regulate serum phosphate.

For patients with ESRD, treatment with standard techniques of haemodialysis or peritoneal dialysis has little impact on phosphate clearance because the majority of body phosphate is intracellular so that clearance is slow. More frequent and longer than usual haemodialysis sessions can help to reduce doses of phosphate binders.

Treatment with vitamin D

Vitamin D therapy works in conjunction with phosphate binder drugs and most renal patients will be prescribed it at some point. As CKD progresses, the quantity of activated vitamin D produced will continue to fall, leading to the complications outlined earlier. Levels of vitamin D in the blood can be measured and this can guide its use as a supplement, particularly in the early stages. However, in most renal units vitamin D is used more as a pharmacological agent than as a simple supplement, and blood levels are rarely checked. The prescription and dose adjustment of vitamin D is based on other parameters of ROD, namely calcium and PTH, to control secondary HPT. The initiation of vitamin D is often in response to a low calcium level but ideally a PTH value should also be available because, once the calcium is corrected, it is the PTH level that is more likely to guide subsequent dose adjustments in the long term. Moreover, unless the serum calcium and PTH are particularly disrupted, prescription of phosphate binders alone in the first instance will often increase calcium and reduce PTH, delaying the need for vitamin D.

Vitamin D supplementation will prevent osteomalacia and has both indirect and direct actions in treating secondary HPT. Gastrointestinal absorption of calcium is promoted, increasing the serum calcium. This in turn stimulates the calcium-sensing receptors on the surface of the parathyroid gland, inducing a drop in PTH secretion. Vitamin D also has a direct effect, suppressing the hormone by inhibiting PTH gene transcription in the parathyroid gland cells.

There are two forms of vitamin D used in patients with CKD:

- Alfacalcidol (1α-hydroxycholecalciferol), usual starting dose 0.25 μg once a day
- Calcitriol (1α,25-dihydroxycholecalciferol), usual starting dose 0.25 μg once a day.

Alfacalcidol still requires activation in the liver, whereas calcitriol is the active form of vitamin D. Both agents are effective at managing secondary HPT but alfacalcidol is more widely prescribed in the UK. Calcium levels can be corrected relatively quickly but PTH correction is a more gradual process. For this reason, vitamin D therapy is adjusted infrequently, every 4–12 weeks in most instances.

The clinically significant side-effects of vitamin D therapy relate to inappropriate changes to the bone biochemistry:

- Exacerbation of hyperphosphataemia (via promotion of phosphate absorption from the gut)
- Hypercalcaemia
- Oversuppression of parathyroid glands (PTH is essential for normal bone turnover so over zealous treatment with vitamin D can reduce PTH to a level at which the patient has a risk of adynamic bone disease).

The first two complications, especially hypercalcaemia, can limit the efficacy of vitamin D therapy. The degree of secondary HPT often dictates a dose increase but the presence of raised calcium can preclude this. Various strategies are employed in an attempt to maximise the effects of vitamin D on the parathyroids while limiting its action on the gut vitamin D receptors. Pulsed doses of vitamin D, given once, twice or three times a week are often given on haemodialysis units. While individual patients may obtain better control of their PTH, there is not a large evidence base to demonstrate superior efficacy over standard daily dosing.[15] However, this approach does have the advantage of guaranteeing concordance with treatment.

Alfacalcidol and calcitriol are also available as intravenous preparations for pulsed treatment. However the benefits of this practice over traditional oral therapy regimens have not been clearly demonstrated.[16] There is also the added factor of greatly increased price compared with the oral formulations. Low bone turnover as a consequence of excessive vitamin D dosage also reduces the buffering action of bone on phosphate and calcium levels because the underactive bone will not take up these minerals, increasing the risk of them being deposited elsewhere as ectopic calcification.

For dialysis patients, adjusting the calcium content of their dialysis fluids can be a non-pharmacological method of improving ROD management. Careful reduction of the calcium content, for example down to 1 mmol/L will reduce the net positive calcium burden to which patients with CKD are frequently subjected. This reduces the risks of hypercalcaemia, allowing greater doses of vitamin D to be employed where necessary to control HPT (Figure 6.5).

The role of parathyroidectomy

For some patients, surgical intervention is eventually necessary to manage the complications associated with ROD. A parathyroidectomy may be indicated in a number of circumstances, for example:

- Presence of tertiary HPT with symptomatic hypercalcaemia that has not responded to avoidance of calcium-based phosphate binders and minimisation of vitamin D dose.
- Resistant HPT that has not responded to high doses of vitamin D and phosphate binders. This could be severe disease that has not been adequately treated or it could be related to poor concordance with drug therapy. As

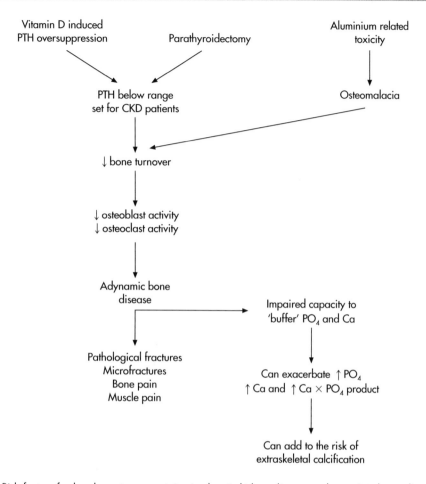

Figure 6.5   Risk factors for low bone turnover states in chronic kidney disease and associated complications.

with the majority of patients considered for parathyroidectomy PTH levels will be very high – typically 10 times above the normal reference or higher.

- Patients with adenomas of the parathyroid glands. These are the more extreme hyperplastic manifestation of HPT, following on from diffuse then nodular hyperplasia of the gland tissue. They are generally resistant to drug therapy due to greatly reduced concentrations of both vitamin D and calcium-sensing receptors on the surface of these nodules compared with normal parathyroid tissue.
- Patients with evidence of significant sequelae of abnormal bone biochemistry, such as calciphylaxis and severe bone damage.

There are three surgical options:

- Subtotal parathyroidectomy
- Total parathyroidectomy
- Total parathyroidectomy with reimplantation.

Removal of all four glands in a total parathyroidectomy will leave the patient devoid of PTH. While this may address the problems that led to the surgery it can present new ones. With no PTH to regulate normal bone cell biochemistry, adynamic bone disease can result, which itself carries an increased risk of fractures. For this reason some parathyroid tissue is often left behind either at the site of the parathyroid glands (subtotal parathyroidectomy) or removed from this site and placed in the forearm (total parathyroidectomy with reimplantation). The resultant risk from either of these techniques is that the remaining parathyroid tissue is still sufficient to cause significant HPT, necessitating further surgery. The latter technique has the advantage of leaving parathyroid tissue in a more accessible site for subsequent operations.

Symptomatic hypocalcaemia is a significant risk in the early post-parathyroidectomy phase and left uncorrected can progress to hypocalcaemic tetany. The risk is higher for total parathyroidectomy and in those patients not prescribed a short course of high-dose vitamin D pre-operatively. Serum calcium should be managed aggressively when it begins to drop after surgery, using high doses of vitamin D (sometimes in the region of 4 µg/day) and calcium supplements (given as large oral doses or intravenously if indicated). Calcium carbonate (e.g. Calcichew) is often used but has the potential to cause confusion for the patient. They may have taken Calcichew as a phosphate binder in the past at mealtimes. They must be informed that it now serves as a calcium supplement and should take it **between** meals to maximise absorption. Vitamin D therapy and possibly calcium replacement may be needed long term, but the risk and magnitude of hypocalcaemia diminishes over time and doses of these drugs should be reviewed regularly to avoid hypercalcaemia.

Therapeutic targets

The benefits of drug therapy to manage ROD may not be immediately obvious to the patient and it is important that they understand their therapy. Phosphate binders and vitamin D are long-term treatments that will gradually correct abnormalities in their blood results, protect the bones and possibly the heart and blood vessels against future damage. Successful drug therapy reduces the morbidity and mortality associated with ROD by reducing fracture incidence, and preventing soft tissue calcification. As the emerging evidence indicates, it also reduces

the massive burden of cardiovascular disease in the CKD population by preventing cardiovascular calcification.

In order for these outcomes to be realised, it is essential that the target ranges for each of the parameters of bone biochemistry are clearly defined and that guidance is available on the most effective pharmacological means to achieve them. In ROD this is crucial, as there are different approaches to drug management and, more importantly, it is not simply a question of returning the serum levels of phosphate, calcium and PTH to the normal reference ranges. The evidence base currently available on these issues is variously regarded as incomplete, inconclusive or conflicting and is complicated by emerging data surrounding cardiovascular calcification. Evidence-based guidance on ROD is published by nephrology groups such as the Renal Association in the UK[17] and the National Kidney Foundation in the USA.[18] The advice may vary depending on the stage of CKD that the patient has reached. The following descriptions of bone biochemistry targets include reference to these guidelines and are generally applicable to the later stages of CKD. Current recommendations are different from those of 5 or 10 years ago. It is worth remembering that in an area such as this where new data are appearing regularly, they could be amended once more in the near future.

Phosphate

For the majority of patients with CKD it is extremely unlikely that a normal serum phosphate will be achieved with binder drugs. In fact, hypophosphataemia in a patient with CKD indicates malnourishment and is an indicator of poor prognosis. Vitamin D therapy, a normal or high-phosphate diet, severe HPT and poor concordance with binder drugs are some of the factors that promote hyperphosphataemia and make successful management very difficult. A more realistic, though still difficult, objective is to bring serum phosphate down below 1.7–1.8 mmol/L and this should have a positive effect on patient mortality rates.

Calcium

Depending on the stage of ROD, either hypo- or hypercalcaemia may be present, so ideally drug treatment should maintain a calcium level in the normal range. Current concerns about calcification risks have led some nephrologists to advocate a serum calcium towards the lower end of normal.

Calcium–phosphate product

Guidance is variable but most suggest a calcium–phosphate product in the region of less than $4.50 \, mmol^2/L^2$ to minimise calcification risks. Aiming to keep the phosphate below 1.7 mmol/L and the calcium in the lower end of the normal range will assist in the achievement of target calcium–phosphate product. Current data indicate that around 50% of dialysis patients have a product greater than $4.44 \, mmol^2/L^2$.[9]

Parathyroid hormone

An important factor to consider with PTH targets is that levels in the normal range are no longer viewed as desirable in most patients with CKD. As described earlier, PTH is a vital component in the physiology of normal bone turnover. Patients with CKD, especially those on haemodialysis, are often described as being in a proinflammatory state and this may be reflected in elevated levels of inflammatory markers such as CRP (C-reactive protein). Inflammatory cytokines (e.g. interleukins 1, 6 and 11 and tissue necrosis factor alpha) can increase bone remodelling. Also, bone growth factors may be deficient or inhibited in CKD and suppressors of bone formation may be present at higher levels than in the general population. Finally, there may be a relative resistance to the actions of PTH in CKD, possibly due to downregulation of PTH receptors. Endogenous factors are induced to attempt to overcome these changes and normalise bone turnover. In CKD, PTH is one of these factors so a degree of hyper-

secretion is necessary[19] and target levels need to be higher than normal, but to what degree is a crucial question. Current theories indicate that a value between three and five times the upper limit of normal should be aimed for in patients with ESRD. This should manage the HPT effectively while avoiding oversuppression of the parathyroid glands and maintaining as near as possible a normal bone turnover state. The incidence of low turnover bone disease has been increasing, partly because of excessive PTH suppression with vitamin D, and this is reflected in the changes to the PTH target range. However, recent worldwide data indicate that around 50% of dialysis patients have a PTH below three times the upper limit of normal (less than 16.2 pmol/L),[9] suggesting that a change in practice is required.

New management strategies and new therapeutic agents for renal bone disease

Phosphate management

One of the current controversies in ROD is the role of calcium intake in the pathogenesis of extraskeletal, especially cardiovascular, calcification. CKD patients have the potential to be in positive calcium balance, both through enhanced gastrointestinal absorption of exogenous calcium from calcium-based phosphate binders and due to vitamin D therapy. Mineralisation of the bone is defective in CKD and the action of elevated PTH will mobilise calcium from the bone. Both of these factors mean that normal physiological utilisation of calcium is impaired. The next question is, where does the positive balance of calcium go if it is not taken up by the bone? Does its utilisation become pathological, with exogenous calcium contributing to extraskeletal calcification? Also, what is the role of ingested calcium in the cellular processes underpinning arterial calcification? Research is ongoing in these areas and more data are needed, especially since opinion is polarised in the nephrology field as to the risks and benefits of prescribing calcium-based phosphate binders.

One problem for clinicians assessing calcification risk is that of the approximately 1000 g of calcium present in the body, serum calcium represents only a tiny proportion of total body calcium (approximately 0.025%). Around 99% of the total body calcium is present in bone. Does serum calcium reflect total body calcium sufficiently well to indicate calcification risk? If not, then could a patient with normal serum calcium still be at risk and could the risk be enhanced by adding to the patient's calcium load with calcium-based phosphate binders?

Various techniques such as echocardiography can visualise calcification to some degree, but obviously in these patients the complication has already manifested itself. A newer technique called EBCT (electron beam computed tomography) can have a role in assessment of coronary artery calcification by providing a calcification score, which can then be matched to a level of cardiovascular risk.[20] EBCT has been used to compare young patients (20–30 years of age, many of them taking calcium-based binders) on haemodialysis with non-dialysis patients with cardiac disease. Coronary artery calcification scores were found to be far higher in the former group.[21] However, EBCT is unable to differentiate accurately between intimal and medial vascular calcification, making it difficult to assign a cause to the calcium deposition. This is important because the former is more closely associated with the traditional cardiovascular risk factor of atherosclerosis than the latter, which may have aetiologies more particular to CKD.

All these factors may in future have a bearing on the prescribing of phosphate binders. Will clinicians continue in the traditional manner using calcium-based agents as first-choice phosphate binders in most instances or will the use of calcium-free phosphate binders as first-line drugs become more commonplace? This could be aluminium-based but is far more likely to be sevelamer. Many nephrologists are already using sevelamer at an earlier stage than previously or even as the first phosphate binder

given to a patient with CKD – for example in younger patients who face years of phosphate binder ingestion, in an effort to avoid or delay calcification. An evidence base needs to be firmly established to compare sevelamer and calcium-based binders with respect to risk of developing cardiovascular calcification, rate of progression of cardiovascular calcification and, crucially, cardiovascular morbidity and mortality. Sevelamer has been compared with calcium-based phosphate binders after 12 months therapy in dialysis patients and elicited an attenuation in cardiovascular calcification as assessed by EBCT score not seen with the calcium-based products.[22]

Lanthanum carbonate (Fosrenol) is a new agent that has just received a European licence. Lanthanum is a rare earth element that binds dietary phosphate so will be prescribed in the same manner as the current range of drugs. Early data suggest that potency could be similar to that of aluminium preparations.

Whatever phosphate binder is used, the accumulating evidence that high serum phosphate levels are linked to increased mortality in patients with CKD (seemingly more so than other measures of bone mineral homeostasis like serum calcium and PTH) means that earlier and tighter control is necessary to achieve target levels and improve outcomes for patients.

New vitamin D analogues

There is a range of alternatives to alfacalcidol and calcitriol either in use or in development. The rationale behind them is to overcome the dose-limiting side-effects associated with standard vitamin D therapy. They purportedly do this through increased selectivity for the parathyroid glands (to maximise PTH suppression) while sparing the actions on the gut vitamin D receptors (to minimise the absorption of calcium). Of these vitamin D analogues only paricalcitol (Zemplar) is currently available in the UK. As with many aspects of drug therapy for ROD there is debate about the role of these new options. However at present there appears to be an absence of good clinical trial data that demonstrate significant advantages in terms of better efficacy or adverse event rate of the new agents over the current management strategies with alfacalcidol or calcitriol.[23]

Moreover, many of the new vitamin D analogues are only available as intravenous formulations, effectively limiting them to patients on haemodialysis only, and they are much more expensive than existing options.

Vitamin D receptors are distributed widely around the body so the effects of alfacalcidol, calcitriol and the newer vitamin D analogues are not restricted to the bone. Examples of postulated extraskeletal actions include:

- Inhibition of renin production and associated reduced angiotensin II levels, which indicates a role in blood pressure homeostasis.
- Possible protective role against mediators of myocardial damage.
- Action on the pancreas to facilitate appropriate secretion of insulin.
- Immunomodulatory effects on various white blood cells.
- Anti-proliferative actions, which could be beneficial for the cardiovascular risk and protect against malignancy.

These and other vitamin D-mediated effects are currently under investigation and if confirmed would suggest a significant and widespread physiological role for vitamin D.

Calcimimetics

Cinacalcet (Mimpara) is the first of a new class of agents called calcimimetics, offering a new approach to the management of ROD. Cinacalcet is an orally active compound which acts on the calcium-sensing receptors on the surface of the parathyroid gland cells, mimicking the action of calcium. This induces a rapid reduction in PTH secretion, offering a useful addition to the range of therapeutic options in the management of HPT.

Cinacalcet will generally be prescribed in addition to rather than instead of phosphate binders and vitamin D. However, the associated effects of calcimimetics (reductions in serum levels of calcium and phosphate) will be of benefit to many CKD patients and may allow for phosphate binder dose reductions, and more importantly, aggressive use of concurrent vitamin D if required to suppress PTH. Patients with adenomas of the parathyroid glands have a deficit of calcium-sensing receptors so are probably less likely to respond to this new therapeutic option. At present due to its high cost, cinacalcet is restricted to the more difficult cases of ROD, for example those with severe HPT resistant to standard treatment, those with HPT complicated by hypercalcaemia or as a pharmacological alternative to parathyroidectomy.

 CASE STUDY

Mrs A is 45 years old and has CKD secondary to hypertension. She has been reviewed in the nephrology clinic and her renal function has now deteriorated from stage 3 to stage 4 CKD.

Blood results:

- Phosphate 1.99 mmol/L (0.8–1.45 mmol/L)
- Corrected calcium 2.10 mmol/L (2.2–2.6 mmol/L).

(continued overleaf)

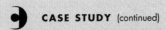

CASE STUDY (continued)

At her last clinic visit three months ago her phosphate was 1.65 mmol/L and corrected calcium 2.28 mmol/L.

Q1.   Why is this patient's hyperphosphataemia worsening?

Q2.   Are there any symptoms she may now experience secondary to her elevated phosphate?
A decision is made to manage the elevated serum phosphate with phosphate binder drugs.

Q3.   What would you advise as first-line phosphate-binding agent for Mrs A? What dose would you recommend? How would you educate the patient on why phosphate binders are important, how they work, when to take them and what side-effects to expect?

Q4.   What do you think is a realistic target serum phosphate level for Mrs A?
A week after the nephrology clinic the junior doctor who reviewed Mrs A is looking for more advice. The patient was commenced on Calcichew (calcium carbonate tablets 500 mg elemental calcium per tablet) at a dose of two tablets three times a day as a phosphate binder, but the doctor is wondering whether vitamin D therapy should also be prescribed (blood results from clinic – phosphate 1.99 mmol/L and corrected calcium 2.10 mmol/L).

Q5.   Is vitamin D therapy indicated for Mrs A at this point? If yes, which vitamin D agent and what starting dose would you recommend? If no, why do you think it is appropriate to leave her on Calcichew alone at present?

Q6.   What other biochemical investigation(s) would you request at this stage in the management of Mrs A's renal bone disease? How would knowledge of the result(s) influence your decision to initiate or hold off vitamin D therapy?
Three years have now passed by and you encounter Mrs A once again. She is now an ESRD patient on regular haemodialysis three times a week. Her current renal bone disease drugs are:

- Calcichew one tablet three times a day
- Alfacalcidol 0.5 µg once a day.

This drug regimen has been stable for the past three months. Her current bone biochemistry profile is:

- Phosphate 2.3 mmol/L
- Calcium (corrected) 2.7 mmol/L
- Parathyroid hormone (PTH) 52 pmol/L (0.9–5.4 pmol/L).

During the last three months, phosphate has been stable but both calcium and PTH have gradually increased.

Mrs A reports that she has been experiencing more muscular aches and pains recently. She concords with her drug therapy and takes her Calcichew appropriately but in view of the mild

→

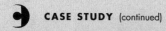 **CASE STUDY** (continued)

(asymptomatic) hypercalcaemia, the nephrology team has decided to stop the Calcichew. Some expert advice is once again needed.

Q7. What are the other two commonly prescribed phosphate binders available to the nephrology team?

Q8. Considering the advantages and disadvantages of each of these agents, which one would you recommend and what would be your suggested starting dose?

Q9. How can vitamin D therapy cause complications in the management of renal osteodystrophy?

Q10. What would you suggest as a vitamin D plan in Mrs A and what are the reasons behind your decision? Stop alfacalcidol? Reduce alfacalcidol dose? Continue alfacalcidol at current dose? Increase alfacalcidol dose?

Later in the year, Mrs A is admitted to the orthopaedic ward with a fractured wrist following a fall. Her bone biochemistry profile is now:

- Phosphate 2.1 mmol/L
- Calcium (corrected) 2.6 mmol/L
- PTH 69 pmol/L.

An alkaline phosphatase of 245 units/L (normal range 30–115 units/L) is also noted from the liver function tests.

Q11. What form of renal osteodystrophy is likely to have contributed to Mrs A's fracture and how does it influence bone turnover?

On admission to the orthopaedic ward, Mrs A was taking the following renal bone disease drug regimen:

- Sevelamer 800 mg three tablets three times a day
- Alfacalcidol 0.75 µg once a day.

The nephrology team have decided to increase her sevelamer to four tablets three times a day and will consider adding in aluminium hydroxide as an additional phosphate binder if hyperphosphataemia not controlled in four weeks. They have told Mrs A that they want to look after her bones better and also reduce her 'calcification risk'.

Q12. Why are the doctors concerned about extraskeletal manifestations of an abnormal bone biochemistry profile (i.e. calcification) in Mrs A? At which sites in the body can calcification occur in a CKD patient? How can calcification impact on the morbidity and mortality of CKD patients?

Q13. What are the benefits of prescribing higher doses of calcium-free phosphate binders (sevelamer and/or aluminium hydroxide) for Mrs A in relation to preventing further bone fractures and reducing her calcification risk?

References

1. Sherrard DJ, Hercz G, Pei Y *et al.* The spectrum of bone disease in end stage renal failure – an evolving disorder. *Kidney Int* 1993; 43: 436–442.
2. Malluche H, Faugere MC. Renal bone disease 1990: an unmet challenge for the nephrologists. *Kidney Int* 1990; 38: 193–211.
3. Davies MR, Hruska KA. Pathophysiological mechanisms of vascular calcification in end stage renal disease. *Kidney Int* 2001; 60: 472–479.
4. Foley RN, Palfrey PS, Saran MJ. Clinical epidemiology of cardiovascular disease in chronic renal disease. *Am J Kidney Dis* 1998; 32: S112–S119.
5. Causes of death. In: *Renal Data System. USRDS 1998 annual data report*. Bethesda, MD: National Institute of Diabetes and Digestive and Kidney Diseases, 1999: 79–90.
6. Gnash SK, Stack AJ, Levin NW *et al.* Association of elevated serum phosphate, calcium × phosphate product and parathyroid hormone with cardiac mortality risk in chronic haemodialysis patients. *J Am Soc Nephrol* 2001; 12: 2131–2138.
7. Lowrie EG, Lew NL. Death risk in haemodialysis patients: the predictive value of commonly measured variables and an evaluation of death rate differences between facilities. *Am J Kidney Dis* 1990; 15: 458–482.
8. Block GA, Hulbert-Sheron TE, Levin NW, Port FK. Association of serum phosphate and calcium × phosphate product with mortality risk in chronic haemodialysis patients: a national study. *Am J Kidney Dis* 1998: 31; 607–617.
9. Young E, Satayathum S, Pisoni RL *et al.* Prevalence of values on mineral metabolism being outside the targets from the proposed new draft NKF-K/DOQI and European Best Practice Guidelines in countries of the dialysis outcomes and practice patterns study (DOPPS). *Nephrol Dial Transplant* 2003; 18 (Suppl 4): 677–678.
10. Janssen MJA, van de Kuy A, ter Wee PM, van Boven WPL. Aluminium hydroxide, calcium carbonate and calcium acetate in chronic intermittent haemodialysis patients. *Clin Nephrol* 1996; 45: 111–119.
11. Altmann P. Aluminium toxicity in dialysis patients: no evidence for a threshold serum aluminium concentration. *Nephrol Dial Transplant* 1993; 8: 25–34.
12. Bleyer AJ, Burke SK, Dillon MA *et al.* A comparison of the calcium free phosphate binder sevelamer hydrochloride with calcium acetate in the treatment of hyperphosphataemia in haemodialysis patients. *Am J Kidney Dis* 1999: 33: 694–701.
13. Block GA, Sakiewicz PG. Serum bicarbonate levels in sevelamer versus calcium containing phosphate binders in haemodialysis patients. *J Am Soc Nephrol* 2001; 12: 761A.
14. Slatopolsky EA, Burke SK, Dillon MA. Renagel, a nonabsorbed calcium and aluminium free phosphate binder, lowers serum phosphorus and parathyroid hormone. *Kidney Int* 1999; 55: 299–307.
15. Herrmann P, Ritz E, Sckmidt-Gayk H *et al.* Comparison of intermittent and continuous oral administration of calcitriol in dialysis patients: a randomised prospective trial. *Nephron* 1994; 67: 48–53.
16. Lee WT, Padayachi F, Collins JF *et al.* A comparison of oral and intravenous alfacalcidol in the treatment of uraemic hyperparathyroidism. *J Am Soc Nephrol* 1994; 5: 1344–1348.
17. Renal Association. *Treatment of Adults and Children with Renal Failure: Standards and Audit Measures*, 3rd edn. London: Lavenham Press, 2002.
18. National Kidney Foundation. K/DOQI clinical practice guidelines for bone metabolism and disease in chronic kidney disease. *Am J Kidney Dis* 2003; 42 (Suppl 3): S1–S201.
19. Hamdy NAT, Kanis JA, Beneton MNC *et al.* Effect of alfacalcidol on natural course of renal bone disease in mild to moderate renal failure. *BMJ* 1995; 310: 358–363.
20. Raggi P, Chertow GM, Bommer J *et al.* Cardiac calcification is prevalent and severe in ESRD patients as measured by electron beam CT scanning. *J Am Soc Nephrol* 2000; 11: 75A.
21. Goodman WG, Golden J, Kuizon BD *et al.* Coronary artery calcification in young adults with end stage renal disease who are undergoing dialysis. *N Engl J Med* 2000; 342: 1478–1483.
22. Chertow GW, Burke SK, Raggi P. Sevelamer attenuates the progression of coronary and aortic calcification in haemodialysis patients. *Kidney Int* 2002; 62: 245–252.
23. Drueke TD. Control of secondary hyperparathyroidism by vitamin D derivatives. *Am J Kidney Dis* 2001; 37: S58–S61.

Further reading

Altmann P. Calcium and phosphate in renal failure: the disease. *Br J Renal Med* 2001; Winter; 6–9.

Altmann P. The control of calcium and phosphate in renal failure. *Br J Renal Med* 2002; Spring: 6–9.

Block GA, Friedrich K. Re-evaluation of risks associated with hyperphosphataemia and hyperparathyroidism in dialysis patients: recommendations for a change in management. *Am J Kidney Dis* 2000; 35: 1226–1237.

Goodman WG, London G. Vascular calcification in chronic kidney disease. Am J Kidney Dis 2004; 43: 572–579.

Hruska KA, Teitelbaum SL. Renal osteodystrophy. *N Engl J Med* 1995; 333: 166–174.

Hudson JQ. Improved strategies for the treatment of renal osteodystrophy. J Pharm Pract 2002; 15: 456–471.

7

Hypertension and hyperlipidaemia

Clare Morlidge

The aim of this chapter is to cover the basics about hypertension and hyperlipidaemia in general, and with respect to a renal patient.

Within hypertension, assessment and diagnosis of the hypertensive patient will be covered, followed by the treatment, both pharmacological and non-pharmacological. The principles for management of hypertension in the non-renal patient apply to the renal patient too, but with a few exceptions, which will be covered.

Within hyperlipidaemia, the causes of dyslipidaemia are examined followed by a risk assessment and treatment options.

Hypertension

Blood pressure distribution within the population displays a bell-shaped curve and there is no clear cut-off point between hypertensive and normotensive subjects. There is, however, considerable evidence that treatment of subjects with a blood pressure (BP) above the thresholds currently used (see below), results in important clinical benefits.

The complications of hypertension include:

- Stroke
- Myocardial infarction
- Other end organ damage (e.g. kidneys)
- Malignant hypertension
- Peripheral vascular disease.

The most common of these are myocardial infarction (MI) and stroke. Small reductions in BP result in substantial reductions in the risk of developing a cardiovascular complication. For example a 5 mmHg increase in diastolic BP results in a 35–40% increase in risk of stroke.[1] A 5 mmHg decrease in BP is associated with a 25% reduction in risk of renal failure.[1] The absolute benefits of lowering BP depend on the underlying level of risk in an individual subject. The majority of end stage renal failure (ESRF) patients will die from a cardiovascular complication.

The kidneys' main function is to remove waste products, toxins and excess fluid from the body. One of their extra functions is in the control of BP. They achieve this by the renin–angiotensin aldosterone cascade, which is important for longer term salt, water and BP control. A high BP can be the cause of renal impairment or a complication of it. It can be difficult to determine whether the high BP has caused the renal impairment or whether the renal impairment has caused the high BP.

The majority of chronic renal failure patients are affected by hypertension, and ischaemic heart disease (IHD) has higher prevalence than in the general population. Both hypertension and chronic fluid overload can lead to left ventricular hypertrophy (LVH), which in turn results in left ventricular failure (LVF). LVH has been shown to be a predictor of mortality in haemodialysis patients.

What is normal blood pressure?

Both systolic and diastolic BPs increase with age, so there is a normal range for each age (Table 7.1).[2] The British Hypertension Society guidelines (2004) state that target BP for diabetics is 130/80 and for non-diabetics is 140/85.[3]

Table 7.1 Normal range of blood pressure at different ages

Age	Blood pressure (mmHg)	
	Systolic	Diastolic
<30 years	100–120	60–70
30–60 years	110–130	70–80
>60 years	120–140	80–90

Data taken from *Kidney Failure Explained.*[2]

Causes of hypertension

In 90–95% of cases of hypertension there is no underlying medical illness to cause the increased blood pressure. The remaining 5–10% of cases are secondary to another disease process, such as renal disease, endocrine diseases (e.g. Conn's syndrome), vascular disease (e.g. renal artery stenosis) or drugs (e.g. oestrogens, ciclosporin, erythropoietin).

Clinical presentation

Hypertension itself causes no symptoms, some people with high BP suffer from a headache, but this is not reliable. Often there are no symptoms until end organ damage occurs (e.g. MI or stroke).

Hypertension usually comes to light at a routine health check or following a hypertensive-related complication (e.g. stroke).

Diagnosis

Blood pressure is measured using a sphygmomanometer (sphyg). Two readings are taken. The first shows the systolic BP (when the heart contracts), and the second shows the diastolic BP (when the heart relaxes), giving a reading of, for example, 140/80. An increase in both systolic and diastolic BPs is a risk factor for stroke and coronary heart disease (CHD).

It is important to use a correctly sized cuff, since one too small will overestimate the patient's BP. As a result, a person may be wrongly diagnosed with hypertension and may receive unnecessary treatment with drugs. To take a reading the arm should be supported level with the heart. BP is measured by listening for the Korokoff sounds. Read systolic BP when sounds first appear and diastolic BP when sounds disappear.

The BP should be measured several times over several visits in order to diagnose hypertension. If the first reading is dangerously high, however, several readings should be taken on the first visit.

Assessment of the hypertensive patient

The patient should be assessed to detect any end organ damage, for example, the optic fundi should be inspected for damage to the eyes, urinalysis and urea and electrolytes (U&Es) carried out for the kidneys, and cholesterol levels should be checked. An electrocardiogram (ECG) should be done to check for ventricular hypertrophy, and echocardiography (ECHO) should be performed if ventricular hypertrophy is suspected after ECG. Abdominal ultrasound should be performed if renal impairment is suspected.

The patient's history should be taken in full to determine if there is a secondary cause for the increased blood pressure. Even in renal patients a careful history should be taken and all the tests performed to help to determine the cause of hypertension. This helps to determine if the renal impairment is the cause of hypertension or a consequence of it. There may be a second cause of hypertension.

The patient should be assessed for contributing factors (e.g. obesity, increased cholesterol). Lifestyle should be addressed and changes made if appropriate. Patients should be advised to:

- Avoid smoking
- Exercise regularly
- Reduce alcohol intake
- Reduce salt intake
- Avoid being overweight
- Stick to fluid restriction if appropriate.

The risks of stroke (sixfold greater in hypertensive patients than in normotensive patients), coronary heart disease (threefold increase) and peripheral vascular disease (twofold increase) are multifactorial.[1] Other risk factors (e.g. smoking, diabetes) act as multipliers determining individual risk. Ischaemic heart disease (IHD) has a much higher prevalence in the renal population than in the general population.

Self-help measures

- **Avoid being overweight** – There is a strong link between being overweight and having hypertension. Patients whose weight is above that advised for their height should be advised to lose weight. Even if not overweight, patients should be advised to follow a low-fat, high-fibre diet. Refer to a dietician if appropriate.
- **Keep alcohol levels down** – There is a strong link between a high alcohol intake and raised BP. Drinking a moderate amount is harmless and may even be beneficial for coronary heart disease (CHD). However excessive alcohol consumption can cause a resistance to antihypertensive drugs.
- **Reduce salt intake** – The relationship between salt intake and BP is difficult to prove, but there is good evidence to suggest that a high salt diet affects your BP. Salt can also increase the amount of fluid that your body retains. Restricting salt intake to 100 mmol (6 g) per day combined with weight reduction does reduce cardiovascular risk in patients with hypertension and this is advised in many renal patients. Salt is hidden in many processed foods. Advise patients to eat mainly fresh, unprocessed foods.
- **Exercise regularly** – Exercise can help to reduce your BP and keep weight down. It is also a good stress reliever. Aim for 20–30 minutes of brisk activity at least three times a week (e.g. brisk walk, swimming, etc.).
- **Stop smoking** – Giving up smoking does not improve BP control, but it does lower the risk of blood vessel damage that can lead to an MI or stroke.

These non-pharmacological interventions can bring down BP a little, but more importantly can reduce the overall risk of end organ damage.

The aims of BP management are to:

- Attain good BP control
- Reduce cardiovascular morbidity and mortality
- Prevent atherosclerosis
- Control other vascular risk factors
- Reverse end organ damage.

These are all important in the renal patient as well as the non-renal patient. In renal patients, especially those on dialysis, chronic fluid overload is treated by fluid removal and optimisation of the patient's dry weight. Patients are advised to stick to their recommended fluid intake and to restrict the sodium in their diet. High-dose loop diuretics help with fluid overload.

Drug treatment

Drugs commonly used in the treatment of hypertension are:

- Thiazides
- Beta-blockers
- Alpha-adrenoceptor blockers
- Calcium channel blockers
- Angiotensin-converting enzyme (ACE) inhibitors
- Angiotensin II receptor blockers
- Centrally acting drugs
- Direct acting vasodilators.

Tight BP control, especially in renal patients, can be difficult to obtain, and may result in patients being on maximum doses of many antihypertensive drugs. In renal patients drugs should be started at low doses and increased cautiously. Refer to the *British National Formulary* or individual summary of product characteristics (SPCs) for dosing information and to the *Renal Drug Handbook*[4] for dosing in renal impairment. Beta-blockers, calcium channel blockers and ACE inhibitors have all been shown to improve LVH in the general population and are safe in chronic renal failure.

The British Hypertension Society recommendations are shown in Figure 7.1.[3]

The ASCOT trial recommends using ACE inhibitors first line for younger patients and

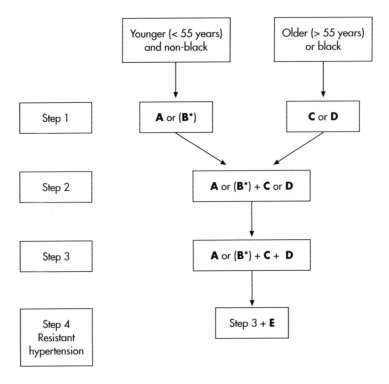

Figure 7.1 British Hypertension Society recommendations for combining blood pressure-lowering drugs. **A** = angiotensin-converting enzyme (ACE) inhibitor or angiotensin II receptor blocker; **B** = beta-blocker; **C** = calcium channel blocker; **D** = thiazide diuretic; **E** = add either alpha-blocker or spironolactone or other diuretic. *Combination therapy involving **B** + **D** may induce more new onset diabetes compared with other combination therapies. Adapted from ref. 3.

calcium channel blockers for older patients.[5] The National Institute for Health and Clinical Excellence (NICE) recommends:

- For patients over 55 years old or black – a calcium channel blocker or thiazide diuretic first line, ACE inhibitor second line, and a calcium channel blocker or thiazide third line whichever was not used first.
- For patients under 55 years old, an ACE inhibitor first line, a calcium channel blocker or thiazide second line and a calcium channel blocker or thiazide third line.
- For all patients an alpha-blocker, further diuretic or beta-blocker as a fourth drug with referral to a specialist.

NICE also recommends that beta-blockers are not used as an initial therapy for hypertension since they have been shown to be less effective at reducing the risk of a major cardiovascular

system event, in particular stroke. Beta-blockers are an alternative to an ACE inhibitor when an ACE inhibitor is contraindicated or not tolerated (e.g. women of childbearing age or those with an increased sympathetic drive).[6]

In patients with renal disease, hypertension can increase the rate of progression to end stage renal disease (ESRD) and therefore the use of drugs can be important in delaying the progression to ESRD. This is the same for all causes of renal impairment. In some cases initiation of dialysis is needed to control hypertension. In diabetics and some other renal diseases (e.g. glomerulonephritis), controlling the BP with an ACE inhibitor or angiotensin II blocker slows the damage to the kidney and therefore delays the time to ESRD. ACE inhibitors should be used with caution in other patients with renal disease since they can increase the damage to the kidney and therefore reduce the time until dialysis is required. In all patients, when starting an ACE inhibitor or angiotensin II blocker, renal function should be measured prior to starting therapy and regularly thereafter to pick up if the drug is affecting the patient's renal function.

In renal artery stenosis (RAS) the main blood vessel running to the kidney becomes blocked – partially or fully – due to atherosclerosis. It usually affects both kidneys. It is a common cause of renal failure in older people, especially those who have suffered an MI or stroke (i.e. are at increased risk of atherosclerosis). In patients with RAS, ACE inhibitors and angiotensin II blockers are generally avoided since they can wipe out renal function completely, accelerating the progression to ESRD. Occasionally, if the benefits outweigh the risks these drugs may be used under the close supervision of a nephrologist.[7]

Thiazide diuretics are ineffective once the glomerular filtration rate (GFR) becomes less than 25 mL/min, and loop diuretics are often used at high doses (e.g. furosemide 500 mg to 1 g daily) to gain an effect. Metolazone is effective when combined with a loop diuretic. Potassium-sparing diuretics such as amiloride are not recommended. Spironolactone is not generally used, but is beneficial in low dose for the treatment of heart failure even in patients on dialysis. Beta-blockers and calcium channel blockers are generally well tolerated. Any ankle swelling with calcium channel blockers must not be confused with fluid overload. Moxonidine, although contraindicated in severe renal impairment, is used in practice.

Hyperlipidaemia

When dietary cholesterol and triglycerides are absorbed from the intestine they are transported in the intestinal lymphatics as chylomicrons. These pass through blood capillaries where the enzyme lipoprotein lipase catalyses the breakdown of triglycerides to free fatty acids and glycerol, which enter adipose tissue and muscle. The cholesterol-rich chylomicron remnants go to the liver where they are cleared from circulation.

High-density lipoprotein (HDL) transports cholesterol from peripheral tissues to the liver, and plays a major role in maintaining cholesterol homeostasis. About 30% of blood cholesterol is carried by HDL. In turn, low-density lipoprotein (LDL) transports cholesterol from the liver via the plasma to those cells that require it. Cholesterol is an essential part of cell membranes and is a precursor of steroid hormones. LDL is the main lipoprotein involved in atherosclerosis.[1]

Elevated concentrations of total cholesterol (TC) and LDLs increase the risk of CHD, while HDLs confer protection. The term dyslipidaemia is a more appropriate term to use when considering the risk of CHD.

An ideal serum lipid profile would be:[1]

- TC <5.0 mmol/L
- LDL <3.0 mmol/L
- Triglycerides <2.3 mmol/L
- HDL >0.9 mmol/L.

Primary dyslipidaemia

This can be genetically determined although expression is influenced by environmental factors. Familial hypercholesterolaemia is the most common inherited dyslipidaemia. It is caused by a mutation in the LDL receptor gene. Patients with the genetic dyslipidaemia will be at increased risk of MI, or stroke, due to elevated concentrations of cholesterol and triglycerides.

Secondary dyslipidaemia

Dyslipidaemia can be secondary to diet, drugs or a number of other disorders. These dyslipidaemias are more easily corrected than primary dyslipidaemia. Common causes of secondary dyslipidaemia include:

- Diabetes mellitus
- Chronic renal failure
- Nephrotic syndrome
- Drugs.

Diabetes

The incidence of CHD is up to four times higher in diabetic patients than in the general population. Many renal patients have diabetes so this is a risk factor for them. In people with diabetes any atherosclerotic disease is often more widespread, and plaque rupture and thrombotic occlusion occur more often. It is the main cause of reduced life expectancy in people with diabetes. The results of the Heart Protection Study suggest that statin therapy reduces vascular events regardless of cholesterol level.[8]

Chronic renal failure

Dyslipidaemia is common in patients with impaired renal function. The hypertriglyceridaemia is associated with reduced lipoprotein lipase activity. In chronic renal failure, diabetes, type of renal disease, transplantation and drugs can all play a part in the dyslipidaemia[9] (see also Chapter 9). Dyslipidaemia often accelerates renal disease partly by promoting renal fibrosis in early atherosclerosis. The pathways for this fibrosis may be reversible and early intervention could preserve the kidney.[10]

Nephrotic syndrome

This is a syndrome in which the kidney's nephrons becomes 'leaky' and allow protein to enter into the urine. There are many causes of nephrotic syndrome, and a biopsy will determine the cause. These patients have an increase in circulating lipoproteins, which is related to the extent of proteinuria and serum albumin level. HDL levels are usually unchanged. The use of steroids may exacerbate the underlying lipoprotein abnormality. Many of these patients require treatment with statins, but intervention is often delayed until after a trial of steroids to see if the disease is controlled, since as the level of proteinuria falls and serum albumin increases the cholesterol level may return to normal. If biopsy shows the nephrotic syndrome is not autoimmune or steroid responsive, then statins may be started immediately. Hyperlipidaemia itself can affect renal function, increase proteinuria and speed glomerulosclerosis, thus determining a higher risk of progression to dialysis. Statin therapy has been shown to prevent creatinine clearance decline and to slow renal function loss, particularly in case of proteinuria and this effect may only partially be due to their favourable effect on hyperlipidaemia.[11,12]

Drugs

Many drugs can adversely affect the lipid profile. Hypertension is a major risk factor for atherosclerosis and there is concern that whilst treating hypertension has reduced the incidence of MI, stroke and renal failure, it has had no major impact on reducing CHD.

Antihypertensive drugs

Many of the antihypertensive drugs themselves have an adverse effect on lipids. Thiazide diuretics and beta-blockers are the main culprits. The benefits of these drugs, for example following MI or in heart failure, outweigh any benefit of withdrawal. However other antihypertensive drugs (e.g. ACE inhibitors or calcium channel blockers) are without adverse effects on lipids and these could be used as alternatives in those patients more at risk.

Ciclosporin

Ciclosporin has been associated with increased LDL. Its use is widespread in renal patients either following transplantation or in certain diseases (e.g. nephrotic syndrome). This adverse effect is often compounded by the concomitant use of prednisolone. This combination contributes to the adverse lipid profile seen following renal transplantation (see Chapter 9). Statins improve the profiles of those atherogenic lipids associated with the hypercholesterolaemia seen in renal transplant patients treated with the immunosuppressants ciclosporin or tacrolimus.[9] The combination of statins with ciclosporin increases the risk of myositis and rhabdomyolysis and therefore should be used with caution (its use is widespread).

Sirolimus

Sirolimus is associated with a marked hyperlipidaemia, including hypercholesterolaemia and hypertriglyceridaemia. Cholesterol levels should be measured prior to starting treatment, and regularly thereafter to monitor extent of hyperlipidaemia, and treatment initiated if necessary.[13]

Risk assessment

The Sheffield table[14] identifies patients who should have their lipid levels measured, and those who would benefit from treatment. The threshold for commencing treatment is a risk of developing CHD of 30% over 10 years. Patients with CHD and levels of TC >5 mmol/L and LDL >3 mmol/L are most likely to benefit from treatment.[14]

Treatment

Before starting drug therapy other risk factors should be tackled, such as obesity, smoking, high alcohol intake and lack of exercise. Underlying disorders, such as hypertension, should be treated. A low-fat diet should be commenced. The patient should be informed that treatment involves a long-term commitment to drug therapy and also appropriate dietary and lifestyle changes.

The two most widely used drugs are statins and fibrates. Doses may need to be adjusted according to renal function.[15]

Statins

Statins inhibit the enzyme 3-hydroxy-3-methyl-glutaryl coenzyme A reductase (HMG-CoA). Their primary site of action is in the liver, where they inhibit the rate-limiting step in the biosynthesis of cholesterol. The effect of statins on lipid profile contributes to their beneficial outcome in reducing morbidity and mortality in CHD. Other mechanisms may also play a part (e.g. plaque stabilisation, inhibition of thrombus formation and anti-inflammatory activity).[1,10,11] All statins have the potential to cause muscle myopathy and this is more prevalent in renal impairment and with concomitant use of ciclosporin.[8] This effect is also seen with tacrolimus and sirolimus. Therefore all statins should be started at low doses and increased with caution in patients with renal impairment.[4]

Fibrates

Fibrates reduce triglycerides and LDL whilst increasing HDL. They also have a beneficial effect on fibrinolytic and clotting mechanisms. Myositis is also associated with fibrates, especially in renal impairment or in combination with statins, and as with the statins doses need to be adjusted with respect to renal function.[4]

Ezetimibe

Ezetimibe inhibits the absorption of cholesterol from the intestine. It can be used either alone or in combination with a statin. It has been well tolerated, with no dosage adjustment required in renal impairment.[4] However, it can affect ciclosporin levels, and ciclosporin can increase ezetimibe levels, so the combination should be used with caution and levels monitored carefully.[16]

In patients with CHD or other occlusive arterial disease (e.g. RAS), treatment should include:

- Statin to lower TC <5 mmol/L
- Advice to stop smoking
- Tight control of BP to <140/90
- Information on risk factors (e.g. diet, alcohol, weight)
- Low-dose aspirin (75 mg daily).

CASE STUDY

Mr BJ is a 50-year-old man whose blood pressure has been consistently above 140/85 for six months although he has not been started on any antihypertensive therapy. He is a type 2 diabetic but has no history of coronary heart disease. On a routine clinic visit he is found to have a blood pressure of 150/95, a creatinine of 160 μmol/L a total cholesterol of 5.5 mmol/L and HDL 0.8 mmol/L.

Q1. What risk factors does he have for CHD?

Q2. What treatment would be suggested with respect to his blood pressure?

Q3. What other advice would be appropriate?

References

1. Walker R, Edwards C. *Clinical Pharmacy and Therapeutics*, 3rd edn. Edinburgh: Churchill Livingstone, 2003.
2. Stein A, Wild J. *Kidney Failure Explained*, 2nd edn. London: Class Publishing, 2002.
3. Williams B, Poulter NR, Brown MJ *et al.* The BHS Guidelines Working Party. British Hypertension Society Guidelines for Hypertension Management, 2004 – BHS IV: Summary. *BMJ* 2004; 328: 634–640.
4. Ashley C, Currie A. *The Renal Drug Handbook*, 2nd edn. Oxford: Radcliffe Medical Press, 2004.
5. Dahlof B, Sever PS, Poulter NR *et al.* for the ASCOT investigators. Prevention of cardiovascular events with an antihypertensive regimen, in the Anglo-Scandinavian Cardiac Outcomes Trial (ASCOT). *Lancet* 2005; 366: 895–906.
6. National Institute for Health and Clinical Excellence (NICE). *Hypertension: Management of Hypertension in Adults in Primary Care*. Clinical Guideline CG34. NICE, June 2006 (accessed from www.nice.org.uk).
7. Stein A, Wild J. *Kidney Dialysis and Transplants*. London: Class Publishing, 2002.
8. Heart Protection Study. MRC/BHF Heart Protection Study of cholesterol lowering with simvastatin in 20536 high risk individuals: a randomised placebo-controlled trial. *Lancet* 2002; 360: 7–22.
9. Imamura R, Ichimaru N, Moriyama T *et al.* Long term efficacy of simvastatin in renal transplant recipients treated with ciclosporin or tacrolimus. *Clin Transplant* 2005; 19: 616–621.
10. Chade AR, Mushin OP, Zhu X *et al.* Pathways of renal fibrosis and modulation of matrix turnover in experimental hypercholesterolemia. *Hypertension* 2005; 46: 772–779.
11. Buemi M, Nostro L, Crasci *et al.* Statins in nephrotic syndrome: a new weapon against tissue injury. *Med Res Rev* 2005; 25: 587–609.
12. Kronenberg F. Dyslipidemia and nephritic syndrome: recent advances. *J Ren Nutr* 2005; 15: 195–203.
13. Wyeth. Summary of product characteristics for Sirolimus. January 2005. http://emc.medicines.org.uk
14. Wallis EJ, Ramsay LE, Haq IU *et al.* Coronary and cardiovascular risk estimation for primary prevention: validation of a new Sheffield table in the 1995 Scottish Health Survey population. *BMJ* 2000; 320: 671–676.
15. Joint Formulary Committee. *British National Formulary*. 53 edn. London: British Medical Association and Royal Pharmaceutical Society of Great Britain, 2007.
16. Kosoglou T, Stalkevich P, Johnson-Leanos AO *et al.* Ezetimibe: a review of its metabolism, pharmacokinetics and drug interactions. *Clin Pharmacokinetics* 2005; 44: 467–494.

8

Renal replacement therapy

Aileen Currie and James Dunleavy

In renal failure the normal function of the kidney deteriorates with time and may be lost completely. In the initial 'pre-dialysis' phase the use of drugs, modification of diet and fluid restriction can delay the patient's progression to stage 5 chronic kidney disease (CKD stage 5), where the glomerular filtration rate (GFR) <15 mL/min. However the resultant loss of homeostatic function results in an accumulation of waste products, fluid retention and abnormal electrolyte levels. Therefore most patients with severe chronic renal failure will eventually require some form of renal replacement therapy, the primary aim being to correct the accumulation of toxins, electrolytes and fluid. In acute renal failure it is also used as a short-term measure to 'rest' the kidneys in the hope they will recover function. These patients may be on it for anything from 1 day to 1 year.

The five main treatment options for CKD stage 5 are:

- Haemodialysis
- Continuous renal replacement therapy, including CVVH, CAVH, CVVHD, CAVHD, CVVHDF, CAVHDF
- Haemodiafiltration
- Peritoneal dialysis
- Transplantation.

The first four will be discussed in this chapter and transplantation is covered in Chapter 9.

Haemodialysis

A Scottish chemist, Thomas Graham, in the 1850s, first discovered the capacity of semi-permeable membranes and diffusion to separate colloids and crystalloids. He termed this process 'dialysis'. Problems in developing suitable vascular access and anticoagulation, however, delayed the introduction of dialysis as a useful treatment. The first successful human dialysis was carried out in Germany in 1924 by George Haas. Willem J Kolff then developed the first dialyser in the Netherlands and used it as a treatment for acute renal failure in 1943. Despite its long history, dialysis has only been available as a treatment for chronic renal disease since the 1960s.[1]

Although haemodialysis is mainly a hospital-based treatment it can also be performed at home, in a nurse-led satellite unit or even on holiday in a unit abroad or in the UK. The majority of patients in the UK are dialysed in hospitals, usually three times a week, although there is interest at the moment in daily dialysis, which has been shown to improve adequacy, hypertension and patient quality of life. Unfortunately there are financial constraints to this at the moment; most units do not have space to dialyse patients every day.[2]

Haemodialysis works by a combination of diffusion (the movement of solutes from fluid with a high to a low concentration across a semi-permeable membrane) and ultrafiltration (the movement of fluid under pressure across a semi-permeable membrane) (Figure 8.1). Excess fluid is removed by ultrafiltration and waste products by diffusion. Essential minerals (e.g. calcium and bicarbonate) are also replaced by diffusion.[3]

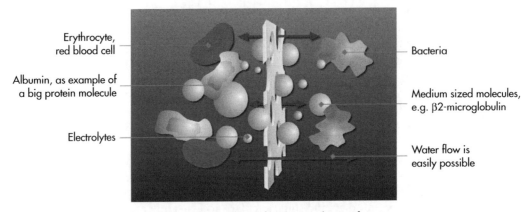

Physical basis of dialysis
Semipermeable membrane

Erythrocyte, red blood cell

Albumin, as example of a big protein molecule

Electrolytes

Bacteria

Medium sized molecules, e.g. β2-microglobulin

Water flow is easily possible

The semipermeable membrane functions similar to a fine sieve, only molecules that are small enough can pass.

Figure 8.1   Diffusion process in relation to dialysis. Copyright and courtesy of Fresenius Medical Care.

Vascular access

There are three methods of vascular access for haemodialysis:

- Fistula
- Catheter
- Graft.

Fistula

A fistula is usually created as a day surgery case under either local or general anaesthesia depending on the patient's medical condition. It is the surgical connection of an artery to a vein by direct surgical anastomosis; some arterial blood will be diverted due to pressure differences into the vein causing the wall to thicken and the lumen to get bigger. This allows blood at arterial pressure into the venous system close to the surface of the skin so the nurses or the patient are able to get needles into the vessel easily. Fistula formation was first introduced in 1966 and is the preferred option for vascular access for haemodialysis.[4] The Renal Association standards state that 80% of people should be dialysed via a fistula (the Scottish Renal Association want at least 70%).[5] Fistulas can

either be created at the wrist (radial artery) or the elbow (brachial artery). Although brachial fistulas have a success rate of 90% with only 60% for radial fistulas, the latter are usually attempted first as once a patient has had a brachial fistula they are unable to have a radial one. It takes about 6–8 weeks in order for the fistula to be ready for use and therefore it is best to be planned in advance, but unfortunately this does not always happen.[6] They last longer than central venous catheters and 60–90% are usually still functioning after 3 years. The patient must also have a good vascular system but 30% of patients do not have suitable veins (e.g. elderly patients or patients with diabetes)[2] (Figure 8.2).

The main complications are thrombosis, which may be due to hypotension, dehydration or prolonged compression of the fistula (either accidentally or on purpose) and steal syndrome, where too much blood is drawn away from the hand and the fistula usually requires to be tied off (more common with brachial fistulas). It is very important that medical and nursing staff do not take blood from or put venflons into any veins which have been used or may later be used for fistulas.[2,7]

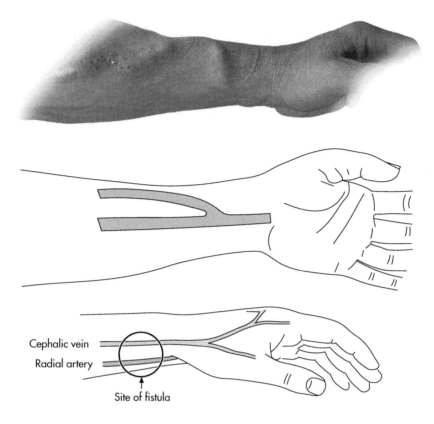

Cephalic vein

Radial artery

Site of fistula

Figure 8.2   Arterio-venous fistula. Copyright and courtesy of Fresenius Medical Care.

Catheter

Temporary or permanent central venous catheters are usually placed into the internal jugular vein. They can also be placed in the femoral vein if there are problems with the internal jugular vein. The main problem with the femoral vein is the high risk of infections and they tend to only be kept in for short periods of time. The subclavian vein is generally not used because of the risk of venous stenosis.[4]

Permanent catheters are inserted in radiology or theatre and are tunnelled and have Dacron cuffs to keep infection at bay and keep them in place. Temporary lines are usually inserted at ward level if dialysis is only required for a few weeks or until a slot for a permanent catheter can be organised (ideally they should not be kept in for more than three weeks). They may be either dual or triple lumen. The main problems with catheters are thrombosis and infections. Lines may be kept patent by locking them with sodium chloride 0.9% or heparin after use. If they become blocked (usually due to fibrin sheath formation) then locks or infusions of urokinase or alteplase may have to be used. Low-dose warfarin therapy may be initiated if it becomes a chronic problem, aiming for an INR of 1.5–2.5.[3,4,7]

Graft

Polytetrafluoroethylene (PTFE) grafts are usually only used in the UK if access is a problem. A plastic tube connects usually the basilic vein to the brachial or radial artery, although they can also be placed in the thigh. They have the advantage that they can be used within 2–4 weeks or if required almost immediately after placement. The disadvantages are that they have an increased infection risk, thrombosis, they are difficult to remove and usually only last for 3–5 years.[2,7]

Process

For haemodialysis, blood is removed from the patient from the arterial site via either the line or fistula and pumped through the dialysis machine via the dialyser where diffusion and ultrafiltration occur. The blood is then returned to the patient via the venous site. The blood and dialysate flow in opposite directions to optimise the removal of waste products. Pumps are needed to produce a high enough flow rate for the blood and dialysate to go round the extracorporeal circuit and to control the ultrafiltration rate, blood pressure and dialysate pressure (Figure 8.3). The blood flow rate is ideally 200–500 mL/min and the dialysate flow rate 500 mL/min, which can be increased to 800 mL/min, although there is not a huge increase in clearance with the latter. As dialysis progresses, the efficiency is decreased because the concentration gradient across the membrane in the dialyser is reduced.[3] The machines are heat sterilised after every patient, chemically sterilised twice a week and heat disinfected and decalcified every second day.

The semi-permeable membrane used for haemodialysis is known as the dialyser or filter or kidney. This is the major high-cost item in haemodialysis. It consists of thousands of long hollow fibres enclosed in a rigid polyurethane shell. There are two ports on each side to allow the blood and dialysate to flow in and out. The blood flows through the fibres and the dialysate surrounds the fibres. The blood and dialysate flow in opposite directions, i.e. countercurrent, allowing diffusion and ultrafiltration to take place more effectively. The dialyser allows the free movement of low-molecular-weight molecules (<5 kDa) but restricts the passage of larger molecules and blood.[3]

Types of dialyser

There are many different dialysers available, the main differences are:[2,7,9,10]

- Shape: Hollow fibre (capillaries) – this is the most common form – or flat plate (parallel plates).

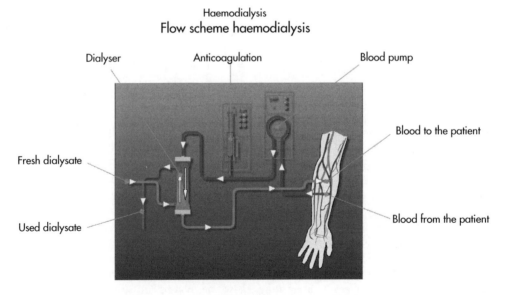

Haemodialysis
Flow scheme haemodialysis

Dialyser   Anticoagulation   Blood pump

Fresh dialysate

Blood to the patient

Used dialysate

Blood from the patient

Figure 8.3   Haemodialysis circuit. Copyright and courtesy of Fresenius Medical Care.

- Surface area: The bigger the surface area the more dialysis the patient receives. A typical dialyser has a surface area of 1–2 m^2.
- Method of sterilisation: Steam, ethylene oxide (this must be rinsed out before use due to its toxicity), gamma-irradiation.
- Material: Cellulose (can cause complement and leukocyte activation) (e.g. cuprophan), modified cellulose (e.g. cellulose acetate, haemophan), synthetic (best for β_2-microglobulin removal) (e.g. polysulfone, polyamide, polyacrylonitrile).
- Membrane permeability: The more permeable the dialyser is to fluid the higher its flux, measured as ultrafiltration coefficient (K_{uf}) and varies from 2 to 85 mL/h/mmHg. Low flux has a K_{uf} of 2–10 mL/h/mmHg and high flux has a K_{uf} greater than 20 to over 60 mL/h/mmHg.
- Clearance: Of urea, creatinine, vitamin B$_{12}$, phosphate, inulin and sieving coefficients for albumin (should be 0) and β_2-microglobulin.

The most biocompatible dialyser is one that has been steam sterilised and is made of a synthetic material (e.g. polysulfone). The more biocompatible the dialyser the fewer long-term side-effects a patient is likely to suffer, although it has not been determined whether the short-term complications (e.g. hypotension, headaches and muscle cramps) are related to bioincompatibility or rate of fluid and urea removal. Biocompatible membranes are most important for people who may be on dialysis long term.[9–11]

Hollow-fibre dialyers can be reused. Initially, this was to save money and to make the dialyser more biocompatible, although they lose their efficiency the more they are reused. In theory, they can be reused up to a maximum of 4–6 times, but none are actually licensed for this in the UK. There are costs involved in reuse, as specialised machinery and personnel are required, as well as storage space where the dialysers are kept labelled for each individual patient. Very few, if any units, reuse them these days due to an increase in morbidity, reduction in costs of new dialysers and improved biocompatibility.[11–13]

Haemodialysis is not as good at removing medium-sized molecules (e.g. β_2-microglobulin) as small molecules. Accumulation of β_2-microglobulin can lead to problems in the long term with amyloidosis that can present as carpal tunnel syndrome, arthropathy and bone cysts.[9,11]

An interesting side-effect occurs between ACE inhibitors and high-flux polyacrylonitrile membranes, where anaphylaxis can occur due to bradykinin formation between the dialyser and the patient's blood. This type of dialyser is no longer routinely used for haemodialysis.[11,14]

Dialysate

The dialysis fluid known as dialysate consists of a concentrated solution of electrolytes dissolved in water. They differ only in respect of the quantities of electrolytes in each (e.g. low or high calcium or potassium concentrations), and which one is chosen depends on the patient's requirements. Some now also come with glucose, which helps prevent hypoglycaemia during dialysis in diabetic patients and can reduce disequilibrium syndrome by maintaining the osmotic pressure. The majority of units will limit the number of different fluids they use; for example, they may keep a low and a high potassium and calcium fluid. The fluid is brought to body temperature by mixing with purified water. Bicarbonate is supplied in dry powder form as it is too unstable to be mixed with the dialysate and the machine calculates the proportion of bicarbonate required.[2]

The water used to dilute the dialysate must be purer than drinking water as patients are exposed to approximately 300–400 L of water each week.[15] Before entering the dialysis machine the water passes through a reverse osmosis system to remove the aluminium and biomaterials (e.g. bacteria and other potential endotoxins) and this is monitored regularly. Aluminium enters the water supply as part of the water treatment process and has been shown to accumulate in people with renal failure. Signs of aluminium toxicity include dementia and bone disease. Aluminium levels can be high in patients who take aluminium hydroxide (AluCap capsules) as a phosphate binder, although they are rarely used now, and when they are it is only for a short period of time. The water supplier limits the aluminium, calcium, chloramines, nitrates, sodium, sulfates, zinc and copper.[2]

Anticoagulation

Anticoagulation is usually necessary to keep the blood flowing through the extracorporeal circuit. Heparin is used to maintain anticoagulation in most patients during dialysis, with the dose being dependent on the response of the patient. The majority of units will use conventional heparin although occasionally low-molecular-weight heparin may be used. Bemiparin, dalteparin, enoxaparin or tinzaparin are licensed in the UK for this use but can make the process of dialysis even more expensive. In patients with bleeding complications, either a continuous infusion of epoprostenol may be used or heparin-free dialysis may be considered. Other drugs used in cases of intolerability to heparin or thrombocytopenia are lepirudin, argatroban and danaparoid, none of which are licensed in the UK for this indication.[2] More information can be found in the *Renal Drug Handbook* by Ashley and Currie.[16]

Time on haemodialysis and adequacy

When people first start on dialysis they have short and frequent sessions as the body has adjusted, or become accustomed to having large quantities of waste products in the blood. If these are removed too rapidly a 'disequilibrium' syndrome occurs which results in headaches, nausea and vomiting, and in severe cases confusion and convulsions.[3]

The length of time on haemodialysis is gradually increased to between 3 and 5 hours three times a week, the length of time depending on the patient's blood results, size and residual urine output.

The patient's weight is measured before and after dialysis, the post weight being as close to their dry weight as possible, which is equivalent to their body weight without excess fluid or causing hypotension. Patients are advised to limit their fluid intake between dialysis sessions to as little as 750–1000 mL per day, depending on their urine output. This can be problematic as fluid includes soup, custard, gravy, etc.

Sometimes if people have problems tolerating fluid removal on dialysis, 'ultrafiltration profiling' or 'sodium profiling' may be attempted. This involves taking more fluid off at the beginning of dialysis so the body has time to normalise before dialysis is finished or altering the sodium content of the dialysate fluid during the dialysis (start with a high sodium concentration then reduce it as the dialysis progresses). It can reduce the incidence of dizziness and cramps due to fluid removal but may exacerbate thirst, which does not help the patient's efforts at fluid restriction.[17]

Inadequate dialysis and poor nutritional intake are associated with increased mortality and morbidity. Inadequate dialysis can also play a major role in erythropoietin resistance, resulting in worsening of anaemia.

There are two main methods of determining the adequacy of dialysis:

- Urea reduction ratio (URR)
- Urea kinetic modelling (UKM) (Kt/V).

URR (as the name suggests) is the difference in urea pre and post dialysis expressed as a percentage. The target URR for adequate dialysis is >65%.[5] This method is not ideal, as it does not take into account the effect of residual renal function or dietary intake.

Urea kinetic modeling (UKM) includes the more complex calculation of urea removal Kt/V, where K is urea clearance per minute, both the patient's and the dialyser's, t is time on dialysis and V is volume of distribution of urea (i.e. the volume of body water in which the urea is distributed). The calculation also takes into account protein catabolic rate, nutritional status and residual renal function so is a more accurate determination of dialysis adequacy. The mathematical equations used may be complex and are best calculated by computer. They can be used to determine how much dialysis a patient requires.[4]

Other factors that can give an indication of adequacy are normalised protein catabolic rate (normalised for weight), acidosis, weight gain and malnutrition.

The Renal Association standards state that an equilibrated *Kt/V* >1.2 equates to a good dialysis for three times a week dialysis. If dialysis is only done twice a week then a *Kt/V* >1.8 is required.[5]

Dialysis adequacy can be increased by:[2,11]

- Higher blood flow rate
- Increasing the dialysate flow rate (does not make a huge difference)
- Increasing the size/surface area of the dialyser
- Longer time on dialysis
- Changing from haemodialysis to haemodiafiltration.

The common complications associated with haemodialysis are listed in Table 8.1.

Continuous renal replacement therapies

Haemofiltration

This method of continuous renal replacement therapy (CRRT) works by convection (movement of solutes in fluid across a membrane under pressure to remove small, medium and large molecules) and ultrafiltration (movement of water across a membrane), which removes extracellular fluid with toxins at the filter and adds haemofiltration fluid to the filtered blood either before (pre-dilution) or after (post-dilution) the haemofilter, so diluting the waste products (Figure 8.4). The ultrafiltration rate can be controlled by pressure or gravity, 25–30 L of fluid may be removed

Table 8.1 Complications of haemodialysis[2,3,7,11]

Complication	Reason	Treatment
Hypotension 'crash' (25–60%)	Too much fluid being removed too quickly e.g. if patients have come in significantly over their dry weight Too many antihypertensives Dry weight too low Autonomic neuropathy	Assess dry weight Perform sodium or ultrafiltration profiling Give at least 100 mL bolus of sodium chloride 0.9% via the haemodialysis machine and raise the patient's feet above the head Reduce the rate of fluid removal Omit antihypertensives on dialysis days Stop the patient eating on dialysis Give midodrine 2.5–30 mg or fludrocortisone, carnitine 20 mg/kg (IV), sertraline 50–100 mg daily
Cramps (5–25%)	This can also be related to hypotension or if the patient has too much fluid removed (e.g. due to an incorrect dry weight) Reduced serum sodium usually near the end of dialysis Carnitine deficiency	Give a bolus of 50–100 mL sodium chloride 0.9% or quinine sulfate tablets Reassess patient's weight Give carnitine, vitamin E supplementation
Pruritis (1–5%)	Dry skin, hyperphosphataemia, uraemic toxins or an allergic reaction to heparin or the dialyser membrane	Give antihistamines and moisturising lotions or change the dialyser
Thrombosis	Especially with dialysis catheters but also can occur with fistulas, usually if the haemoglobin is too high	Usually give urokinase/alteplase locks or infusions according to local policy. Urokinase infusions can vary from 10 000 to 250 000 IU over 1–24 hours People with fistulas may be on prophylactic aspirin or low-dose warfarin Reduce/stop ESA and iron

(continued overleaf)

Table 8.1 (continued)

Complication	Reason	Treatment
Infections	Especially at the exit site of dialysis catheters or fistulas due to an increase in manipulations and skin penetration Dialysis patients also have an impaired immune response The main organisms involved are *Staph. aureus* or *Staph. epidermidis*. Rarely they can be due to Gram-negative organisms, mainly with femoral haemodialysis catheters. They can be very serious and lead to infections like septic shock, endocarditis or discitis Hepatitis B and C outbreaks can also very rarely occur	Low threshold for commencing patients on antibiotics, mainly anti-staphylococcal agents (e.g. flucloxacillin, vancomycin or gentamicin). Continue for 2–3 weeks. Antibiotic locks of gentamicin/heparin, vancomycin/heparin, taurolidine or citrate may also be used May require replacement of catheter if it becomes colonised Nasal mupirocin may be used for nasal *Staph.* carriers To prevent hepatitis B, units should vaccinate their patients and staff and any infected patients should be isolated Isolate hepatitis C patients Screen for both viruses on a regular basis
Anaemia	Blood loss, inadequate dialysis, excessive bleeding post dialysis, iron or erythropoietin deficiency	Give ESA and intravenous iron Reduce the heparin dose
Hair loss	Heparin Low zinc levels	Try low-molecular-weight heparin or one of the other agents used for anticoagulation Zinc supplements
Dialysis-related migraine/headache (5–10%)	Minor effect of disequilibrium syndrome possibly due to excess urea removal	Give low-dose clonidine 25–75 µg pre-dialysis
Arrhythmias (5–60%)	Can be linked with hypokalaemia	Increase dialysate potassium concentration
Nausea and vomiting (5–15%)	Associated with hypotension and disequilibrium syndrome	Give antiemetics Reduce blood flow rate at the start of dialysis.
Recirculation	This is the repeated uptake of blood which has already been dialysed. Usually leads to poor adequacy and/or biochemistry	Access may need to be reviewed

per treatment.[2,18,19] Haemofiltration can be either continual or intermittent depending on the stability of the patient, although continual is best for very unstable patients.

The post-dilution method is most common now but has problems with clotting if the blood becomes too concentrated in the filter due to a reduction in blood flow. Therefore the ultra-filtration rate should be less than 20% of the blood flow rate to help prevent this happening or the blood flow rate can be increased. It does give a more accurate fluid balance as the replacement fluid is returned after all the fluid has been removed at the filter.

Pre-dilution is slightly less efficient for removal of larger molecular weight compounds than for small molecules; it is the best treatment if you have to remove more than 25 L a day or

Haemodialysis
Flow scheme haemofiltration

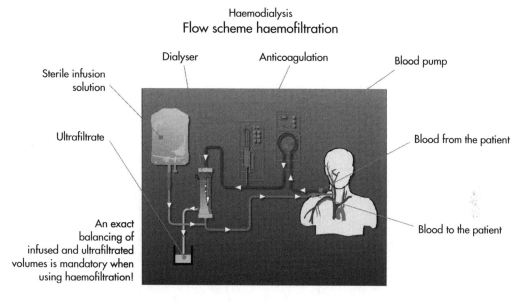

Figure 8.4   Haemofiltration circuit. Copyright and courtesy of Fresenius Medical Care.

if the patient has a high haemoglobin as the blood is diluted before the filter and therefore there is reduced clotting and the filter lasts longer. More fluid is needed compared with post-dilution.[18–20]

The advantages of convective and continuous treatment are as follows:[2,3,21,22]

- It improves cardiovascular stability, possibly due to convection producing a cooling effect in the extracorporeal circuit and by the removal of inflammatory mediators and the more biocompatible membranes that are used.
- It gives better control of blood pressure.
- More physiological fluid removal is possible due to a reduction in hypovolaemic effects.
- It can remove larger quantities of fluid (up to 3–6 L/day) as it is also usually carried out over a longer time interval so there is a reduced risk of disequilibrium syndrome. Also it can be used to create 'space' in fluid-restricted patients who need enteral or parenteral nutrition or are receiving intravenous antibiotics.
- It produces a higher rate of removal of molecules with a middle (500–15 000 Da) or large (>15 000 Da) molecular weight (e.g.

β_2-microglobulins, advanced glycation end-products).
- Continuous renal replacement therapy is better for cardiovascular and intracranial stability, especially in patients at risk of cerebral oedema (e.g. after neurosurgery or acute liver failure) due to slower fluid shifts and a more gradual change in electrolytes. If fluid is removed too rapidly, as in intermittent haemodialysis, it would result in a reduction in cardiac filling pressures and cardiac instability. Body water is unable to move fast enough from the intracellular and interstitial spaces to the plasma.[2,22]

The disadvantages of convective and continuous treatment are as follows:[11,22,23]

- It is more expensive than haemodialysis as more fluid and more expensive filters are required. Because of this it is used as a short-term treatment in the acute situation.
- It is a more complex treatment so extensive training of staff is required.
- There is no definite measure of adequacy as yet.
- Small molecule clearance (e.g. urea) is reduced.

Continuous arterio-venous haemofiltration

Continuous arterio-venous haemofiltration (CAVHF) was the first haemodialysis system developed in the 1960s. It uses the patient's blood pressure to drive the filtration so no blood pumps are needed. Blood leaves by the arterial line and returns by the venous line. It had the disadvantage of a high risk of clotting in hypotensive patients and was not very efficient – only between 10 and 20 L of plasma water could be removed a day, so dialysis would still sometimes be required to remove the small molecules. It was good for anaemic patients and those with low protein levels as it depended on the movement of plasma water i.e. the thinner the blood the easier the patient was to treat (similar to pre-dilution haemofiltration, when the replacement fluid dilutes the blood before the filter).

CAVHF then led to CAVHD (continuous arterio-venous haemodialysis), which improved small solute clearance and resulted in better cardiovascular stability than intermittent haemodialysis. CAVHDF (continuous arterio-venous haemodiafiltration) is better still for haemodynamically unstable patients and is more efficient than CAVHD, but unless you have on-line fluid production it can be very expensive.[11,19,22]

Pumped circuits were then developed which only needed venous access so removed some of the problems associated with arterial access (e.g. elderly atherosclerotic patients who have poor access). This is known as CVVHF (continuous veno-venous haemofiltration). It is more efficient than CAVHF because the blood pumps controlled the ultrafiltration and so it can be used in people with low blood pressure, but it is not as good for haemodynamically unstable patients. CVVHD (continuous veno-venous haemodialysis) improves efficiency once again, and CVVHDF (continuous veno-venous haemodiafiltration) improves efficiency and stability.[11,19,22]

Slow continuous ultrafiltration (SCUF) usually uses arterial access and can remove between 3 and 6 L of fluid a day. It is preferred for fluid-overloaded patients, such as patients with heart failure but without renal failure, as excess fluid can be removed gradually. Replacement fluid is not usually required. There can be problems though with lines clotting due to low blood flow and haemoconcentration.[2,11]

The dialysers used for haemofiltration are known as haemofilters and are high flux, usually synthetic hollow-fibre dialysers.[2] They have to be very permeable to both fluids and solutes, as extensive ultrafiltration has to take place. There is significant clearance of both phosphate and amino acids; about 10% of intravenous amino acids from parenteral nutrition may be removed by haemofiltration.[22] Biocompatibility issues with the filters are similar to those for haemodialysis.

Haemofiltration fluid is a balanced electrolyte solution of sodium, calcium, magnesium and chloride, which usually comes in 5 L bags. The rate of haemofiltration fluid flow rate is usually 1–2 L/h increasing to 3–4 L/h for high-volume haemofiltration with an ultrafiltration rate of at least 35 mL/kg/h.[3] The rate is usually decided by how much fluid has to come off the patient per day compared with how much fluid to return to the patient. The fluid is available with or without potassium, and 1–4 mmol/L of potassium are usually added per bag if they are potassium free; the amount added depends on the patient's blood results. The fluid is usually buffered with lactate as lactate is metabolised to bicarbonate, which is used to correct the patient's underlying metabolic acidosis. If patients have problems metabolising lactate (e.g. patients with hepatic failure, severe sepsis or cardiogenic shock) then lactate-free or bicarbonate solutions should be used as they can increase cardiovascular stability, improve dialysis symptoms (nausea, vomiting, headache, and hypotension) and patient well-being.[2,22]

Anticoagulation has to be balanced with excess bleeding in acute renal failure patients. If at all possible it is best to avoid anticoagulating the patient and just flush the lines with heparin, but this is not always possible. Heparin is usually used, but if there are complications then epoprostenol can be used. It should be noted that epoprostenol can cause severe hypotension and the dose must be adjusted depending on the patient's response; 40% of epoprostenol will be removed by haemofiltration. The other anticoagulants used in haemodialysis may also be chosen, but heparin and epoprostenol are most commonly used.[2,11,22]

Access is mainly via dual or triple lumen central lines inserted into the internal jugular or femoral vein for CVVHF/CVVHD/CVVHDF. The lines are not usually tunnelled as they are normally inserted at ward level so are generally changed every 4–5 days and can achieve a blood flow rate of around 150–300 mL/min.[2]

Haemodiafiltration

Although the use of haemodialfiltration as a long-term treatment is still in the early stages in the UK, it was first done in 1976 and is very common in Germany.[24] Interest waned in the 1980s, due partly to the cost of the replacement fluid compared with dialysis fluid and also because of developments in haemodialysis, such as bicarbonate dialysis, sodium profiling, accurate volume monitoring to allow weight loss to be controlled, all of which could improve cardiovascular stability. Interest picked up again as people realised the long-term complications and increased mortality of haemodialysis due to the accumulation of middle and large-molecular-weight molecules (e.g. β_2-microglobulins) and also with the ability to produce on-line haemofiltration fluid (also known as substitution or replacement fluid). β_2-Microglobulin is associated with complications such as amyloidosis and carpal tunnel syndrome. Some studies have shown a reduction of 70% in β_2-microglobulin, which may reduce these complications of long-term dialysis.[23,25–27]

Approximately 3.5% of patients on dialysis are on haemodiafiltration, and if high-flux dialysis (i.e. dialysis using high-flux dialysers but no convection) is included the total is taken up to 25%.

As the name suggests, haemodiafiltration is a combination of haemodialysis and haemofiltration (simultaneous diffusion, ultrafiltration and convection).[3] This gives clearance of small, middle and large molecules. Blood is withdrawn as for haemodialysis and passes through a very permeable dialyser where diffusion occurs. This is known as a high-flux dialyser and has the ability to remove large volumes of extracellular fluid and molecules up to 30 kDa. Replacement fluid and the filtered blood are then returned to the patient.[3,25]

Dialysers that are used for haemodiafiltration must have an ultrafiltration coefficient of at least 55 mL/h/mmHg but this must be balanced with excess albumin loss if the dialysers are too leaky.

In order to make haemodiafiltration affordable it is necessary to have on-line substitution fluid production from dialysis fluid. To do this ultra pure water is required as the fluid goes directly to the patient. The water goes through 2–3 extra filters compared with haemodialysis, one each for the water, the dialysate and the substitution fluid and can be within the machine or external depending on the machine.[18] The high-flux dialysers required can also be very expensive but they are slowly coming down in price.

Advantages of haemodiafiltration are improved cardiovascular tolerance to fluid removal, removal of middle molecules, inflammatory markers and advanced glycation endproducts (AGEs) and better blood pressure control.[26,27]

One of the problems with haemodiafiltration is the increased removal of drugs, especially vitamins, antibiotics and low-molecular-weight heparins. This must be taken into consideration, and if using low-molecular-weight heparins as anticoagulation for haemodiafiltration an additional dose is sometimes required half way through the dialysis. Care must also be taken with vancomycin, as up to 50% of vancomycin may be lost during haemodiafiltration, necessitating increased doses.

Efficiency

Efficiency can be affected by:[24]

- Dialyser membrane and surface area
- Blood flow rate – Q_B (range is 300–500 mL/min; an increase in Q_B can increase small solute clearance)
- Dialysis fluid flow rate – Q_D (range is 500–800 mL/min)

- Substitution fluid volume – Q_S (standard is 60 mL/min, range 0–150 mL/min for post-dilution and 0–250 mL/min for pre-dilution and can affect β_2-microglobulin removal)
- Treatment duration
- Haemoglobin concentration (β_2-microglobulin is mainly found in plasma and there is an inverse correlation with its removal and the patient's haemoglobin)
- No one is quite sure how to measure adequacy in haemodiafiltration as conventional measurements (e.g. Kt/V) only take small molecule clearance into account.

In pre-dilution haemodiafiltration the blood is diluted by the substitution fluid before going through the dialyser. This was the original form of haemodiafiltration.

Its advantages are that:

- It is better tolerated than post-dilution haemodiafiltration
- Less heparin is required
- Blood is less likely to clot in patients with a good haemoglobin or access problems.[21,26]

The disadvantages of pre-dilution haemodiafiltration are that:

- Small solute clearance is reduced as the substitution fluid has diluted the blood before the diffusion has taken place in the dialyser so there is a reduced equilibrium gradient. Higher infusion rates of substitution fluid are possible to compensate for this (not too important as small molecules will be removed by diffusion)
- β_2-Microglobulin clearance is reduced
- Approximately twice as much substitution fluid is needed compared with post-dilution haemodiafiltration (i.e. higher dialysate flow rates are needed).[18]

Post-dilution haemodiafiltration is the more usual method now; blood is diluted by substitution fluid after going through the dialyser. The advantages with this method are that:

- Smaller volumes of fluid are required
- It is more efficient, getting the best removal of small and large molecules.

The disadvantages are that:

- A good blood flow is required in order for it to be efficient, or else the number of hours on dialysis must be increased
- More anticoagulation is required
- There may be problems with the lines clotting and efficiency if the haemoglobin is too high and the blood is too viscous, as the blood concentrates in the dialyser
- Treatment is of longer duration as small molecule clearance is not as good.[24,28]

There is some work being done at the moment looking at mid-dilution haemodiafiltration which gives better removal of the middle and large molecules but is worse for small molecules (e.g. urea and creatinine) compared with post-dilution. Here you get post-dilution occurring first and then pre-dilution within the dialyser. A special dialyser is required, which is split into two internally. Problems encountered with this method are increased albumin loss (equivalent to peritoneal dialysis), increased clotting and increased removal of low-molecular-weight heparins.[28]

Peritoneal dialysis

Although the principle of peritoneal dialysis had been considered as early as 1923, it was not until 1959 that it was first used because procedural problems held up development. In 1968 Tenckhoff and co-workers developed suitable access for peritoneal dialysis and then in 1976 Popovich and colleagues developed an ambulatory dialysis system. It has had varying popularity due to consultant bias, haemodialysis availability and financial constraints.[30] By the end of 2002 there were 130 000 people on peritoneal dialysis worldwide, representing 15% of the total dialysis population.[31] It is a good choice for diabetic patients (as people with diabetes tend to have more vascular access problems and heparin on dialysis can increase the risk of retinopathy), children, people with unstable cardiovascular disease and those who are well motivated and still pass urine, or patients who live a significant distance from the dialysis centre.[30]

Peritoneal dialysis works on the three main principles of diffusion, osmosis and convection. A solution is infused into the peritoneal cavity where the patient's own peritoneum acts as the semi-permeable membrane. The peritoneal membrane is a thin, highly vascular, stretchable membrane, with a surface area of approximately 2 m². Diffusion and convection of solutes occurs between the capillary blood and the dialysis solution in the peritoneal cavity, with excess fluid being removed by osmosis.[30,32] There is less clearance of the small solutes (e.g. urea and creatinine) but this tends not to be too big a problem as the patients usually still pass urine.[30]

Peritoneal dialysis is good for initial therapy as it preserves vascular access, there is a reduced risk of contracting hepatitis B and C, reduced cardiac dysfunction, reduced anaemia and doses of erythropoiesis-stimulating agents (ESA); it is also less expensive than haemodialysis.

Access

Access is via a small (6 mm in diameter), soft, flexible catheter (e.g. Tenckhoff catheter), usually made of silicone rubber, inserted into the peritoneum at the midline below the umbilicus and tunnelled through the abdominal wall to emerge on one side of the abdomen (15 cm of the catheter remains outside the body). The catheter can be inserted under general or local anaesthesia and can be put in laparoscopically. This has a success rate of 75% and the addition of one or two Dacron cuffs helps to secure the catheter in place by facilitating fibrous growth in the tunnelled section, which helps reduce infections.[7,32] (Figure 8.5).

It is advised that patients should receive prophylactic antistaphylococcal agents (e.g. vancomycin or flucloxacillin) before insertion of the catheter to reduce the risk of infection.[33] Some units may also advise a 5-day course of nasal mupirocin for people who are staphylococcal carriers. The catheters are usually not used for two weeks after insertion. During this time the exit site should be kept dry.[33] It is also very important that the patient does not become constipated either before the catheter is in situ or once it is in place, as that can then cause problems with the dialysis. Post care of the exit site is usually with a liquid antibacterial soap or Betadine or saline solutions.[32]

Peritoneal dialysis is not as aggressive as haemodialysis and does not leave the patient feeling washed out at the end of each session, as disequilibrium syndrome is rare compared

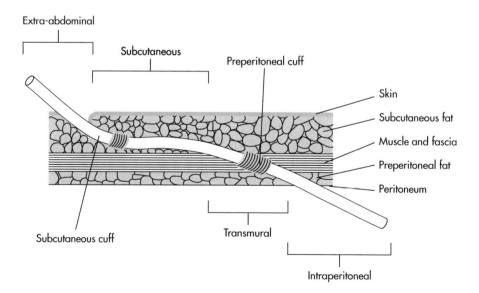

Figure 8.5   Positioning of peritoneal dialysis catheter. Copyright and courtesy of Baxter Healthcare Ltd.

with haemodialysis. It can also preserve residual renal function.[30] Dietary and fluid restrictions tend not to be as strict as on haemodialysis because patients usually still pass some urine and because dialysis is done every day rather than three times a week as with haemodialysis.

Peritoneal dialysis is not recommended for people who:[32]

- are homeless
- have breathing problems
- have diverticular disease
- have had previous abdominal surgery
- have problems with body image
- lack storage space for supplies
- are anuric
- have hernias.

(These are not all necessarily contraindications.)

The dialysate prescribed uses mainly glucose as the osmotic agent and traditionally comes in three strengths: weak, medium and strong. The solution also contains lactate, sodium, potassium, calcium and magnesium. Weaker solutions are used if the patient is dehydrated and stronger ones if the patient is fluid-overloaded. The consultant and peritoneal dialysis nurse decide the prescription that is most suitable for the patient depending on the result of adequacy tests, fluid balance and the patient's blood results. The prescription may need to be changed during periods of peritonitis as the peritoneum becomes more permeable.

The characteristics of several commonly used peritoneal dialysis fluids are summarised in Table 8.2.

Types of peritoneal dialysis

There are two main forms of peritoneal dialysis:

- Continuous ambulatory peritoneal dialysis
- Automated peritoneal dialysis.

Continuous ambulatory peritoneal dialysis

The patient usually performs this form of dialysis manually 4–5 times each day although carers can also be trained to do it. Continuous ambulatory peritoneal dialysis (CAPD) has the advantage that it is easy to teach people how to use it as no machine is involved.

The dialysate is warmed to body temperature by bag warmers and run into the patient/peritoneal cavity via the catheter by gravity (this usually takes about 10 minutes) and remains in the peritoneum for about 4 hours, known as the dwell time. After 4 hours the patient connects their catheter to a drainage bag and a fresh bag of fluid. The fluid in the peritoneal cavity is drained out, this usually takes about 10–20 minutes, and a fresh bag is then drained in. This is known as the 'flush before fill' system and can reduce the risk of infections. The optimum dialysate fill volume that the body can tolerate is 2.5 L for a 1.73 m^2 body surface area; the average volume used is 2 L (range 1.5–3 L). If the body surface area is greater than 2 m^2 then a fill volume of 3–3.5 L can be tolerated. The volume of fill is reduced if there is a history of hernia, pleural leak or if the patient experiences abdominal pain.[30,32,34]

Automated peritoneal dialysis

This follows the same principles as CAPD except the exchanges are done by a machine during the night over 8–10 hours (usually six exchanges). In automated peritoneal dialysis (APD) 1.5–3 L of fluid are drained into the peritoneum by a machine, left for about 1–3 hours when it is then drained out and fresh dialysate drained in. This process is repeated throughout the night until the total prescription volume has been reached (e.g. 10 L).

This is a more expensive procedure than CAPD but many patients find it more socially acceptable as the patient can lead a normal life during the day, free from dialysis exchanges. As the dwell times are shorter than traditional CAPD, an extra bag of fluid may need to be run in at the end of dialysis and kept in during the day to improve the efficiency of the dialysis. This can be either glucose or starch-based (icodextrin).[34]

Another advantage is that larger total fill volumes can be used as the intraperitoneal pressure is reduced when lying down. This is good for bigger patients as they can get more exchanges and for high transporters (see later) who tend to

Table 8.2 Characteristics of some peritoneal dialysis fluids[31,35–37]

Fluid	Advantages	Disadvantages
Basic glucose fluid[a] (e.g. Dianeal 1.36%, 2.27%, 3.86%, Gambrosol 1.5%, 2.5%, 3.9%)	Good osmotic agent Can control ultrafiltration by changing the glucose concentration Cheap	Weight gain Short-lived ultrafiltration (6 hours) GDPs produced during heat sterilisation can increase the production of AGEs, which can damage the peritoneum and is associated with atherosclerotic cardiovascular disease in diabetics Increased insulin requirements Hyperlipidaemia Pain on filling due to low pH
Glucose-based with bicarbonate buffer[a] (e.g. Physioneal, pH 7.4, Balance, pH 7)	Reduced pain on instillation Reduced GDPs More physiological	Need to mix before using due to instability Weight gain Short-lived ultrafiltration (6 hours) Increased insulin requirements
Amino acid-based (e.g. Nutrineal, pH 6.7, 1.1% amino acid solution, 15 amino acids (64% essential))	Maintains nutritional balance Can give 25% of daily protein intake Reduced weight gain from glucose therefore better for diabetics No GDPs Less hyperlipidaemia	Not very efficient at improving nutrition Can only be used once a day due to increase in urea nitrogen concentrations and mild metabolic acidosis No evidence it can prevent malnutrition
Starch-based polymers (e.g. icodextrin (Extraneal))	Longer ultrafiltration life (8–12 hours) Improved diabetic control Reduced weight gain from glucose therefore better for diabetics Reduced GDPs Can be used to increase the adequacy of patients on APD if they require a daytime exchange Achieves better ultrafiltration than 2.27% glucose bag Reduced hyperlipidaemia	Sterile peritonitis Rash Pain due to low pH (especially if patient is used to the bicarbonate-based bags) Can only be used once a day due to maltose accumulation (unknown long-term problems) Both maltose and icodextrin metabolites can give falsely high glucose levels in monitors that use dehydrogenase pyrroloquinolinequinone Expensive

[a]Differences in calcium concentration, usually 1.25 or 1.75mmol/L.
Some bags are available as 'specials' with lower calcium and magnesium concentrations.
GDP, glucose-degradation product; AGE, advanced glycation end-products.

be fluid-overloaded with CAPD due to reduced ultrafiltration; this is overcome by the short dwell times with APD. This form of treatment can also reduce the incidence of peritonitis, as there are fewer connections to be made by the patient, so reducing the risk of contamination.

Tidal peritoneal dialysis is a variant of APD. Dwell times are considerably shorter and only about half of the fluid is drained out and replaced with clean fluid at each exchange, which occurs every 30–60 minutes. It can also be used in patients who complain of pain with traditional APD. The high flow rate with this form of treatment leads to better diffusion, as the equilibrium gradient is always present.[34] One of its disadvantages is that large volumes of dialysate are required, up to 30–36 L per session.[32]

Adequacy

Adequacy depends on the permeability and efficiency of the membrane, net ultrafiltration rate, peritoneal blood flow rate and the dialysate flow rate and is related to small solute clearance. This is calculated as either a creatinine clearance or Kt/V estimation. Both of these take into account any residual renal function as well as the clearance from the dialysis. To measure adequacy you need a 24-hour urine collection to measure urea and creatinine and also the volume of urine and a blood sample at the end of the collection. This gives an indication of the patient's residual renal function. To calculate the clearance from the dialysis you collect all the drain samples for 24 hours and combine them, from this you take a 10 mL sample to measure urea, albumin, glucose and creatinine. You also need to measure the volume drained in and the volume drained out. Both of these measurements are put into a computer program, which calculates the patient's adequacy. It should be checked every six months, if the patient is fluid-overloaded or symptomatic and one month after a regimen change.

The British Renal Association Standards document states that renal units should aim for a Kt/V greater than 1.7 and a creatinine clearance of at least 50 L/week/1.73 m².[5] In the USA, the National Kidney Foundation KDOQI Guidelines have suggested a target Kt/V of at least 2 and a creatinine clearance greater than 60 L/week/1.73 m².[2,31] These targets are for CAPD. Higher targets should be aimed for in the APD population.

Some methods of enhancing adequacy are:[30,31]

- Increase bag volumes for CAPD
- Increase frequency of exchanges for CAPD
- Increase the strength of the bag
- Increase the dwell time
- Use icodextrin during the day for APD or overnight for CAPD. This is a glucose polymer product which produces high ultrafiltra-

tion rates over a longer period while reducing the patient's glucose exposure.

Some factors that can affect adequacy are:

- No residual renal function
- Large body weight
- Hypo- or hyper-permeable membranes
- Overhydration
- Peritonitis episodes.

The transport status of a patient (i.e. the permeability of their peritoneal membrane) is determined using a peritoneal equilibrium test (PET), this can also give an indication as to whether the patient is best suited to APD or CAPD. This will normally be measured at the beginning of peritoneal dialysis (within 4–8 weeks), if there have been a number of peritonitis episodes that may have damaged the peritoneum, or if there have been a lot of mechanical problems.[5]

Procedure

1 Usually a 2.27%, 2 L bag is kept in overnight. The next morning it is drained out and the volume measured.

2 Another bag of the same strength and volume is drained in with the patient lying down, every 400 mL (usually drained in over 2 minutes) the patient is rolled from side to side to ensure that the whole peritoneum is coated.

3 Then 10 mL samples are taken at 0, 2 and 4 hours. This is done by withdrawing 200 mL and taking 10 mL from that sample and returning the remaining 190 mL to the patient. These are sent to the lab to measure for urea, creatinine and glucose.

4 A venous blood sample is taken at 2 hours to measure urea and electrolytes, bone profile and glucose.

5 After 4 hours, the dialysate is drained out and the volume measured.

This procedure measures the ratio between dialysate to plasma (D/P) urea, creatinine and glucose for a set period of time compared with the volume drained out after 4 hours and is used to assess the loss of ultrafiltration, transport status or under-dialysis. The D/P creatinine

Table 8.3 Transport status	
High transporters	Very efficient membrane
	Solutes are transported quickly
	Increased glucose absorption
	Poor ultrafiltration
	Risk of hypoalbuminaemia
	Best on APD with shorter dwell times
Low transporters	Inefficient membrane
	Very good ultrafiltration
	Solutes are transported slowly
	Best on CAPD with longer dwell times

APD, automated peritoneal dialysis; CAPD, continuous ambulatory peritoneal dialysis.

at 4 hours is used to classify the patient as a 'high', 'high average', 'low average' or 'low' transporter. Ten per cent of the population are high transporters, 53% high average, 31% low average and 6% low (Table 8.3).

Peritoneal dialysis tends to have a limited survival, up to 8 years with only 20% remaining at 10 years. Repeated peritonitis episodes account for 36% of dialysis failure, due to the peritoneal membrane becoming fibrosed, adhesions forming and it becoming inefficient for dialysis. These patients then transfer to the haemodialysis programme. 'Burn out' can be another problem in peritoneal dialysis as some people find that they can only cope with it for a few years before it becomes too much for them.[31]

Complications of peritoneal dialysis

The main complications with peritoneal dialysis are associated with the insertion of the catheter and infections.[33]

Peritonitis

The Renal Association standards state that less than one episode per 18 patient months is an acceptable peritonitis rate for a unit with an initial cure rate greater than 80% without the catheter needing to be removed.[5] There is a supposedly reduced incidence with APD although this was not shown in an audit in Scotland between 1999 and 2002.[35] Repeated infections can lead to damage to the peritoneal membrane, leading to technique failure and hospital admission.

Good hygiene is one of the most important factors to prevent exit site infections and peritonitis. If the catheter is dropped or the protective cap falls off then prophylactic antibiotics should be given to prevent peritonitis, this is usually a stat dose of vancomycin or a course of oral flucloxacillin.

The main causes of peritonitis are poor hygiene (usually due to a skin contaminant), exit site or tunnel infections, colonoscopy, diarrhoea, constipation or diverticular disease (due to movement of bowel bacteria – known as enteric peritonitis).[33]

Peritonitis presents as abdominal pain, nausea, vomiting, diarrhoea, pyrexia, flu-like symptoms and cloudy peritoneal dialysis effluent bags, usually with a white cell count >100 mm^3 and at least 50% polymorphonuclear neutrophil cells.[7,33]

White cell counts, culture sensitivities and Gram stains are sent off although antibiotics should be started empirically while waiting for the results and changed if required. Antibiotics to cover both Gram-positive (vancomycin or a cephalosporin) and Gram-negative (aminoglycosides or third-generation cephalosporin, e.g. ceftazidime or oral ciprofloxacin) organisms should be started. If the bags are cloudy then 500–1000 units/L of heparin should be added to each bag to dissolve the fibrin in the peritoneum until the bags are clear.

It is possible to get culture-negative results sometimes due to the culture process or the patient may be on antibiotics. The Renal Association states that you should have less than 15% of culture-negative episodes.[5,33]

The antibiotics are usually administered intraperitoneally (IP) together into the peritoneal dialysis fluid bags, although penicillins and aminoglycosides should not be mixed together due to incompatibility. The antibiotics should be added to a bag that will have a dwell time of at least 6 hours.

The antibiotics can be administered daily or with each exchange; vancomycin is usually only required weekly depending on levels. Very good systemic absorption is obtained from IP antibiotics; some units monitor aminoglycoside levels but others do not. There are opposing views on whether the small amount of aminoglycoside we give can affect the patient's residual renal function; some units use cephalosporins instead, although they may not be as effective for peritonitis. The antibiotics should be continued for at least 2–3 weeks depending on the severity of the infection. The peritonitis will usually start to resolve after 48 hours. If the catheter has to come out it should be out for 6–8 weeks, but this may depend on the patient and the medical and nursing staff.

There are various terms linked with peritonitis episodes:[33]

- Refractory peritonitis: condition does not improve after 5 days of antibiotics and usually will require the catheter to be removed
- Recurrent peritonitis: repeat episode within four weeks with a different organism
- Relapsing peritonitis: repeat episode within four weeks with the same organism or sterile peritonitis
- Repeating peritonitis: repeat episode after more than four weeks with the same organism.

Death is more likely with Gram-negative bacilli and fungi. The organisms associated with peritonitis include:

- Coagulase-negative staphylococcus (CNS) (e.g. *Staphylococcus epidermidis*, which accounts for 50% of cases) is usually from touch contamination and is often quite straightforward to treat.[30] It can even be treated at home if the patient is taught how to administer the antibiotics to the peritoneal dialysis bags.
- *Staphylococcus aureus* infections can be severe and are also due to touch contamination or more usually from exit site infections. Infection is also associated with nasal carriage of *Staph. aureus* and prophylactic nasal and/or topical mupirocin or cyclical rifampicin have been shown to reduce exit site and peritonitis infections. This is advised by the Renal Association.[5,31,33] Methicillin-resistant *Staph. aureus* (MRSA) is more difficult to treat.

These two *Staph.* species are the most common organisms implicated in peritonitis; Gram-positive infections account for 75% of cases.

- Enterococcal infections (from the gastrointestinal tract) and streptococcal infections are usually associated with a greater morbidity and are often linked with exit site or tunnel infections.
- Gram-negative infections are usually caused by *Escherichia coli*, *Klebsiella* and *Proteus* organisms, and are usually transmural due to constipation, colitis, touch contamination or exit site infections. Treatment is with cephalosporins (e.g. ceftazidime); there is a high incidence of treatment failure.
- *Pseudomonas* infections are usually due to skin contamination and are linked to exit site and tunnel infections. They are treated with two different antibiotics as they can result in quite a severe peritonitis; one is usually a quinolone and the other, for example, ceftazidime. The catheter may need to be removed.
- *Mycobacterium tuberculosis* or non-TB peritonitis can be very difficult to diagnose. There is an increased incidence in Asia. It is treated with conventional antituberculosis drugs.[33]

Fungal peritonitis is usually preceded by prolonged or multiple courses of antibiotics and has an incidence of 2–7%. Treatment in this case is usually IP, IV or oral with either single or combination treatment with amphotericin, fluconazole, flucytosine, voriconazole or caspofungin, depending on sensitivities and local protocol. Usually the catheter needs to be removed. If the catheter is not removed quickly there is a high risk of mortality, with death occurring in 25% of patients. Intraperitoneal amphotericin can cause chemical peritonitis and is also quite painful on administration. However, when amphotericin is given intravenously, there is poor penetration into the peritoneum. With flucytosine it is important to monitor levels to limit the risk of bone marrow toxicity developing. Antifungal therapy should be continued for 10 days after the catheter has been removed.[33]

Sclerosing peritonitis is irreversible sclerosis of the peritoneal membrane and usually occurs after patients have been on peritoneal dialysis for a long period of time. It can be related to continual inflammation, and the risk increases after 4 years on peritoneal dialysis. Sclerosing peritonitis can be difficult to detect and CT and ultrasound scans are required.[38] Chlorhexidine gluconate, which is sometimes used for cleaning the exit site, and long-term damage to the peritoneum by AGEs have been associated with sclerosing peritonitis.

Treatment can be with prednisolone at a dose of 0.5 mg/kg/day and tamoxifen 10–40 mg daily and/or other anti-inflammatory or immuno-suppressive drugs (e.g. azathioprine) or surgery, although there is no definite treatment.[39,40]

Removal of the catheter is essential and peritoneal dialysis must be discontinued, as it can be fatal.

Other complications of peritoneal dialysis are listed in Table 8.4.

Table 8.4 Other complications of peritoneal dialysis[2,7,11,29,31,33]

Other complications	Reason	Treatment
Exit site infections (usually *Staph. aureus* or *Pseudomonas* infections)	Can be due to poor technique Environmental (e.g. showers) If not treated may result in tunnel infections, peritonitis Diagnosis: purulent drainage from exit site, erythema alone not necessarily an indication of infection	Treat with antibiotics for at least two weeks (e.g. flucloxacillin for *Staph. aureus* or quinolones for *Ps. aeruginosa*) Hypertonic saline dressings may also be used (1 tablespoon of salt to 500 mL water, apply to gauze), wrap around catheter for 15 minutes Enhanced training can reduce recurrent infections Prophylactic mupirocin or gentamicin cream may be used but there is a concern about resistance developing. (Mupirocin ointment should not be used as it may corrode polyurethane catheters) Staph nasal carriers may be given mupirocin nasal cream prophylactically
Flow or drainage problems with the catheter	Constipation (can be due to drugs, reduced motility or hypokalaemia which can reduce bowel motility) Catheter misplacement, migration or kinking Fibrin deposition	Laxatives. In severe cases drugs like Picolax may be required Replacement/manipulation of catheter in theatre Urokinase lock of 5000 IU Add heparin 500 units/L to dialysis fluid for a few days
Peritoneal leaks	Catheter used too soon Badly positioned catheter Can leak into tissues, lungs and scrotum	Rest the catheter and temporary haemodialysis In extreme cases catheter may require to be removed
Technique/ultrafiltration failure (3% after 1 year, 30% after 6 years)	Due to repeated occurrences of peritonitis, this can cause damage to the peritoneum leading to ultrafiltration failure and inadequate dialysis Fibrosis due to AGEs	Increase strength of bag but this can lead to damage of the peritoneum Reduce the dwell time Add in icodextrin Change to haemodialysis

(continued overleaf)

Table 8.4   (continued)

Other complications	Reason	Treatment
Hernia	Due to the force of the fluid in the abdomen Can cause flow problems if they are large	Surgery and temporary haemodialysis
Blood in dialysate	If patients are menstruating Peritonitis present Heparin is being added to the bags Strenuous exercise	Treat peritonitis Investigate other causes
Malnutrition (severe 8–10% and mild 30%)	Possibly associated with chronic inflammation and is associated with poor prognosis, more research is needed in this area Due to albumin and amino acid loss in the dialysate, reduced intake and appetite, abdominal fullness, delayed gastric emptying and glucose absorption	Use an amino acid based dialysis fluid Refer to a dietitian for supplements and advice

AGE, advanced glycation end-products.

 CASE STUDIES

Q1. At the monthly multidisciplinary meeting, a haemodialysis patient's urea reduction ratio is only 50%. What can be done to improve their adequacy?

Q2. Miss RB is an 80-year-old woman recently started on haemodialysis. After about an hour on dialysis she becomes hypotensive. What can be done about it?

Q3. Mr MP has recently started on CAPD and has been having problems with pain on draining in his fluid. What could be the reason for his pain and what dialysis fluid should he use?

Q4. Mr BA is a 45-year-old man on peritoneal dialysis. He was admitted with abdominal pain the previous evening. What are the possible causes of his abdominal pain and what should be done?

Q5. On checking the notes it appears that Mr BA has had a couple of peritonitis episodes in the past few months and is a known staph carrier. What would you recommend?

Q6. Miss RB did not have good enough veins for a fistula so has a permanent catheter in place. She has come in today and the line is not working. What can be done?

Q7. Mr MC has only been on haemodialysis a few weeks and it was noticed that his platelet count has fallen quite dramatically. Heparin-induced thrombocytopenia (HIT) has been diagnosed. What can be used as an anticoagulant for his dialysis?

References

1. Fleming L. A view of dialysis through the ages. *Br J Ren Med* 1999/2000; 4: 20–22.
2. Levy J, Morgan J, Brown E, eds. *Oxford Handbook of Dialysis*. London: Oxford University Press, 2004.
3. Fraser D, Venning M. Principles of haemodialysis. *Medicine* 1999; 27: 44–46.
4. Ringrose T. What's new in vascular access? *Br J Ren Med* 1998; 3: 6–8.
5. Renal Association and Royal College of Physicians of London. *Treatment of Adult Patients and Children with Renal Failure: Standards and Audit Measures*, 3rd edn. Renal Association and Royal College of Physicians of London, 2002.
6. Rodger RSC, Briggs JD. Renal replacement therapy in the elderly. *Scot Med J* 1997; 42: 143–144.
7. Stein A, Wild J, Cook P, eds. *Vital Nephrology*. London: Class Health, 2004.
8. Chesser AMS, Baker LRI. Temporary venous access for first dialysis is common, undesirable and usually avoidable. *Kidney Int* 1997; 52: 267.
9. Hoenich N. Choosing a haemodialyser. *Br J Ren Med* 1997; 2: 15–18.
10. Hoenich N, Graham K. Membranes for renal replacement therapy. *Br J Ren Med* 1996; 1: 18–21.
11. Daugirdas JT, Blake PG, Ing TS, eds. *Handbook of Dialysis*, 3rd edn. Philadelphia: Lippincott Williams & Wilkins, 2001.
12. Shaldon S. Dialyser reuse: A practice that should be abandoned. *Semin Dialysis* 1993; 6: 11–12.
13. Lowrie EG, Zhensheng L, Ofsthun N *et al.* Reprocessing dialysers for multiple uses: recent analysis of death risks for patients. *Nephrol Dial Transplant* 2004; 19: 2823–2830.
14. Tielemanns C, Madhoun P, Lenaers M *et al.* Anaphylactoid reactions during hemodialysis on AN 69 membranes in patients receiving ACE inhibitors. *Kidney Int* 1990; 38: 982–984.
15. Hoenich N. Quality of water in dialysis. *Br J Ren Med* 1999; 4: 21–22.
16. Ashley C, Currie A. *The Renal Drug Handbook*, 2nd edn. Oxford: Radcliffe Medical Press, 2004.
17. Peticlerc T, Jacobs C. Dialysis sodium concentration: what is optimal and can it be individualized. *Nephron Dial Transplant* 1995; 97: 596–599.
18. Ledebo I. On-line hemodiafiltration: Technique and therapy. *Adv Ren Replace Ther* 1999; 6: 195–208.
19. Challinor P. Acute renal failure. In: Challinor P, Sedgewick J, eds. *Principles and Practice of Renal Nursing*. London: Stanley Thornes, 1998: 74–89.
20. David S, Tagliavini D, Cambi V. Pre-post dilution haemofiltration. *Nephrol Dial Transplant* 1989; 4: 37–40.
21. David S, Cambi V. Haemofiltration: predilution versus postdilution. *Contrib Nephrol* 1992; 96: 77–85.
22. Kirby S, Davenport A. Haemofiltration/dialysis treatment in patients with acute renal failure. *Care Crit Ill* 1996; 12: 54–58.
23. Locatelli F, Di Filippo S, Manzoni C. Removal of small and middle molecules by convective techniques. *Nephrol Dial Transplant* 2000; 15 (Suppl 2): 37–44.
24. Wizemann V, Kulz M, Techert F *et al.* Efficacy of haemodiafiltration. *Nephrol Dial Transplant* 2001; 16 (Suppl 4): 27–30.
25. Ledebo I. Principles and practice of hemofiltration and hemodiafiltration. *Artif Organs* 1998; 22: 20–25.
26. Canaud B, Bosc JY, Leray-Moragues A *et al.* On-line haemodiafiltration. Safety and efficacy in long-term clinical practice. *Nephrol Dial Transplant* 2000; 15 (Suppl 1): 60–67.
27. Padrini R, Canova C, Conz P *et al.* Convective and adsorptive removal of beta2-microglobulin during predilutional and postdilutional haemofiltration. *Kidney Int* 2005; 68: 2331–2337.
28. Krieter DH, Falkenhain S, Chalabi L *et al.* Clinical cross-over comparison of mid-dilution hemodiafiltration using a novel dialyzer concept and postdilution hemodiafiltration. *Kidney Int* 2005; 67: 349–356.
29. Gokal R. Peritoneal dialysis and complications of technique. In: Davison M, Cameron AM, Grunfield *et al.*, eds. *Oxford Textbook of Clinical Nephrology*, 2nd edn. London: Oxford University Press, 1998.
30. Gokal R. Peritoneal dialysis. *Medicine* 1999; 27: 47–49.
31. Gokal R. Peritoneal dialysis in the 21st century: An analysis of current problems and future developments. *J Am Soc Nephrol* 2002; 13: S104–S116
32. Graham C. Principles of peritoneal dialysis. In: Challinor P, Sedgewick J, eds. *Principles and Practice of Renal Nursing*. London: Stanley Thornes, 1998: 167–183.
33. Piraino B, Bailie GR, Bernardini J *et al.* ISPD Guidelines/Recommendations: Peritoneal dialysis-related infections recommendations: 2005 update. *Perit Dial Int* 2005; 25: 107–131.
34. Williams P. Automated peritoneal dialysis – new targets. *Br J Ren Med* 1997; 2: 17–19.

35. Kavanagh D, Prescott GJ, Mactier RA. Peritoneal dialysis-associated peritonitis in Scotland (1999–2002). Nephrol Dial Transplant 2004; 19: 2584–2591.

36. Marshall J, Jennings P, Scott A *et al.* Glycaemic control in diabetic CAPD patients assessed by continuous glucose monitoring system (CGMS). *Kidney Int* 2003; 64: 1480–1486.

37. Dasgupto MK. Strategies for managing diabetic patients on peritoneal dialysis. *Adv Perit Dial* 2004; 20: 200–202.

38. Campbell S, Clarke P, Hawley C *et al.* Sclerosing peritonitis: identification of diagnostic, clinical, and radiological features. *Am J Kidney Dis* 1994; 24: 819–825.

39. Del Peso G, Bajo MA, Aguilera A *et al.* Clinical experience with tamoxifen in peritoneal fibrosing syndromes. *Adv Perit Dial* 2003; 19: 32–35.

40. Evrenkaya TR, Atasoyu EM, Unver S *et al.* Corticosteroid and tamoxifen therapy in sclerosing encapsulating peritonitis in a patient on continuous peritoneal dialysis. *Nephrol Dial Transplant* 2004; 19: 2423–2424.

9

Renal transplantation

Andrea Devaney and Mark Lee

Replacing a failed organ of the body with another from a human or animal donor has long been desired as an effective method of curing disease. The first report of a human renal transplant was in 1936.[1] However, in the absence of effective immunosuppressive agents, organs were rapidly rejected unless the donor was an identical twin to the recipient.[2] Allografts (hereafter termed grafts) are organs from non-identical members of the same species. Several series of allograft transplants were reported in the 1950s with the advent of methods of suppressing the immune system. Only after the introduction of azathioprine in 1961 did one-year graft survival rates significantly improve. Azathioprine was usually used in combination with corticosteroid. Anti-lymphocyte globulins also became available in the 1960s and were used both in short courses around the time of transplant (induction immunosuppression) and to treat the frequent rejection episodes. Co-morbidities were significant from the high doses of induction and maintenance immunosuppression.

It was not until the introduction of ciclosporin in the early 1980s that both graft and patient one-year survival rates dramatically improved to figures comparable with today's clinical practice (one-year graft survival of 85–95% and patient survival of 95–100%). Maintenance triple therapy with ciclosporin combined with lower doses of corticosteroid and azathioprine became the standard until the introduction of tacrolimus, mycophenolate and sirolimus in the 1990s.[3]

The late 1990s saw the launch of engineered monoclonal antibodies as alternative induction agents to the non-specific anti-thymocyte globulins. However, despite the marked improvement seen in one-year graft survival with current immunosuppressive regimens, the incidence of graft loss over time remains significant.[4] This is principally due to chronic allograft nephropathy (CAN). It is also the case that most recipients die with a functioning graft, typically from cardiovascular causes. Thus, the focus over the last decade has shifted from reducing the frequency of acute rejection to minimising both CAN and patients' cardiovascular risks.

Renal transplantation is significantly more cost effective to the health service than any form of dialysis and offers a patient the opportunity of a normal lifestyle.[5,6] There are not enough donor kidneys, however, to fulfil demand: 5773 patients were registered on the UK transplant waiting list for a renal transplant as of April 2006. This has increased by around one-third between 1996 and 2005 and now represents almost 100 patients per million of population.[7]

The donor organ

Transplant organs are obtained either from a cadaveric donor (heart beating or non-heart beating/asystolic) or a living donor (related or unrelated). Recipients receive a solitary kidney unless, rarely, the donor is a small child and there is not a suitable paediatric recipient. In this case both donor organs may be transplanted into the adult recipient in an en bloc operation. Some diabetic patients with end stage renal disease (ESRD) will receive a simultaneous kidney and pancreas transplant from a cadaveric donor which will also cure their diabetes. A patient's native kidneys are left in situ unless they have previously been removed (for example because of recurrent infection, hypertension or, in the case of cystic kidneys, to make space for the transplant). The graft is usually placed extraperitoneally in the right ileac fossa for ease of surgical access to the iliac arteries, veins and the bladder.

Most patients are transplanted whilst stabilised on dialysis; however, some patients may receive a pre-emptive transplant, usually within 6–12 months of their anticipated need for dialysis. With the fall in numbers of cadaver organs, living donor transplant programmes have expanded in the UK and this now represents one-third of the total kidney transplant activity. Kidney transplants currently account for four out of every five solid transplants in the UK, but despite efforts to increase donation, overall activity remains static (Table 9.1).[7]

Graft function

Urine volumes and daily measurement of a recipient's serum creatinine levels are the standard ways of monitoring transplanted graft function. The incidence of delayed graft function (DGF), where the recipient continues to require dialysis for a period after the operation, is higher with cadaveric grafts, particularly those from asystolic donors. The term DGF is usually reserved for the temporary, recoverable situation when the kidney presents histologically with acute tubular necrosis in the absence of signs or symptoms of other causes of early non-function. Assuming that the cross-match is negative, then the other probable cause of early non-function is usually surgical, for example renal artery thrombosis or a tamponade resulting from a ureteric or blood vessel anastomotic leak.

Transplant rejection and its prevention

Transplant rejection is mainly the result of responses by the recipient's adaptive immune system once donor antigens on the kidney have been recognised as non-self. Typically the patient will feel unwell with a temperature and tenderness over the kidney, urine output will diminish and serum creatinine will rise by more than 25% over 24–48 hours. The effect is mediated by the recipient's T- and B-lymphocytes. Some of the potential for rejection can be minimised by carefully matching donor and recipient characteristics (human leukocyte antigens (HLAs) and ABO blood group antigens are the most relevant) but immunosuppressive medicines, taken vigilantly for the life of the graft, are the mainstay of prevention.

Ensuring ABO blood group compatibility is a matter of routine across all transplanted organ types to prevent hyperacute rejection. Hyperacute rejection, which ensues within minutes and hours of unclamping the blood vessels to the graft, will irreversibly damage the kidney, leading to its loss if a recipient has pre-formed antibodies to donor antigens. In addition to ABO blood group incompatibility a recipient might have pre-formed antibodies from exposure to non-self antigens (for example HLAs) from a previous blood transfusion, transplant or pregnancy. To prevent this a cross-match of

Table 9.1   Comparative kidney transplant numbers for the UK 2003–2006

Transplant	2003–2004	2004–2005	2005–2006
Total kidneys	1849 (65%)	1783 (65%)	1799 (82%)
Total pancreas (including kidney and pancreas)	59 (2%)	86 (3%)	126 (6%)
Total solid organ transplants	2867	2724	2196

donor lymphocytes with recipient serum is undertaken when the recipient is called for surgery and a negative result is required for the transplant to proceed.

Acute rejection is most commonly seen in the first few months after a transplant but can occur at any time. The standard is for diagnosis to be confirmed by histological examination of core biopsy tissue, which often shows T-lymphocyte infiltration underlining the importance of this type of response in rejection. The Banff classification is the histological standard for excluding or the differential diagnosis of the type and severity of rejection.[8]

To understand how acute rejection can be prevented both by HLA matching and the action of immunosuppressive drugs, a mechanistic overview of the provoked immune response is needed.

Donor antigens on the surface of graft cells (for example, HLA-A) are presented to resting T-helper (Th) lymphocytes by macrophages and other antigen-presenting cells (APCs). The recognition process activates the Th-cells to produce and secrete chemical messenger cytokines (e.g. interleukin 2 (IL-2)) and activate cell surface receptors for them (e.g. IL-2R). This line of T-cells now differentiates and proliferates under the influence of the chemical messengers. Cytotoxic Tc-cells are activated and begin to lyse the donor cells. At the same time B-lymphocytes are activated by cytokines, eventually leading to antibody formation against the antigen. The intense, localised immune activity prompts the involvement of the innate immune system with its phagocytes and enzyme systems, such as 'complement'. In higher grade acute vascular rejections a greater degree of antibody deposition is seen. Untreated acute rejection results in graft loss within a few days.

Reduced rates of rejection and improved long-term graft survival is seen if the 'foreignness' of donor kidney cells to the recipient is reduced by histocompatibility testing and matching. Humans inherit two antigens from each of the HLA-A, -B and -DR groups, one haplotype from each parent. An HLA identical match, sometimes called a zero mismatch, will only be present if all six specific HLA antigens (two HLA-A, two HLA-B and two HLA-DR) are the same for the donor and recipient. That there are, for example, over 120 HLA-DR antigens alone makes clear the need for the national registration and donor kidney allocation scheme as undertaken by the UK Transplant Special NHS Health Authority. In practice, few cadaveric grafts are HLA identical and the total number of mismatches is taken into account when deciding the immunosuppressive regimen for that patient.

Chronic allograft nephropathy is also sometimes termed chronic rejection. It can present as early as just a few months post transplant, but is most common after a number of years. Compared with acute rejection, the progress of deterioration of kidney function is slow and largely relentless. The aetiology is not understood but there are thought to be many factors that contribute to the response (for example cytomegalovirus infection and the nephrotoxicity of calcineurin inhibitors). Episodes of acute rejection are risk factors for the subsequent development of chronic rejection.[9,10]

Transplant immunosuppression

To maintain longevity of the transplant, patients are required to take immunosuppressive drugs to attenuate the natural immune response to the allograft. Immunosuppressive drugs can be categorised by pharmacological class or by when and how they are used. Induction therapy refers to those drugs used peri-operatively (for example high-dose, intravenous corticosteroid or a short course of IL-2R-blocking antibodies). Maintenance immunosuppression usually consists of two or three drugs with different and complimentary mechanisms of action at lower individual dosages to achieve a cumulatively adequate immunosuppression. It is usual to aim for greater exposure to maintenance immunosuppression in the first few months after a transplant (for example, higher corticosteroid doses or higher target tacrolimus trough levels). The secondary aim of the maintenance regimen is to minimise individual drug adverse effects, including their contribution to cardiovascular risk, and the risk of infection and malignancy which strongly correlates with the degree of overall immunosuppression.

The third category of immunosuppression is that used to treat acute rejection should it occur. The first-line treatment is usually a short course of high-dose, intravenous corticosteroid. Acute rejection can also be resolved by changing the maintenance immunosuppression and this might be undertaken alongside pulsed steroid. Histologically higher grade rejections might require a course of antithymocyte globulin (for example, Thymoglobulin) or muromonab CD3 (OKT3), either first line or if a pulse of corticosteroid fails.

During the first year post transplant, graft survival rates are similar for most modern immunosuppressive regimens. All transplant centres will have their own preferred induction and maintenance regimens for different scenarios. Unless agreed otherwise with local commissioners, regimens in the UK will be National Institute of Health and Clinical Excellence (NICE) compliant.[12] There is a tension between applying a consistent, standardised and auditable approach and yet still tailoring the choice of drugs to the collective assessment of donor and recipient risk factors. Some of the many factors that might affect the choice of drug include the donor's age, organ origin, the recipient's age, ethnicity, concordance and transplant history, titre of antibodies against a standard panel (panel reactive antibodies or PRA) and the degree of HLA mismatching.

Long-term patient and graft survival is the new Holy Grail of transplantation. The goal of maintenance immunosuppression is to optimise these outcomes and to help maintain a high quality of life.

Induction immunosuppression

Much research continues around induction therapy in an effort to find the ideal regimen to minimise or avoid maintenance steroids and calcineurin inhibitors with the goal of improving long-term outcomes in renal transplantation. Several induction antibody agents are available, including: rabbit anti-thymocyte globulin (rATG,

Thymoglobulin), the humanised anti-interleukin-2 receptor (IL-2R) antibodies basiliximab and daclizumab, alemtuzumab and rituximab. Each antibody will be discussed in turn.

Rabbit anti-thymocyte globulin (rATG, Thymoglobulin)

Thymoglobulin remains unlicensed in the UK. It is a rabbit polyclonal antibody directed at a wide variety of human T-cell surface antigens, including major histocompatibility complex (MHC) antigens and adhesion molecules. It is a depleting antibody and thus confers long-lasting immunosuppression.

Some units use it as induction on a daily basis for a short course of specified duration. Other centres choose to administer doses on an intermittent basis with the decision to dose being based on CD3[+] count, total lymphocyte count or absolute T-cell count. One study found patients receiving daily ATG had a longer and more profound duration of lymphocyte depletion than those receiving intermittent dosing.[11] A test dose of 5 mg infused over 1 hour is given prior to administration of the first full dose to check for any sensitivity to rabbit protein. If a patient suffers an untoward reaction during the test dose then this contraindicates any further treatment with Thymoglobulin. The usual daily dose is 1.25–2.5 mg/kg. Central venous administration, by a slow infusion over 6–12 hours, is preferred as phlebitis and inflammation can be a problem; however, there is growing experience with peripheral administration. Intravenous corticosteroids, antihistamine and oral paracetamol should be given 30 minutes before administration of the first full dose, and subsequent doses if necessary, to reduce the cytokine release syndrome which most patients experience to a greater or lesser degree.

Basiliximab, daclizumab

These antibodies were approved by the NICE review on immunosuppression[12] as an option for induction therapy as part of a calcineurin inhibitor-based immunosuppressive regimen. Both are monoclonal human/mouse antibodies manipulated to disguise the mouse region and so minimise antibody formation in the recipient. They bind very specifically to a part of the IL-2R found only on the surface of activated T-lymphocytes and reduce the sensitivity of the receptor to the cytokine IL-2. Unlike ATG they do not affect the inactivated or resting T-cell population. The effect persists for 2–3 months.

NICE specified that the drug with the lowest acquisition cost should be used and most units have elected to use basiliximab on this basis. A phase IV trial evaluated the effectiveness and safety of basiliximab when added to a regimen consisting of ciclosporin (Neoral), azathioprine and corticosteroids.[13] When compared with placebo, and as observed in other trials,[14] the basiliximab group showed a lower incidence of acute rejection without increasing adverse effects, notably infection or post-transplant lymphoproliferative disease (PTLD). One-year patient and graft survival rates were similar in the two groups. These findings were corroborated in a 2004 meta-analysis involving 38 trials that enrolled nearly 5000 patients.[15]

No trials to date have directly compared basiliximab and daclizumab. Individually they have similar patient and graft outcomes but they have different pharmacokinetic profiles and, at licensed doses, differ in cost and frequency of administration.

Alemtuzumab

Alemtuzumab is unlicensed in transplantation. It is a humanised monoclonal antibody directed against the CD52 cell surface receptor that is expressed on most T- and B-lymphocytes, eosinophils and on some populations of monocytes, macrophages and dendritic cells. Like ATG it is a depleting antibody and confers long-lasting immunosuppression. It is used in induction with the aim of allowing steroid-free and/or calcineurin-free/sparing maintenance immunosuppressive protocols. A recent systematic review of alemtuzumab's use in organ transplantation concluded there is a need for more and larger randomised trials, with long-term follow-up, before its role can be established in practice.[16] The dose, route and frequency of administration of alemtuzumab, and optimal maintenance immunosuppressive regimen to

be utilised with this agent remain to be determined.

Rituximab

Rituximab is unlicensed in transplantation. It is a high-affinity mouse–human chimeric monoclonal antibody directed against the human anti-CD20 antigen, which is a cell surface receptor found mostly on B-lymphocytes. It inhibits B-cell proliferation while inducing cellular apoptosis. It may reduce pre-existing PRA titres and has been shown to assist in overcoming positive cross-matches in planned 'incompatible' transplants. It has a long-lasting duration of action. A recent report[17] found that 15 months after a single induction dose of rituximab, B-cells were still considerably reduced in peripheral blood and there was complete elimination within the graft. The exact place of rituximab in immunosuppressive therapy is yet to be established, however, and again there is a need for controlled trials to support its use in transplantation.

Maintenance immunosuppression

The optimal maintenance immunosuppressive therapy in renal transplantation has not been established. Conventional maintenance regimens consist of a combination of agents that differ by mechanism of action. This strategy minimises the morbidity associated with each drug while maximising effectiveness. By the early 1990s a combination of ciclosporin, azathioprine and steroid was accepted as the standard maintenance regimen. We now have more drugs and many more possible combinations and so preferred regimens vary between each UK transplant centre and indeed across the world. The major immunosuppressive agents that are currently used in various combinations are:

- Corticosteroids (primarily oral prednisolone)
- Antimetabolites, such as azathioprine, mycophenolate mofetil (CellCept), mycophenolate sodium (Myfortic)
- Calcineurin inhibitors, such as ciclosporin, tacrolimus

- mTOR inhibitors, such as sirolimus, everolimus
- Investigational maintenance immunosuppression agents.

The NICE appraisal on immunosuppressive therapy in renal transplantation in adults[12] made specific recommendations about when certain agents should be used. They acknowledged that some of these recommendations would result in medicines being prescribed outside the terms of their marketing licence:

- Tacrolimus could be used as an alternative to ciclosporin based on the relative importance of each drug's side-effect profile for individual people
- Mycophenolate should only be used

  - where there is proven intolerance to calcineurin inhibitors, such as nephrotoxicity leading to risk of chronic allograft dysfunction, and
  - where there is a very high risk of nephrotoxicity necessitating minimisation or avoidance of a calcineurin inhibitor

- Sirolimus should only be used in cases of proven intolerance to calcineurin inhibitors (including nephrotoxicity) necessitating complete withdrawal of these treatments.

For the purposes of this chapter we will provide information on each immunosuppressive agent rather than the variety and efficacy of the numerous drug combinations. Suffice to say in the UK, unless medicines are being used in the context of a clinical trial, the combinations used will generally be compliant with the NICE guidelines. Most transplant centres still use a triple therapy immunosuppressive regimen with a calcineurin inhibitor, an antimetabolite and prednisolone. An element of individualisation may occur, taking into account specific patient characteristics. Many Trusts audit against their guidelines.

Corticosteroids – prednisolone

The effects of corticosteroids in transplantation are complex and multiple. In addition to powerful, general anti-inflammatory properties, steroids have more known specific effects such as inhibiting interleukin 1, preventing T-lymphocyte proliferation and altering lymphocyte response to antigen at an intracellular level.

Initial regimens will involve doses of prednisolone 15–20 mg/day which will then be reduced to a lower maintenance dose (e.g. 5 mg/day) over a few weeks and months. In some cases recipients may be weaned off steroid where no acute rejection episodes have occurred, rejection risks are lower and steroid co-morbidity is an issue (for example, hypertension or new onset diabetes). The long-term side-effects of corticosteroids are diverse and well known. Patients maintained on even low-dose steroids for longer than 6–12 months should have their bone mineral density assessed and will often require treatment with bisphosphonates and adjunctive calcium and vitamin D to reduce the risk of fractures from the associated osteoporosis.

Antimetabolites – azathioprine, mycophenolate mofetil (CellCept), mycophenolate sodium (Myfortic)

Azathioprine is a precursor of 6-mercaptopurine, which is further metabolised to thioguanine nucleotides which disrupt cellular DNA and RNA production, prevent mitosis and so inhibit the proliferation of activated T- and B-lymphocytes.

Mycophenolic acid is the active moiety of both the mofetil salt and the enteric-coated sodium salt. It also impairs lymphocyte proliferation by blocking purine biosynthesis through reversible inhibition of the enzyme inosine monophosphate dehydrogenase.

Given current evidence, azathioprine and mycophenolate mofetil when used with micro-emulsion ciclosporin appear to be similar in terms of acute rejection and medium-term graft survival rates.[18] Analysis of the large US Renal Transplant Registry database indicates that patients prescribed mycophenolate mofetil experience a significantly lower incidence of CAN compared with those taking azathioprine.[19] Further prospective studies are required to determine whether outcomes such as long-term allograft survival differ with these antimetabolites. Current UK practice is that mycophenolates are used de novo primarily in patients at higher risk of acute rejection (re-transplants, high PRA or immunological cause of renal disease). Mycophenolate presentations are markedly more expensive than azathioprine and it is safe to assume that economic issues will play a larger role in choosing between the two.

The usual starting dose of azathioprine is 1–2 mg/kg once daily. Mycophenolate mofetil is started at 1 g twice daily if the patient is on con-comitant ciclosporin. If, however, the baseline immunosuppression is tacrolimus or sirolimus, the starting dose is often reduced to 500–750 mg twice daily as ciclosporin is known to inhibit the entero-hepatic recirculation of the active metabolite of mycophenolate. In terms of active mycophenolic acid 1 g of mycophenolate mofetil is the near molar equivalent to 720 mg of mycophenolate sodium.

Leucopenia is one of the most common side-effects for both drugs and may necessitate a dose reduction. Anaemia may occur more frequently with mycophenolate than with azathioprine. Excluding infection, the most frequent adverse effects associated with the mycophenolates are gastrointestinal, usually manifested as nausea, gastritis and diarrhoea. There is not yet con-vincing evidence of any significant difference in gastrointestinal side-effects between the mofetil salt and the enteric-coated sodium salt. Myco-phenolic acid blood levels can be measured as a means of establishing the optimum dose of mycophenolate, however the evidence for the usefulness of this is inconclusive.

Calcineurin inhibitors

Both ciclosporin and tacrolimus are calcineurin inhibitors. As such, their immunosuppressive action is mediated via blockade of calcineurin-mediated T-cell receptor signal transduction and inhibition of IL-2 transcription. By inhibiting cytokine gene transcription, they suppress T-cell and T-cell-dependent B-cell activation. They differ in the target cytoplasmic protein (immunophilin) they bind to: ciclosporin binds to ciclophilin and tacrolimus to FKBP-12. Tacrolimus is the preferred calcineurin inhibitor, principally because several studies have reported that it is associated with fewer acute rejection episodes than ciclosporin and is possibly associ-ated with improved allograft survival.[20,21] In addition, it does not cause the cosmetic adverse effects associated with ciclosporin (e.g. hirsut-ism and gum hypertrophy), which are known to effect compliance. Tacrolimus is more likely to increase the risk of post-transplant diabetes mellitus, which may then result in decreased allograft survival among affected patients.

Both agents are nephrotoxic and this is one known contributing factor to CAN. Doses are initiated on a weight basis and then adjusted according to blood trough levels as shown in Table 9.2. Because of the pharmacokinetics of tacrolimus ($t_{\frac{1}{2}}$ = 12–14 hours), it is prudent to only measure blood levels a maximum of three times a week when a patient is in hospital.

Tacrolimus is more water soluble than ciclosporin and is not dependent upon bile salts for absorption. However food intake can reduce the extent and rate of absorption of tacrolimus. In practice, patients are advised to either con-sistently take tacrolimus with food or away from food. Most patients choose to take it with food, at the same time as all their other medications. On days when patients come to hospital for a blood test they are asked to not take their morn-ing dose of calcineurin inhibitor. Instead they should take all their other medication at the usual time but bring their morning dose of cal-cineurin inhibitor to hospital with them and

Table 9.2 Calcineurin inhibitor initial doses and target blood levels

Calcineurin inhibitor	Common initial oral doses doses (mg/kg twice daily)	Typical target blood levels (ng/mL)	
		0–6 months	Over 6 months
Ciclosporin (Neoral)	4	150–300	75–150
Tacrolimus	0.05–0.1	10–15	5–10

take it after their blood test. This is to ensure the blood test taken is a trough level.

Reported difference in toxicity with tacrolimus as compared to ciclosporin include:

- More prominent neurological side-effects, such as tremor and headache
- More frequent incidence of post-transplant diabetes mellitus
- Less frequent incidence of hirsutism, gingival hyperplasia and hypertension
- More frequent diarrhoea, dyspepsia and vomiting
- More frequent alopecia
- Increased predisposition to polyoma virus infection.

Generic ciclosporin

Although not yet available in the UK at the time of writing, generic ciclosporin will probably be licensed in the near future. Ciclosporin is a critical dose drug and absorption can be highly dependent upon formulation in some patients. It has a narrow therapeutic index and the potential consequences of a variance in bioavailability associated with unplanned generic substitution are very significant (e.g. graft rejection or nephrotoxicity). To this end the *British National Formulary* (*BNF*) states that 'because of differences in bioavailability, the brand of ciclosporin to be dispensed should be specified by the prescriber'.

Inhibitors of mammalian target of rapamycin (mTOR)

Sirolimus and everolimus are the two agents in this, the newest class of immunosuppressants. At the time of writing, only sirolimus is currently available in the UK. These two drugs have a unique mechanism of action and add another therapeutic category to the immunosuppression armamentarium. Sirolimus and everolimus do not share a mechanism of action with calcineurin inhibitors but, like tacrolimus, they are only active after binding to FKBP-12. Rather than inhibiting IL-2 production they work further downstream to block cytokine-driven proliferation of T-cells, B-cells and vascular smooth muscle cells. The drug–FKBP complex

works on mTOR to inhibit the activation of protein kinase S6 (p70S6k), interfering with protein synthesis and preventing cell cycle progression from the G_1 phase to the S phase.

The main advantage of this class of drugs is that they are not nephrotoxic. In practice, sirolimus is used mostly outside of its licensed indication.[22] This is largely due to its adverse effects profile, which is dissimilar to that of other agents.

Early use of sirolimus, as described in the licensed indication, can impair wound-healing, with dehiscence and breakdown of anastamoses described. Given the high incidence of lymphocele formation there is a strong case for delaying initiation of sirolimus until after the early post-operative period. Acne type rashes, mouth ulceration and peripheral oedema are particularly common and may be severe enough to warrant drug withdrawal. Hyperlipidaemia appears to be dose related and most patients taking sirolimus will require treatment with a statin. Arthralgia and interstitial lung disease will generally be an indication for this drug's withdrawal. Anaemia and thrombocytopenia are more commonly seen than leucopenia or neutropenia and particularly if sirolimus is combined with another antiproliferative drug such as mycophenolate.

The majority of sirolimus side-effects are related to greater exposure to the drug. Many units now aim for maintenance trough levels of 5–8 ng/mL, which are about one-quarter of the initial target ranges in phase III trials.

NICE recommends that sirolimus is only used for proven cases of calcineurin inhibitor intolerance, where either ciclosporin or tacrolimus have to be withdrawn.[12] The possible niche for sirolimus is in patients where the calcineurin inhibitor component of the immunosuppressive regimen is beginning to compromise renal function.[23]

Sirolimus has a long half-life (about 60 hours[24]). There is controversy as to whether or not a loading dose is necessary when therapy is initiated. Supporters believe a loading dose is required to ensure that the patient reaches steady state quickly. Opponents believe the high peak levels associated with loading dose can worsen early side-effects and tolerability.

Sirolimus and ciclosporin taken together interact to increase exposure to, and raise serum levels of, sirolimus. The drugs should be given at least 4 hours apart until ciclosporin is withdrawn.[25] There is no similar interaction with tacrolimus and sirolimus. Monitoring sirolimus trough levels is not required as frequently as with calcineurin inhibitors as steady state will take 10–14 days. Doses often need to increase once the calcineurin inhibitor is eliminated and are adjusted according to target serum levels. In common with the calcineurin inhibitors, sirolimus is metabolised by cytochrome P450 3A4 and is subject to many drug interactions which are detailed later in the chapter.

Experimental maintenance immunosuppression

The only noteworthy drug being pursued in clinical trials at present is belatacept. This is a selective blocker of CD28 co-stimulation. Co-stimulation is required for full activation of T-cells by the antigen on the antigen presenting cell. Belatacept marks a new approach to maintenance immunosuppression as it is only available as an intravenous formulation. In current phase II clinical trials maintenance doses are administered every 4 or 8 weeks as a 30-minute intravenous infusion. Preliminary 12-month data from an on-going study report that belatacept did not appear to be inferior to ciclosporin as a means of preventing acute rejection after renal transplantation.[26] All patients received induction therapy with basiliximab, mycophenolate mofetil and corticosteroids. Patients were randomised to receive one of two doses (low/high intensity) of belatacept or ciclosporin (control arm). Belatacept may preserve the glomerular filtration rate (GFR) and reduce the rate of chronic allograft nephropathy and, if licensed, the challenge will be to incorporate regular intravenous infusions in the renal units transplant follow-up.

Treatment of rejection

Treatment of rejection is influenced by the histological findings on the biopsy.

Acute rejection

Methylprednisolone is used first line in the treatment of acute rejection. It is given as an IV infusion on a daily 'pulse' basis for 3 days, usually at a dose between 500 mg and 1 g/day. Its anti-inflammatory action profoundly alters the effector phases of graft rejection, including macrophage function. As a means of comparison, 500 mg methylprednisolone is an equivalent anti-inflammatory dose to 625 mg prednisolone. Patients often experience dyspepsia and become emotionally labile over the period of the pulse. Diabetic patients receiving a course of methylprednisolone will require an IV insulin sliding scale in order to normalise their blood sugars. At the end of the methylprednisolone course, oral prednisolone may be added or the baseline maintenance dose increased for a short time as a further additional increase in overall immunosuppressive load.

Maintenance immunosuppression may also be altered (e.g. replacing ciclosporin with tacrolimus or azathioprine with mycophenolate) usually alongside a course of high-dose intravenous steroids or antibody therapy.

Steroid-resistant acute rejection is so named because it refers to on-going rejection despite one or more courses of high-dose, IV steroids. Anti-T-cell antibody therapy, such as rabbit anti-thymocyte globulin (already described) or muromonab-CD3 (OKT3), may then be used. There is controversy about how to manage maintenance immunosuppression during concomitant antibody therapy. Some advocate stopping all maintenance immunosuppression and then re-introducing calcineurin inhibitor a few days before the end of the antibody course. Others would support continuing maintenance immunosuppression unchanged throughout.

Muromonab-CD3 (OKT3) is unlicensed in the UK. It is a mouse-derived monoclonal antibody directed against the CD3 antigen complex found on all mature human T-cells. No test dose is necessary. However, patients should be premedicated with 500 mg IV methylprednisolone prior to the first dose to reduce the cytokine release syndrome. It is given as a daily peripheral bolus dose over a 7–14 day period depending on patient's response. Some units administer muromonab-CD3 intermittently according to absolute lymphocyte count.

Antibody-mediated rejection (AMR or humoral or vascular rejection) is estimated to occur in 3–10% of all renal transplants.[27] It is now a more clearly defined phenomenon and its detection is classically based on three key factors: characteristic histological findings (severe vascular changes), positive C4d staining on the biopsy and the presence of donor-specific antibodies (DSA). There are emerging case reports describing numerous treatment options for AMR but none are clinically proven. The options include: plasma exchange, intravenous immunoglobulin, immunoabsorption, antilymphocyte therapy (anti-T-cell: Thymoglobulin, anti-B-cell: rituximab), altered maintenance immunosuppression (usually to combination of tacrolimus and mycophenolate) and finally a combination of those above.

Chronic allograft nephropathy

Chronic allograft nephropathy (CAN) was referred to previously as chronic rejection or chronic renal allograft dysfunction or transplant glomerulopathy. Unfortunately there are no universally accepted diagnostic criteria for CAN but there are characteristic histological changes present on biopsy. The clinical diagnosis is usually suggested by gradual deterioration of renal function over time, increasing proteinuria and worsening hypertension. The causes of CAN are multifactorial and include both immunologic (e.g. cell-mediated immune responses, incidence of acute rejection, presence of growth factors such as transforming growth factor-β) and non-immunologic factors (e.g. occurrence of delayed graft function, on-going hypertension, hyperlipidaemia, cytomegalovirus (CMV) infection).

The prevention and management of CAN remains one of the major challenges. Intervention usually results in changes to immunosuppressive medication. Usual practice would be stop the calcineurin inhibitor and maintain patients either on a mycophenolate or sirolimus based regimen. There is no clinical evidence to support one drug being better than the other. However caution should be exercised

when switching to sirolimus to ensure that the GFR is greater than 40 mL/min. Patients with a GFR less than 40 mL/min experienced a higher rate of serious adverse events in clinical trials.

Drug interactions

Most of the immunosuppressants can be adversely affected by other drugs and some can, themselves, interact with common medicines. The importance of interactions with immunosuppression results from these drugs having a relatively narrow therapeutic window where excess exposure leads rapidly to adverse effect and reduced exposure risks acute rejection.

Use of live vaccines (e.g. measles, mumps and rubella (MMR), yellow fever or bacille Calmette-Guérin (BCG)) is contraindicated in immunosuppressed individuals. This is particularly important when considering paediatric recipients and those planning more exotic foreign travel. It is also possible that patients will exhibit diminished response to killed and polysaccharide vaccines.

Colestyramine, magnesium and aluminium are all known to reduce absorption of mycophenolate. Agents that interfere with enterohepatic recirculation should, where possible, be avoided. As described earlier, replacing ciclosporin with tacrolimus is believed to increase enterohepatic recirculation of mycophenolic acid, increasing exposure to the active drug by about 30%. Taking some immunosuppressive drugs with food is known to alter the rate and extent of absorption, although the general advice for renal transplant patients is to be consistent about dose timing with respect to meals rather than complicating otherwise difficult regimens. A potassium-rich diet should be avoided and potassium-conserving medicines should be used cautiously in patients taking calcineurin inhibitors, in particular tacrolimus which has a propensity to lead to hyperkalaemia.

The major categories of immunosuppressant interaction are those that disrupt metabolism. Xanthine oxidase activity is inhibited by allopurinol, slowing conversion of biologically active 6-thioinosinic acid to its inactive metabolite. Thioinosinic acid is a metabolite of

Table 9.3 The effect of metabolic interactions on calcineurin inhibitor and m-TOR inhibitor levels

Interacting drug	Effect on blood level
Erythromycin and clarithromycin	Increased
Diltiazem, nicardipine, verapamil	Increased
Fluconazole, itraconazole, ketoconazole, voriconazole	Increased
Rifampicin	Decreased
Carbamazepine	Decreased
Phenobarbital	Decreased
Phenytoin	Decreased
St John's wort	Decreased

azathioprine, so when allopurinol is given concomitantly with azathioprine, the dose of the latter should be reduced to one-quarter of the original. Ciclosporin, tacrolimus and sirolimus are metabolised by the cytochrome P450 3A4 family of isoenzymes. If known inducers or inhibitors (Table 9.3) cannot be avoided then the immunosuppressant level must be frequently monitored and the dose adjusted to maintain a safe effect.

Tacrolimus is itself known to inhibit P450 3A4 and care should be taken when other medicines metabolised by the liver are co-prescribed (for example, oral contraception). Ciclosporin has been demonstrated to increase the exposure to concomitant diclofenac, a non-steroidal anti-inflammatory drug (NSAID) with a high degree of first-pass metabolism. It has been recommended that the dose of diclofenac is halved in combination with ciclosporin. In practice all NSAIDs (including topical) are usually avoided in renal transplant recipients as they can impair function. A risk/benefit assessment must be made before they are used in any circumstance and renal function monitored closely if they are deemed necessary.

Probenecid and other drugs which might compete for excretion with the glucuronide metabolite of mycophenolic acid (for example, aciclovir) should be used cautiously where a patient has impaired renal function and where tubular secretion is likely to account for a significant proportion of the clearance.

Care should also be taken when combining other nephrotoxic drugs such as aminoglycosides, NSAIDs and amphotericin with calcineurin inhibitors. Additive neurological effects are more likely to be seen when drugs with such adverse effects are combined with tacrolimus. Myelosuppression is also more likely when drugs known to depress bone marrow function are used with the antimetabolites.

Lipid-lowering agents tend to cause problems in practice. Many patients with kidney transplants require concomitant use of HMG-CoA reductase inhibitors (statins) either to treat hypercholesterolaemia or as prevention of cardiovascular morbidity. It must be borne in mind that ciclosporin can increase the risk of muscle toxicity of statins, simvastatin in particular. A maximum daily dose of 10 mg simvastatin is recommended in combination. Ciclosporin also greatly increases exposure to ezetimibe, though the significance of this is as yet unclear.

Interactions are not confined to licensed medicines. Grapefruit juice will inhibit the metabolism of tacrolimus, ciclosporin and sirolimus, leading to greater exposure. The herbal remedy St John's wort is a potent enzyme inducer and can rapidly reduce plasma levels of the aforementioned drugs. Echinacea is claimed to stimulate the immune system, which would be counterintuitive for a patient on immunosuppression. General advice for transplant recipients is to avoid additional herbal remedies unless the safety is well established.

Post-transplant complications

The patient's state of health before the transplant, and especially that of their cardiovascular system, is the key to a long-term successful outcome. However the consequences of surgery and immunosuppression per se are far from benign and offer many potential complications. The management of these in terms of prevention, prophylaxis and treatment is discussed below. Adverse effects of the individual immunosuppressants, whilst clearly a complication, are discussed earlier in the chapter and not revised below.

Surgical complications tend to occur early, often during the transplant admission. They can include such seemingly contradictory problems as disastrous renal artery thrombosis and life-threatening bleeding from the graft site. Most patients will receive prophylaxis for graft thrombosis with either lower doses of low-molecular-weight heparins (e.g. enoxaparin 20 mg daily) or low-dose aspirin (e.g 75 mg daily). Lymphoceles and collections requiring drainage are not uncommon and recipients occasionally develop a temporary, unilateral leg oedema caused by impaired lymphatic drainage secondary to compression by the transplanted kidney. Urethral catheterisation for the first few days after surgery relieves pressure on the ureter/bladder anastamosis. Ureteric strictures can largely be avoided by the placement of a double J stent for the first few weeks.

Infection

Some immunosuppressants are associated with higher rates of infection than others but such complications should be considered as a function of the overall immunosuppressive load the patient has received since the transplant. This will increase the risk of bacterial, viral, fungal and parasitic disease.

Bacterial urinary tract infection (UTI) is common, particularly whilst a ureteric stent is in situ, and most patients receive some antibiotic prophylaxis in the early months after surgery. UTI in an immunocompromised patient often requires longer than 3 days of antibiotic treatment. Trimethoprim can be used empirically but resistance is not uncommon where a patient is already taking co-trimoxazole prophylaxis. It should also be noted that use of trimethoprim can itself elevate serum creatinine.

Life-threatening fungal infections such as aspergillosis are rare in renal transplant recipients. Much more common are *Candida* infections of the mouth, oesophagus and genito-urinary tract. Many units will offer prophylaxis in the early period post transplant, when the immuno-suppressive burden is greatest.

Cytomegalovirus

This virus from the Herpes family is common in the general population, and in the developed world four out of five have been exposed to it by the age of 60. It usually causes minor flu-like illness, but infection in immunosuppressed patients can cause life-threatening disease. Those most at risk of disease are recipients naïve to the virus (CMV negative) whose primary infection is from the organ of a CMV-positive donor. It is UK practice that such recipients either receive prophylactic treatment against CMV or are monitored, pre-emptively for early signs of developing infection and then treated. CMV-positive recipients risk reactivation of their own virus or super-infection with a different strain from the donor and prophylaxis or pre-emptive treatment is often offered if the immunosuppressive load is high (for example, if rATG has been used). The agents commonly used for prophylaxis are aciclovir, valaciclovir and valganciclovir, the latter two being licensed for this indication. Prophylaxis is usually given for around the first three months post transplant. All three drugs are renally excreted and dose adjustment according to changing renal function is crucial[28].

CMV disease can be delayed and occur at the end of the prophylaxis. Signs and symptoms of disease include rigors, night-sweats, pneumonitis and deranged renal and liver function. Disease usually responds to antiviral therapy with intravenous ganciclovir. A clinical trial is on-going into the use of oral valganciclovir to treat CMV disease.

BK virus

BK virus is so-named after the initials of the patient from whom it was first isolated. It is a member of the polyomavirus family and, although prevalent in humans, it appears to only cause disease in immunocompromised individuals. Primary infection usually occurs in childhood (via oral and/or respiratory exposure) and once infected the virus remains dormant in renal epithelium and lymphoid cells. Clinical manifestations in renal transplant recipients include: asymptomatic haematuria, haemorrhagic and non-haemorrhagic cystitis, ureteric stenosis and tubulo-interstitial nephritis. Some units now perform BK virus screening of urine and blood. BK viral DNA is first detected in the urine followed by the plasma and finally the kidney. BK virus infection in transplant recipients is directly related to the patient's immunosuppressive load rather than use of any one specific agent. Optimum management is unproven but the usual first-line measure is to reduce immunosuppression. The goal of decreased immunosuppression is to minimise viral replication without triggering rejection. There are reports of alternative approaches in the literature, including treatment with intravenous immunoglobulins, cidofovir or leflunomide.

Pneumocystis carinii pneumonia

Pneumocystis jiroveci (*Pneumocystis carinii*) is a parasitic organism which invades and infects the alveolar space in the immunosuppressed. Most of the Western population is exposed to *P. jiroveci* by the age of 10 but only the immunocompromised develop life-threatening pneumonia. Many transplant units in the UK prescribe co-trimoxazole 480–960 mg daily for at least the period whilst induction and early maintenance doses are providing a high immunosuppressive burden. Those intolerant of co-trimoxazole can receive intermittent nebulised pentamidine isetionate or daily dapsone.

In active infection there may be as many as 10^9 organisms per gram of lung tissue, preventing oxygen transfer and leading to hypoxaemia. Signs are mainly tachypnoea and hypoxia, with approximately half of patients developing a fever and/or cough. Prompt treatment with high-dose, intravenous co-trimoxazole, augmented with high-dose oral corticosteroid, is required if severe disease is not to be fatal.

Tuberculosis

Reactivation of latent tuberculosis (TB) is a particular risk for those recipients from communities where this infection is endemic (e.g. black African and South-East Asian communities in Britain). The relative risk of developing active TB has been judged to be 37 times higher in renal transplant recipients than in non-immunosuppressed individuals.[29] Patients with a history of TB or thought to be at risk of reactivation will generally be prescribed a course of isoniazid 200–300 mg daily for between 6 and 12 months after the surgery. In such patients, who have often received a suboptimal diet before transplant, it is necessary to co-prescribe pyridoxine 10 mg daily to prevent peripheral neuropathies.

Malignancy

Long-term immunosuppression confers on transplant recipients a greater risk of certain malignancies than the general population. A recent analysis of over 35 000 American renal transplant recipients provides us with the largest experience on the relative incidence and types of malignancy in this population.[30] It should be considered when reviewing this data that American immunosuppressive protocols are typically more aggressive than European protocols. The analysis showed:

- A twofold increase in common tumours including colon, lung, prostate, stomach, pancreas, oesophagus, ovary and breast
- A threefold increase in testicular and bladder cancer
- A fivefold increase in melanoma, leukaemia, hepato-bilary, cervical and vulvo-vaginal cancers
- A fifteenfold increase in renal cell carcinoma
- A twentyfold increase in non-melanoma skin cancers, Kaposi's sarcoma and non-Hodgkin's lymphoma.

The British Association of Dermatologists has designed a helpful patient information leaflet specifically for recipients with an organ transplant.[31] This leaflet addresses the three key issues of skin cancer: early detection, early treatment and ways to decrease the risk.

Post-transplant lymphoproliferative disorders

Post-transplant lymphoproliferative disorders (PTLDs) are often the most serious and potentially fatal complication of long-term immunosuppression. In 2003, Andreone *et al.*[32] reported the incidence of PTLD to be 1%, with an over-all increasing frequency, which is 30–50 times higher than in the general population. The main contributing factors for development are the immunosuppressive load and the Epstein–Barr virus (EBV) status of the donor/recipient (seropositive donor/seronegative recipient con-ferring greatest risk). EBV is the primary agent of infectious mononucleosis (glandular fever) and is a widely disseminated herpesvirus. The human host cells for EBV are limited to B-lymphocytes, T-lymphocytes, epithelial cells and myocytes. The majority of PTLDs are EBV-driven B-cell lymphomas. Once diagnosed, there are a number of possible treatment options. The usual first step is to reduce the immunosuppression in a step-wise manner, monitoring the patient for signs of tumour regression (shrinkage of lesions, reduced EBV

Table 9.4   Common changes to prescribed medicines on transplant

Pre-transplant medication	Action
Antihypertensives (e.g. diuretics, ACE inhibitors and angiotensin II receptor blockers, calcium channel blockers, alpha-blockers)	Stop immediately pre-transplant and only re-introduce if BP persistently >130/80 mmHg
Beta-blockers and other anti-anginals (e.g. nitrates and nicorandil)	Continue (rebound tachycardia and angina risk). Review indication and dose post transplant
Statins, fibrates and ezetimibe	Review indication, dose and possible drug interactions. Where appropriate continue
Antiplatelets and oral anticoagulants	Temporarily withhold and re-introduce before discharge. Some patients will require full anticoagulation with unfractionated heparin (easily reversed if biopsy necessary)
Erythropoietins and iron	Stop pre-transplant
Phosphate binders	Stop pre-transplant
Vitamin D metabolites	Continue if previous parathyroidectomy – review serum calcium daily (dose increase ± calcium supplement often necessary) Stop for all other indications
Quinine preparations	Stop pre-transplant
Hypnotics and agents for restless leg syndrome (e.g. clonazepam, gabapentin)	Continue with a view to withdrawing slowly after discharge
Enzyme-inducing antiepileptics (e.g. carbamazepine, phenytoin)	Continue. Empirically double starting dose of calcineurin inhibitor and monitor levels closely
Other antiepileptics and drugs for neuropathic pain (e.g. gabapentin, pregabalin)	Continue and consider need for dose increases where drug is renally cleared
Antidepressants	Continue
Allopurinol	Stop pre-transplant unless cause of renal failure familial hyperuricaemia (rare). If continued with azathioprine—reduce azathioprine dose by half and monitor WCC closely. Consider using mycophenolate instead
Gastro-protection (e.g. H_2 antagonists, protein pump inhibitors)	Clarify indication and continue post-transplant
Insulin and oral hypoglycaemics	Early post-transplant sliding scale insulin and re-instate with regular review of blood sugars (dose may need to increase)

viral load). If there is poor response or additional therapy is required (based on the severity of the disease) then chemotherapy may be administered.[33] Anti-B cell antibody therapy with rituximab may also be indicated.[34]

The pharmacist's role in caring for transplant patients

Most of the surgical transplant units have access to a specialist pharmacist who will take responsibility for medicines management issues perioperatively. Likewise the renal pharmacists at secondary referral hospitals will see significant numbers of transplant recipients, usually as outpatients. Pharmacists' remits will differ from centre to centre and the roles mentioned below should be considered as a guide only.

At the time of transplant all medications should be critically reviewed. Analgesia (e.g. morphine PCA), regular aperients and thrombosis prophylaxis will be prescribed and are crucial for an acceptable and safe inpatient experience. Many medicines that are essential for good health whilst approaching or receiving dialysis will no longer be required and may be discontinued. Some agents will need to be weaned slowly to prevent withdrawal effects. There will be an enduring need for others, sometimes at higher dosage, sometimes temporarily withheld. Table 9.4 offers some guidance on typical medicine changes made at the time of transplant.

Vigilance is required during the early post-transplant period of improving renal function and stabilisation of immunosuppressant dosing to ensure medicine use is safe, effective and evidence-based. If there is DGF, and continued dialysis is required, then the pharmacist must consider the timing of the newly prescribed drugs around this and, occasionally, their fluid volumes. The need for some antimicrobial prophylaxis (e.g. CMV disease prevention) may not be immediately clear and may require some research (e.g. with the UKT Core Donor Details form held by the transplant coordinators and the patient's transplant CMV IgG status).

With the newly prescribed regimen of immunosuppression the need for adjunctive medication (for example, early use of calcium and vitamin D ± bisphosphonates) should be considered, but care should be taken to ensure that it is suitable for long-term concordance.

Promoting adherence to the medicine regimen is one of the most important roles for the renal pharmacist. We know that the prevalence of 20–32% non-adherence in renal transplant recipients is directly related to the incidence of late acute rejection and graft loss.[35] Pharmacists can work to reduce this by informing recipients about their medicines to the level they desire (verbally and with written information) and responding positively to self-reported side-effects and concerns. Where possible, limiting medicine-taking to twice daily, tagging this to another life function such as eating and providing a medicine record prompt card can be facilitated by the pharmacist working within the larger team.

Like concordance issues, avoidance of drug interactions is an ongoing role and many patients will contact their hospital pharmacist before taking any prescribed or over-the-counter medicines. At the very least all recipients should have a point of contact for advice. This is likely to extend beyond patients to other healthcare professionals with many pharmacists actively managing either ongoing immunosuppression prescribing/supply or shared-care across the primary/secondary care interface.

Transplantation is the most cost-effective treatment option for chronic kidney disease (CKD). The CKD patient pathway aims to optimise the patient's general health at all time points and this is continued with a transplant. With modern immunosuppression, early acute rejection rates are low, one-year patient and graft survival rates are excellent but the biggest cause of graft loss is death with a functioning graft. This, and management of chronic allograft nephropathy constitute the current Holy Grail in transplantation. Over coming years eagerly awaited long-term (>5 years) data on immunosuppressive therapies will be published.

There also exists a dichotomy between too little immunsuppression predisposing to rejection and too much immunosuppression causing infection and malignancy. This situation is carefully balanced for each individual patient, taking into account donor and recipient details and the merits/negatives of each immunosuppressive agent.

The renal pharmacist can make a vital contribution on safe, effective and evidence-based use of medicines and should be an integral member of a multidisciplinary team involved in the care of transplant patients. In addition, the pharmacist has a positive role in educating the patient to aid long-term concordance and adherence.

 CASE STUDY

JL is a 60 kg, 45-year-old, white, British woman diagnosed with insulin-dependent diabetes mellitus (DM) at the age of 17. She is treated for hypertension and is registered as blind secondary to diabetic retinopathy. Her IDDM has recently been very well controlled (HbA1c 6.4% last month). She is single and has three children, the youngest of whom was delivered by caesarean section 10 years previously, and after which she received a blood transfusion. She started peritoneal dialysis 4 years ago but, following two episodes of peritonitis which required peritoneal dialysis catheter removal, she is now on haemodialysis. She passes less than 50 mL of urine from her native kidneys each day. She was CMV negative when listed with UK Transplant 38 months ago.

Q1. What recipient factors may have led to JL remaining on the waiting list for over 3 years?
JL is called for a kidney transplant. At this point she takes the following medicines each day:

- Calcium acetate 1 g three times a day with meals (phosphate binder)
- Alfacalcidol 0.5 μg daily (secondary hyperparathyroidism)
- Vitamin B Co Forte 2 daily (supplements)
- Folic acid 5 mg daily
- Aspirin dispersible 75 mg daily (primary cardiovascular prevention)
- Simvastatin 40 mg at night
- Ramipril 5 mg daily (hypertension)
- Epoetin beta 1000 units SC twice weekly (anaemia)
- Carbamazepine 200 mg twice daily (neuropathic pain)
- Insulin glargine 28 units SC each evening (IDDM)
- Insulin lispro 6–10 units SC with meals.

Q2. Which medicines should be stopped at this point and which would normally continue to be prescribed?
On day 0 she receives a CMV-positive renal transplant from a 29-year-old, cadaver donor to which she has a 2,1,1 HLA mismatch. She receives methylprednisolone 1 g in theatre. The transplanted kidney perfuses well on the operating table but does not have primary function. Urine output is minimal (<4 mL/h). Ultrasound scans show the graft is perfused and there are no obvious surgical complications. JL is prescribed an immunosuppression regimen of tacrolimus, azathioprine and prednisolone. Her prescribed medicines are as follows:

- Aspirin dispersible 75 mg once daily (currently withheld)
- Simvastatin 40 mg at night

→

CASE STUDY (continued)

- Carbamazepine 200 mg twice daily
- Enoxaparin 20 mg SC once daily
- Morphine sulfate 50 mg/50 mL IV 1 mg bolus patient-controlled analagesia with 5-minute lockout
- Paracetamol 1 g four times daily
- Senna 15 mg at night
- Human soluble insulin 50 units/50 mL IV sliding scale based upon hourly blood sugar
- Tacrolimus 3 mg twice daily
- Azathioprine 100 mg once daily
- Prednisolone 20 mg in the morning
- Co-trimoxazole 480 mg at night
- Cefradine 500 mg IV twice daily for 2 days post-op.

Q3. What other antirejection strategy might have been considered?
She requires haemodialysis on day 1, continues to be effectively anuric and on day 3 her tacrolimus trough level is 6 ng/mL.

Q4. Is this tacrolimus level usually considered adequate?

Q5. What might be contributing to this level?
Her tacrolimus dose is doubled to 6 mg twice daily. She has further dialysis on day 3 and day 5. On day 6 her tacrolimus level is 12 ng/mL. She is now back on regular SC insulin albeit requiring higher doses. On day 6 she passes more urine (80 mL/24hr) and on day 7 more again (400 mL/24 h). For the first time her plasma creatinine level has not risen significantly over the previous day. Medicines discharge training is commenced.

Q6. What input can the pharmacist make to maximise the chances of medicine regimen adherence?
On day 8 her urine output slows, she spikes a temperature of 38.1°C and is tender over her left iliac fossa. JL's transplanted kidney is biopsied under ultrasound guidance and, before the result is available, she is given an infusion of methylprednisolone 500 mg. A 'sliding scale' IV insulin infusion is prescribed simultaneously and the regular SC insulin prescription is stopped. Biopsy results the following day suggest a low-grade acute cellular rejection and a further 2 days' doses of methylprednisolone 500 mg infusion are prescribed. Day 9 tacrolimus trough levels are 18 ng/mL and the dose is reduced to 4.5 mg twice daily.

Q7. If the transplanted kidney continues to function poorly what could be the possible reasons?

Q8. What treatment options would be typical?
On day 11 JL's urine output has increased to 1.5 L and her creatinine level has fallen from 450 to 375 µmol/L.

(continued overleaf)

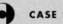

CASE STUDY (continued)

By day 13 her creatinine has fallen to 198 μmol/L and she is passing 2 L urine each day, her tacrolimus level is 12 ng/mL, blood sugars are controlled on SC basal/bolus insulin and she is deemed medically ready for discharge with thrice weekly follow-up.

Q9.   In addition to co-trimoxazole, what other prophylaxis might you expect to see on the TTA?

References

1. Voronoy YY. *El siglo Med* 1936; 97: 296.

2. Merrill JP, Murray JE, Harrison JH. Successful homotransplantations of the human kidney between identical twins. *JAMA* 1956; 160: 277–282.

3. Kuss R, Bourget P. *An Illustrated History of Organ Transplantation. The Great Adventure of the Century*. Rueil-Malmaison: Sandoz, 1992: 45.

4. Meiser-Kriesche HU, Schold ID, Srinivas TR *et al*. Lack of improvement in renal allograft survival despite a marked decrease in acute rejection rates over the most recent era. *Am J Transplant* 2004; 4: 378–383.

5. Evans RW, Manninen DL, Garrison LP *et al*. The quality of life of patients with end stage renal disease. *N Engl J Med* 1985; 312: 553–559.

6. Aranzabal J, Perdigo L, Mijores J, Villar F. Renal transplantation costs: an economic analysis and comparison with dialysis costs. *Transplant Proc* 1991; 23: 2574.

7. UK Transplant Activity. http://www.uktransplant. org.uk/ukt/statistics/statistics.jsp (accessed 12 July 2006).

8. Racusen LC, Solez K, Colvin RB *et al*. The Banff 97 working classification of renal allograft pathology. *Kidney Int* 1999; 55: 713–723.

9. Matas AJ. Acute rejection is a major risk factor for chronic rejection. *Transplant Proc* 1998; 30: 1766–1768.

10. Pirsch JD, Ploeg RJ, Gange S *et al*. Determinants of graft survival after renal transplantation. *Transplantation* 1996; 61: 1581–1586.

11. Agha IA, Rueda J, Alvarez A *et al*. Short course induction immunosuppression with thymoglobulin for renal transplant recipients. *Transplantation* 2002; 73: 473–475.

12. National Institute for Health and Clinical Excellence (NICE). Technology appraisal 85: Immunosuppressive therapy for renal transplantation in adults; September 2004. http://www. nice.org.uk/TA085guidance (accessed 15 July 2006).

13. Ponticelli C, Yussim A, Cambi V *et al*. A randomised, double-blind trial of basiliximab immunoprophylaxis plus triple therapy in kidney transplant recipients. *Transplantation* 2001; 72: 1261–1267.

14. Lawen JG, Davies EA, Mourad G *et al*. Randomised double-blind study of immunoprophylaxis with basilixmab, a chimeric anti-interleukin-2 receptor monoclonal antibody, in combination with mycophenolate mofetil-containing triple therapy in renal transplantation. *Transplantation* 2003; 75: 37–43.

15. Webster AC, Playford EG, Higgind G *et al*. Interleukin 2 receptor antagonists for renal transplant recipients: a meta-analysis of randomised trials. *Transplantation* 2004; 77: 166–176.

16. Morris PJ, Russell NK. Alemtuzumab (Campath-1H): a systematic review in organ transplantation. *Transplantation* 2006; 81: 1361–1367.

17. Genberg H, Hansson A, Wernerson A *et al*. Pharmacodynamics of rituximab in kidney allotransplantation. *Am J Transplant* 2006; 6: 2418–2428.

18. Remuzzi G, Lesti M, Gotti E *et al*. Mycophenolate mofetil versus azathioprine for prevention of acute rejection in renal transplantation (MYSS): a randomised trial. *Lancet* 2004; 364: 503–512.

19. Ojo AO, Meier-Kriesche H, Hanson JA *et al*. Mycophenolate mofetil reduces late renal allograft loss independent of acute rejection. *Transplantation* 2000; 69: 2405–2409.

20. Kramer BK, Montagnino G, Del Castillo D *et al*. Efficacy and safety of tacrolimus compared with cyclosporine A microemulsion in renal trans-

plantation: 2 year follow-up results. *Nephrol Dial Transplant* 2005; 20: 968–973.

21. Margreiter R. European tacrolimus versus ciclosporin microemulsion renal transplantation study group. Efficacy and safety of tacrolimus compared with ciclosporin microemulsion in renal transplantation: a randomised multicentre study. *Lancet* 2002; 359: 741–746.

22. Wyeth. Summary of product characteristics for Rapamune. http://emc.medicines.org.uk/emc/industry/default.asp?page=displaydoc.asp&documentid=5747 (accessed 26 September 2006).

23. Watson CJE, Firth J, Williams PF *et al.* A randomized controlled trial of late conversion from calcineurin inhibitor-based to sirolimus-based immunosuppression following renal transplantation. *Am J Transplant* 2005; 5: 2496–2503.

24. Zimmerman JJ, Kahan BD. Pharmacokinetics of sirolimus in stable renal transplant patients after multiple oral dose administration. *J Clin Pharmacol* 1997: 37: 405–415.

25. Baxter K, ed. *Stockley's Drug Interactions*, 7th edn. London: Pharmaceutical Press, 2006.

26. Vincenti F, Larsen C, Durrbach A *et al.* Costimulation blockade with belatacept in renal transplantation. *N Engl J Med* 2005; 353: 770–781.

27. Watschinger B, Pascual M. Capillary Cd4 deposition as a marker of humoral immunity in renal allograft rejection. *J Am Soc Nephrol* 2002; 13: 2420–2423.

28. Newstead CG. *Guidelines for the Prevention and Management of Cytomegalovirus Disease after Solid Organ Transplantation*, 2nd edn. London: British Transplantation Society, 2004.

29. Lichtenstein IH, MacGregor RR. Mycobacterial infections in renal transplant recipients: report of five cases and review of the literature. *Rev Infect Dis* 1983; 5: 216–226.

30. Kasiske BL, Snyder JJ, Gilbertson DT, Wang C. Cancer after kidney transplantation in the United States. *Am J Transplant* 2004; 4: 905.

31. Information about skin cancer for patients with an organ transplant. http://www.bad.org.uk/public/leaflets/transplant.asp (accessed 15 July 2006).

32. Andreone P, Gramenzi A, Lorenzini S *et al.* Post-transplantation lymphoproliferative disorders. *Arch Intern Med* 2003; 163: 1997.

33. Paya CV, Fung JJ, Nalesnik MA *et al.* Epstein-Barr virus-induced posttransplant lymphoproliferative disorders. ASTS/ASTP EBV-PTLD Task Force and The Mayo Clinic Organized International Consensus Development Meeting. *Transplantation* 1999; 68: 1517.

34. Choquet S, Leblond V, Herbrecht R *et al.* Efficacy and safety of rituximab in B-cell post-transplantation lymphoproliferative disorders: results of a prospective multicenter phase 2 study. *Blood* 2006; 107: 3053.

35. Schafer Keller P, Lyon S, Van Gelder F, De Geest S. A practical approach to promoting adherence to immunosuppressive medication after renal transplantation. *Curr Opin Nephrol Hypertens* 2006; 15 (Suppl 2): S1–S6.

10

Drug dosing in patients with renal impairment and during renal replacement therapy

Anne Millsop

The kidney plays an important role in the handling of drugs in the body. Patients with renal impairment may therefore require different dosage regimens to patients with normal renal function. Unfortunately, there are no absolute guidelines on how to adjust doses in renal impairment, and pharmaceutical company literature often excludes patients with renal impairment in the dosage guidelines.[1] Even when information can be found the advice may not be specific and different texts may give different advice.[2] It is important, therefore, for pharmacists to have an understanding of the potential pharmacokinetic and pharmacodynamic changes in renal impairment so that appropriate dosing decisions can be made.

Drug handling considerations in patients with renal impairment

Changes to the way drugs are handled in the presence of impaired kidney function will affect both the choice of drug and the method of administration. Renal impairment can affect the absorption, distribution, metabolism and elimination of a drug. There may also be pharmocodynamic changes.

Absorption

Absorption of orally administered drugs may be reduced in patients with renal impairment as a result of:

- Nausea, vomiting or diarrhoea associated with uraemia[3]
- Hypoproteinaemic oedema of the gastro-intestinal tract (e.g. in nephrotic syndrome)[3]
- Reduced intestinal motility and gastric emptying time (e.g. in uraemic neuropathy)[3], which can reduce the time taken for the drug to be absorbed but does not generally affect the extent of absorption[4]
- An increase in pH in the gut from increased gastric ammonia production in uraemia, which reduces the bioavailability of drugs requiring an acidic environment for absorption[3,4]
- Co-administration of drugs which increase gastric pH (e.g. H_2-antagonists)
- Co-administration of chelating agents such as those used for binding phosphate (see Chapter 6).

It is also speculated that the absorption of some drugs is increased as a result of:

- Reduced activity of drug-metabolising enzymes in the intestine, although this effect may be offset by increased first-pass metabolism in the liver[4]
- Co-administration of drugs that increase gastric pH, which will increase the bioavailability of weakly acidic drugs.[4]

Drug doses are not routinely altered to allow for these factors alone but must be considered in the whole picture. If therapeutic levels of drugs are not being achieved or if a fast onset of action is required, a change of dose or a different route of administration may be required.

Distribution

Changes to the distribution of drugs in the body in patients with renal impairment may occur as a result of:

- Changes in the hydration state of the patient
- Alterations in protein binding
- Alterations in tissue binding.

Changes in the hydration state of the patient

The state of hydration of a patient is only important for drugs with a small volume of distribution (V_d) (<50 L), such as gentamicin.[5] In the presence of oedema the V_d will be increased and in the presence of dehydration the V_d will be reduced. It is important to note the state of hydration when blood samples are taken for therapeutic drug monitoring (TDM) and to use this knowledge when interpreting the results. This is particularly important when the state of hydration is fluctuating with the use of intravenous fluids, diuretics or intermittent renal replacement therapy (RRT).

Alterations in protein binding

Protein binding is altered due to:

- Hypoalbuminaemia
- Uraemia and the accumulation of metabolites and endogenous substances, which will compete with the drugs for binding to albumin
- Altered structural arrangement of albumin possibly reducing the affinity or number of binding sites for drugs.[3,4]

Alterations in protein binding are clinically important for highly protein-bound drugs (>80%).[3] A reduction in bound drug in the plasma will result in a higher proportion of

unbound, and therefore active, drug in the plasma. However, as there is more unbound drug available for metabolism this effect is usually transient.

For highly bound drugs care must be taken in interpreting TDM results as total drug concentrations (bound and unbound) are usually reported and not free active drug. In this instance low TDM levels may not necessarily be subtherapeutic. The most important example of this is phenytoin. Free phenytoin levels should be measured where possible. However, as free levels are not usually readily available it is important to know how to interpret a total plasma level. Equation 10.1 from *Basic Clinical Pharmacokinetics*[6] may be used to adjust a total plasma level:

$$C_{p \text{ Normal binding}} = \frac{C_p{}'}{(1 - \alpha) \ [P'/P_{NL}] + \alpha}$$

where $C_{p \text{ Normal binding}}$ is the plasma drug concentration that would have been observed if the patient's serum albumin concentration had been normal; $C_p{}'$ is the observed plasma concentration reported by the laboratory; α is the normal free fraction of phenytoin (0.1 for non-renal failure patients and 0.2–0.35 for patients with renal failure, quoted as creatinine clearance <25 mL/min); P' is the patient's serum albumin in units of g/dL; and P_{NL} is the normal serum albumin (4.4 g/dL).

Where creatinine clearance is <10 mL/min and the patient is undergoing haemodialysis treatment an equation incorporating a factor which takes into account both altered serum albumin concentration and decreased binding affinity for this patient group should be used:

$$C_{p \text{ Normal binding}} = \frac{C_p{}'}{(0.48)(1 - \alpha) \ [P'/P_{NL}] + \alpha}$$

For this equation α has a value of 0.1.[6] Although these equations can help us determine TDM results more accurately they are still only an estimation. Clinical signs and symptoms must also be used, and free levels of phenytoin should be specifically requested.

Before taking samples for TDM consideration must be given to the time taken for equilibrium to be reached ($4\frac{1}{2}$ half-lives), as for some drugs the half-life is increased in renal impairment.

Alterations in tissue binding

Alterations in tissue binding may affect the volume of distribution (V_d) of a drug. For the majority of drugs this is not clinically relevant.[4] One drug for which it is relevant is digoxin. The V_d of digoxin may be reduced by up to 50% in established renal failure patients. Reduced loading doses will need to be given to prevent toxicity. Maintenance doses of digoxin are also markedly reduced because it is predominantly renally excreted.

Metabolism

Phase I and phase II metabolism is slower in chronic kidney disease.[4,7] The effect of this is to increase serum drug concentrations of the parent drug. This may lead to higher prevalence of adverse effects and toxicity where drugs are usually metabolised to inactive metabolites. The kidney itself is also the site of metabolism for some drugs. Two important examples are the hydroxylation of 25-hydroxycholecalciferol to active vitamin D (1α,25-dihydroxycholecalciferol) and the metabolism of insulin. For patients requiring vitamin D, either the active drug (calcitriol) or a preparation requiring metabolism to active drug by the liver (alfacalcidol) should be used. For diabetic patients insulin requirements will be reduced.

Elimination

The kidney is involved in the elimination of drugs and metabolites by glomerular filtration, renal tubular secretion and resorption.[4] In renal impairment all these functions are reduced. The reduction in glomerular filtration and tubular secretion results in higher plasma levels of drug and the reduction in resorption results in higher concentrations of drug in the urine. The extent to which drugs are affected depends on the percentage of active drug or active metabolite that would normally be excreted by this route. For some drugs accumulation of active metabolites with different properties to the active parent may change the pharmacological response in renal impairment. An example of this is pethidine. An excess of pethidine produces CNS depression, but an accumulation of the renally excreted metabolite norpethidine produces CNS stimulation and seizures.[7]

In order to make decisions on doses of drugs excreted by the kidney an assessment of renal function needs to be made (see below).

Pharmacodynamic alterations

Although there is not as much literature on changes in the body's response to drugs in renal impairment it is known that patients with uraemia have:

- An increased sensitivity to drugs acting on the central nervous system such as benzodiazepines
- A reduced sensitivity to some endogenous hormones such as growth hormone
- An increased sensitivity to cholinesterase inhibitors
- An increased risk of gastrointestinal bleeding with irritant drugs such as non-steroidal anti-inflammatory drugs
- An increased risk of hyperkalaemia with drugs such as potassium-sparing diuretics.[8]

Assessment of renal function

Assessing the degree of renal impairment usually involves a measurement of glomerular filtration rate (GFR). GFR cannot be measured directly so it is estimated from the clearance of a solute present in a stable concentration in the plasma and freely filtered by the kidney.[9] The solute ideally should not be secreted or reabsorbed by the renal tubule. Naturally occurring solutes which have been used are urea, creatinine and cystatin C. Exogenous products which have been used include inulin, isotopes and iohexol. The merits of each will be considered in turn.

Endogenous solutes

Urea

Urea is used with other results as a guide to the severity of renal impairment but its use to calculate GFR is limited by external factors that affect urea production. These include alterations in protein intake by the patient (which alters production throughout the day); catabolism caused by sepsis or treatment with corticosteroids; hyperthyroidism; liver disease; gastrointestinal bleeding and muscle injury. Another problem with using urea as a filtration marker is that it undergoes resorption by the renal tubules as well as being filtered, therefore it gives an underestimate of GRF and at low urine flow rates its clearance is independent of GFR.[9]

Creatinine

Creatinine is a product of muscle breakdown formed by non-enzymatic degradation of muscle creatinine.[9] Creatinine production is relatively constant in any individual with a stable diet, making it a good filtration marker. The production of creatinine varies between individuals as it is proportional to muscle mass and meat intake. It is therefore important to take into account the age, sex, race and weight of each individual, and to ensure the individual has a stable diet. Creatinine is actively secreted in the proximal tubule as well as being filtered, so measuring creatinine clearance leads to an overestimate of GFR by 10–20 mL/min/1.73 m^2.[10] Creatinine secretion in the tubules is blocked by some drugs (e.g. cimetidine, trimethoprim, probenecid, amiloride, spironolactone, triamterene). Administration of these drugs in patients with renal impairment can produce an increase in serum creatinine without altering the GFR. Despite these limitations, creatinine is the most commonly used marker

for GRF assessment. The ways creatinine clearance (CrCl) by the kidneys can be estimated are given below.

Cystatin C

Cystatin C is a low-molecular-weight protein that is produced at a constant rate and freely filtered by the glomerulus.[9] After filtration it is reabsorbed and catabolised by the tubular epithelial cells which means that it is only present in the urine in small amounts. Plasma levels of cystatin C correlate well with GFR and may be more accurate than creatinine estimations in mild renal impairment.[10] Cystatin C levels are not routinely used at present.

Exogenous solutes

Inulin

Inulin was considered the gold standard in measuring GFR.[9] It is an inert polymer of fructose that is freely filtered and is neither secreted nor reabsorbed by the tubules. Measurement was by infusion of inulin to produce steady state plasma levels and an accurately timed urine collection. Inulin is no longer used as it is not readily available in the UK and is difficult to assay.

Isotopes

Radioactive chromium-51-ethylenediaminetetra-acetic acid (EDTA) can be injected and accurate blood samples taken following injection to estimate GRF. The method measures disappearance from the plasma rather than renal clearance but the results correlate well with inulin studies.[9] The disadvantage is that the patient is exposed to radiation. Technetium-99-diethylenetriamine pentaacetic acid (DTPA) can also be used. GRF can be measured by dynamic renal scanning to measure the rate of disappearance of the isotope or by blood samples or collection of urine samples. Currently these assay methods are not in routine use.

Iohexol

Iohexol is a contrast medium that can be measured with high-performance liquid chromatography. It shows good correlation with inulin techniques as a filtration marker. Currently this assay method is not in routine use.

Estimation of renal function

Calculation of creatinine clearance

If a 24-hour urine collection has been carried out then a creatinine clearance can be calculated using the following equation:[5]

$$\text{CrCl (mL/min)} = \frac{UV}{S}$$

Where U is the urine creatinine concentration in µmol/L; V is the urine flow rate in mL/min (i.e. volume of urine collected divided by the time over which it was collected) and S is the serum creatinine concentration (sample taken midway through the 24-hour collection period) in µmol/L.

When conducted properly this is a very accurate way of determining creatinine clearance, however inaccuracies in collection often occur and it is cumbersome to perform.

An alternative method is to calculate the creatinine clearance using serum creatinine levels. The most widely used calculation for this is the Cockcroft and Gault equation:

$$\text{CrCl [mL/min]} = \frac{F \times (140 - \text{age [years]}) \times \text{ideal body weight [kg]}}{\text{Serum creatinine [µmol/L]}}$$

where F is 1.23 for men and 1.04 for women.

The ideal body weight is used for patients who are obese and is calculated as follows:

Ideal body weight (men) = 50 kg + 2.3 kg for every inch over 5 feet in height

Ideal body weight (women) = 45.5 kg + 2.3 kg for every inch over 5 feet in height.

This equation takes into consideration the differences in muscle mass (and therefore creatinine production) between men and women and for different age groups. However it does not take into account variations between different races. It can only be used if the renal function is stable, and it becomes inaccurate as the GFR falls because creatinine excretion is not solely by filtration (see above). It should not be used for patients in end stage renal failure or receiving RRT. Also the equation is reliant on accurate serum creatinine measurement and studies have shown that these results vary between laboratories.[11] Despite all of these points the Cockcroft and Gault equation is widely used because it can be quickly calculated at the patient's bedside using readily available laboratory results.

Estimated GFR

The Modification of Diet in Renal Disease (MDRD) study group compared different methods for calculating GRF and found the following equation to give a good prediction of GFR:[12]

$$\begin{aligned} \text{eGFR} = \ &170 \times (P_{cr})^{-0.999} \times (\text{age})^{-0.176} \times \\ &(0.762 \text{ if female}) \times (1.180 \text{ if African} \\ &\text{American}) \times [\text{SUN}]^{-0.170} \times [\text{Alb}]^{+0.318} \end{aligned}$$

where eGFR is expressed in mL/min/1.73 m², P_{cr} is plasma creatinine concentration in mg/dL, age is in years, SUN is serum urea nitrogen concentration in mg/dL and Alb is serum albumin concentration in g/dL. The equation was developed in patients with chronic kidney disease, who were predominantly white and did not have diabetic kidney disease or a kidney transplant. The equation has been validated for African Americans but no other ethnic groups. The authors report that this method is more accurate at estimating GFR than the Cockcroft and Gault equation.[12] However the equation assumes that all patients have a body surface area (BSA) of 1.73 m². For patients with a BSA less than 1.73 m² the eGFR is likely to overestimate their kidney function and for patients with a BSA greater than 1.73 m² the eGFR is likely to underestimate their kidney function. Use of the patient's actual BSA will overcome this problem, but this requires the patient's height and weight to be available. Simplified versions of the equation using four rather than six variables are also in use.[10] In units where the MDRD prediction equation is being used the eGFR is calculated automatically by the reporting laboratory.

When considering drug doses it is important to remember that most standard texts use creatinine clearance as an estimation of renal function and not eGFR.[13] For most drugs there is a broad range for guidance on dosage and so in practice the variations of measurement will not change the recommendations,[14] but it is important to consider the implications of under- and overdosing for patients whose calculated GFR varies according to which formula has been used.

Classification of renal function

Some texts giving advice on drug doses in renal impairment classify renal impairment in terms of creatinine clearance values and some texts use qualitative measurements such as 'mild', 'moderate' or 'severe' renal impairment.[2] The classification for each literature source should always be followed but dosage decisions are more difficult when quantitative values are not given.

Adjusting doses for patients with renal impairment

It can be seen from the information above that assessing the degree of renal impairment is not an exact science. The same is applicable to the dosing of these patients. There are many literature sources available with suggested doses for patients with renal impairment (see Further reading) but the advice in different sources is not always consistent.[2] It is important therefore to be able to apply your pharmaceutical knowledge to each individual case.

The first step is the choice of drug to use. In

order to limit the potential problems with adverse effects and toxicity, as far as possible drugs with the following characteristics should be used:

- Not nephrotoxic
- Has a large therapeutic index
- Does not require renal metabolism to an active form
- Does not require renal excretion of active drug or active metabolites
- Has a low adverse effect profile
- Is not highly protein bound
- Has an action unaffected by altered tissue sensitivity
- Is unaffected by fluid balance changes
- Is able to reach the site of action in high enough concentrations in the presence of renal impairment.

In addition, if a drug is to be given by the intravenous route it is preferable to use a drug with a low sodium content and requiring a small infusion volume.

It is rarely possible to find a drug fitting all these criteria, but where a drug has potential renal adverse effects, serious dose-related adverse effects, or a narrow therapeutic range with no potential to monitor, an alternative drug should be sought.

Once a drug has been selected, a decision on the dose needs to be made. Ideally one or more of the available renal drug dosing reference sources should be consulted along with the summary of product characteristics (SPC), and advice sought from a renal pharmacist who may have clinical experience of using the drug. When interpreting the dose recommendations, remember that eGFR and creatinine clearance values are not interchangeable (see Calculation of renal function above). The following principles should also be applied:

- If the drug is unaffected by renal impairment it may be used in usual doses and the patient should be monitored for signs of increased sensitivity to the effects of the drug or to the adverse effects.
- Drugs that require therapeutic levels quickly may require a loading dose as the time taken to reach steady state will be prolonged for

drugs where the metabolism and excretion is slowed in renal impairment.

- Maintenance doses and frequency will depend on the extent of renal impairment and the drug to be used.

Loading doses

The following equation can be used to calculate a loading dose:

Loading dose (mg) = Target plasma concentration (mg/L) × Volume of distribution (L/kg) × Ideal body weight (kg)

There will be variations in the loading dose calculated depending on the target concentration chosen (most drugs have a target range) and depending on the volume of distribution figure used (this can vary between literature sources and may again be quoted as a range). Knowledge of the adverse effect and toxicity profile will be important in choosing the loading dose.

Maintenance doses

The following equation can be used to calculate maintenance doses:[5]

$$DR_{rf} = DR_n \times [(1 - Feu) + (Feu \times RF)]$$

where DR_{rf} is the dosing rate in renal failure, DR_n is the normal dosing rate, RF is the extent of renal failure (calculated as patient's CrCl (mL/min) divided by the ideal CrCl of 120 mL/min) and Feu is the fraction of drug normally excreted unchanged in the urine (available in literature sources and the SPC).

Once a dosing regimen has been decided it is important to monitor the patient's progress. For drugs with a narrow therapeutic range serum drug levels should be monitored and the physiological response to the drug should also be monitored. The patient and his or her carers should be informed of potential adverse effects or signs of toxicity so that they can report any they may experience.

Drug handling considerations in patients undergoing renal replacement therapy

Once a patient requires RRT their own kidney function is negligible and so removal from the body of a drug dependent on renal excretion is also negligible. It is therefore important to know whether a drug is likely to be removed by RRT. The factors to consider during RRT fall into two categories:

- The drug characteristics that will affect drug removal
- The RRT characteristics that will affect drug removal.

Drug characteristics affecting drug removal in RRT

The following drug characteristics are likely to affect drug removal by RRT:

- Molecular weight
- Percentage of drug bound to plasma proteins
- Volume of distribution
- Water solubility
- Percentage of renal clearance in normal subjects
- Steric hindrance.

Knowledge of the molecular weight is more important for drug removal by intermittent haemodialysis than for continuous haemofiltration or haemodiafiltration. For haemodialysis, molecules with a molecular weight >500 Da are not likely to be removed, whereas for haemofiltration using a highly permeable membrane molecules with a molecular weight of up to 30 000 Da may be removed.[15,16] As only unbound drug will be available for removal by RRT, knowledge of the percentage of drug that is protein bound is important. Drugs with low protein binding potential are more likely to be removed. It is also important to remember that changes in protein binding occur in patients with low serum albumin levels and uraemia as discussed above. The volume of distribution of each drug is important as only free drug in the plasma is available for removal by RRT. Drugs with a $V_d < 1$ L/kg are more likely to be removed by dialysis.[17] Care must be taken in interpreting literature on V_d as alterations in protein binding in renal impairment will alter the volume of distribution of highly protein-bound drugs (see above). For intermittent haemodialysis only small fractions of drugs with a high V_d will be removed. For continuous RRT, drugs with a high V_d will be more effectively removed because the equilibrium between the plasma and tissue levels will be constantly changing. The water solubility of a drug will reflect the level of drug usually in the plasma and therefore available for removal by RRT. The higher the water solubility the more likely the drug is to be removed.[17]

Another reflection of a drug's likelihood of being removed is the amount of drug usually removed by the kidneys. Although RRT cannot mimic completely the role of the kidneys, it is more likely to remove drugs usually filtered by the kidney in normal subjects. Lastly steric hindrance is important. Even if a molecule appears small enough to be removed by the RRT process the atomic arrangement of the drug molecule will affect its ability to pass through the RRT membrane.

RRT system characteristics affecting drug removal

The system characteristics affecting drug removal will vary depending on the type of RRT used. The characteristics important to each system are listed in Table 10.1.

For intermittent haemodialysis, the duration of dialysis will affect drug removal. For example, more drug will be removed in a 4-hour session than a 3-hour session. The flow rate of both the blood and dialysate is important. Drug removal by haemodialysis is predominantly by diffusion, increasing the flow rate will therefore result in a higher concentration gradient between the two and more drug being removed. The composition of the dialysate will also affect the diffusion process. Lastly, there are different membranes available for dialysis, the type of membrane will affect drug removal because of changes in permeability and composition which favour removal of different drugs.[16]

Table 10.1 System characteristics important for drug removal by haemodialysis, continuous peritoneal dialysis or continuous haemofiltration

	System characteristics important for drug removal
Haemodialysis	Duration of the dialysis procedure
	Blood flow rate in the dialyser
	Dialysate flow rate
	Composition of the dialysate
	Type of membrane used
Peritoneal dialysis	Volume of exchange of dialysate
	Frequency of exchange of dialysate
	Composition of the dialysate
	Osmotic gradient between dialysate and plasma
	Pathology of the peritoneum
Continuous haemofiltration	Type of membrane used
	Selection of A-V or V-V system used
	Pump pressure (if used)

For continuous peritoneal dialysis the membrane used is the peritoneal membrane and the health of this membrane is important for drug removal. During peritonitis the membrane becomes more porous and will remove a larger proportion of drugs and solutes. Larger volumes of exchange and frequent changes will increase the concentration gradient and aid diffusion of drugs out of the plasma. The composition of the dialysate used will also affect the rate of diffusion. Lastly the osmotic gradient is important, a high gradient will remove more water and therefore more water-soluble drugs with it.

The most important factors influencing drug removal in continuous haemofiltration are the membrane permeability and the system pressure (which depends on whether an arteriovenous or venovenous system is used and the pump pressure, see Chapter 8). This is because convective transport and ultrafiltration are the predominant factors for drug removal in haemofiltration. For continuous haemodiafiltration a combination of the haemodialysis and continuous haemofiltration factors will apply. For any system using a membrane, interactions between the drug and membrane may occur. Adsorption onto the synthetic polymer membrane will reduce the drug clearance. Adsorption is dependent on blood pH, drug and membrane. These are complex interactions and cannot always be predicted.

Adjusting drug doses for patients undergoing renal replacement therapy

For patients receiving RRT a creatinine clearance cannot be calculated using the equations discussed above. Table 10.2 gives a guide to the clearance provided by each system.

However, it is important to know the type of dialysis and membrane used as clearances will vary as described above. The manufacturer of the machine and filters should be able to give an estimate of creatinine clearance by their system. Haemodialysis is more effective than peritoneal dialysis at removing fluid and solutes. However, because the procedure is intermittent (often every 2–3 days) drugs should be dosed as if for a creatinine clearance of <10 mL/min unless the SPC or other specialist texts state differently. If a drug is likely to be removed by dialysis it should be given after the procedure and not before. For continuous peritoneal dialysis doses for creatinine clearance <10 mL/min are also used. Continuous renal replacement therapy not involving the use of a pumped circuit (CAVHF, CAVHDF) will allow drug doses for a clearance in the range of 10–20 mL/min to be used. However, those utilising pumped systems (i.e. CVVHF and CVVHDF) have an even better solute clearance, and in the case of CVVHDF, clearances can be in the range of 30–40 mL/min, allowing for much larger drug doses to be prescribed.

Dosage decisions can also be made using a calculation involving the sieving coefficient of the drug. The sieving coefficient is a measure of the proportion of drug that will pass through the haemofiltration membrane during ultrafiltration.[3] A drug which passes freely through the membrane will have a sieving coefficient of 1 and a drug which does not pass through the membrane will have a sieving coefficient of 0. A knowledge of the machine clearance and the sieving coefficient can be combined to calculate the drug clearance for that system:

$$\text{Drug clearance} = \frac{\text{Machine clearance} \times}{\text{Sieving coefficient}}$$

The sieving coefficient can be found in specialist texts but is dependent on the type of haemofiltration and membrane used. Once an idea of the rate of drug clearance in RRT has been established, literature sources such as renal drug dosing textbooks and the SPC may be consulted to find information on dosing.

Table 10.2 Creatinine clearance for different systems of renal replacement therapy	
Renal replacement therapy	Typical theoretical GFR achieved during therapy (mL/min)
Intermittent haemodialysis	150–200 during dialysis (0–10 between dialysis periods)
Continuous arterio-venous haemofiltration (CAVHF)	0–15
Continuous veno-venous haemofiltration (CVVHF)	15–25
Continuous arterio-venous haemodiafiltration (CAVHDF)	20
Continuous veno-venous haemodiafiltration (CVVHDF)	30–40
Continuous ambulatory peritoneal dialysis (CAPD) (4 exchanges daily)	5–10

Data from Industry Submission, Renal National Service Framework (Acute Renal Failure), October 2003.[17]

Loading doses

For drugs requiring therapeutic levels quickly and with a prolonged half-life in renal failure a loading dose may be required. The equation above can be used to calculate the loading dose.

Supplementary doses for intermittent renal replacement therapy

Some texts quote supplementary doses to be given after intermittent RRT. These will only be important for drugs with a low V_d and a narrow therapeutic range. It is better to adjust the timings of the regular doses so that the next dose falls after the RRT session rather than add in extra doses.

Summary

Drug dosing in patients with impaired renal function is a complex area. It is important to have an understanding of how drug handling may be altered in renal impairment and RRT and on the limitations of the calculations used to estimate renal function in order to help make informed decisions on drug doses. Where possible, textbooks on drug dosing in renal impairment should be consulted and also make use of the pharmacists with a special interest in the field who have clinical experience with these patients. In all cases once a drug regimen has been prescribed monitor the patient for efficacy, adverse effects and signs of toxicity.

 CASE STUDY

Mr PT is a haemodialysis patient. He dialyses three times a week via a tunnelled line. The haemodialysis registrar has admitted him to the renal ward suffering with rigors and fever (39°C) and has prescribed him IV flucloxacillin.

Current medication:

- Flucloxacillin IV 1 g four times daily
- Alfacalcidol 0.25 µg three times weekly
- Calcium acetate 2 tablets with meals
- Atenolol 50 mg daily
- Lisinopril 5 mg daily
- Erythropoietin 2000 units SC three times weekly
- Iron sucrose 100 mg IV weekly.

Blood results pre-dialysis on the day of admission:

- Creatinine 505 µmol/L (70–120 µmol/L)
- Urea 26 mmol/L (3.7–8.4 mmol/L)
- Sodium 138 mmol/L (134–148 mmol/L)
- Potassium 5.5 mmol/L (3.5–5 mmol/L).

Q1. Is the dose of flucloxacillin reasonable for a haemodialysis patient?

Q2. Should supplementary doses be given on dialysis days?

Q3. How should Mr PT be monitored?

References

1. Martin-Facklam M, Rengelshausen J, Tayrouz Y *et al.* Dose individualisation in patients with renal insufficiency: does drug labelling support optimal management? *Eur J Clin Pharmacol* 2005; 60: 807–811.
2. Vidal L, Shavit M, Fraser A *et al.* Systematic comparison of four sources of drug information regarding adjustment of dose for renal function. *BMJ* 2005; 331: 263–266.
3. Aweeka F T. Dosing of drugs in renal failure. In: Koda-Kimble MA, Young LY, eds. *Applied Therapeutics: The Clinical Use of Drugs*, 7th edn. Philadelphia: Lippincott Williams & Wilkins, 2001: 32.1–32.21.
4. Gabardi S, Abramson S. Drug dosing in chronic kidney disease. *Med Clin N Am* 2005; 89: 649–687.
5. Harper A. Acute renal failure. In: Walker R, Edwards C, eds. *Clinical Pharmacy and Therapeutics*, 2nd edn. London: Churchill Livingstone, 1999: 215–229.
6. Winter ME. *Basic Clinical Pharmacokinetics*, 3rd edn. Vancouver: Applied Therapeutics Inc., 1994.
7. Matzke GR, Frye RF. Drug administration in patients with renal insufficiency: Minimising renal and extrarenal toxicity. *Drug Safety* 1997; 16: 205–231.
8. Aronson JK. Drugs and renal insufficiency. *Medicine* 2003; 31: 103–109.
9. Mole DR, Mason PD. Assessment of renal function. *Medicine* 2003; 31: 5–10.
10. Stevens LA, Levey AS. Measurement of kidney function. *Med Clin N Am* 2005; 89: 457–473.
11. Schneider V, Henschel V, Tadjalli-Mehr K *et al.* Impact of serum creatinine measurement error on dose adjustment in renal failure. *Clin Pharmacol Ther* 2003; 74: 458–467.
12. Levey AS, Bosch JP, Lewis JB *et al.* A more accurate method to estimate glomerular filtration rate from serum creatinine: a new prediction equation. Modification of Diet in Renal Disease Study Group. *Ann Intern Med* 1999; 130: 461–470.
13. Bauer L. Creatinine clearance versus glomerular filtration rate for the use of renal drug dosing in patients with kidney dysfunction. *Pharmacotherapy* 2005; 25: 1286–1287.
14. Thompson CA. Better renal-function estimates not expected to alter drug dosing right away. *Am J Health-Syst Pharm* 2005; 62: 2442–2444.
15. Davies JG, Kingswood JC, Street MK. Drug removal in continuous haemofiltration and haemodialysis. *Br J Hosp Pharm* 1995; 54: 524–528.
16. Giles L. Renal replacement therapy. In: Elliott R, ed. *Critical Care Therapeutics*. London: Pharmaceutical Press, 1999: 49–56.
17. Industry Submission, Renal National Service Framework (Acute Renal Failure) October 2003.
18. Ashley C, Currie A, eds. *Renal Drug Handbook*, 2nd edn. Oxford: Radcliffe Medical Press, 2004.

Further reading

Ashley C, Currie A, eds. *Renal Drug Handbook*, 2nd edn. Oxford: Radcliffe Medical Press, 2004.
Bennett WM, Arnoff GR, Berns JS *et al. Drug Prescribing in Renal Failure: Dosing Guidelines for Adults*, 4th edn. Philadelphia: American College of Physicians, 1999.
Dollery C. *Therapeutic Drugs*, 2nd edn. London: Churchill Livingstone, 1999.
Sweetman, SC ed. *Martindale: The Complete Drug Reference*, 35th edn. London: Pharmaceutical Press, 2007.

11

Drug-induced kidney disease

Jane Pearson

Acute renal failure (ARF) is generally defined as a sustained rise in serum creatinine of at least 50 µmol/L, or greater than 20% rise above baseline (if the baseline is 250 µmol/L), that occurs over a period of days to several weeks. It is usually accompanied by a fall in urine output. This may present as anuria or oliguria. Anuria is a complete lack of urine output and oliguria is low urine output of less than 15–20 mL/h or about 500 mL in a normal adult.

ARF is common, but the incidence depends on the definition being used. It is quoted in the literature as being anything between 72 to 620 cases per million. As many as 30% of all cases of ARF are thought to be secondary to drugs and 2–5% of hospital inpatients develop drug-induced renal failure.[1]

Drug-induced ARF can occur with or without oliguria and different mechanisms are used to determine the patterns of drug-induced renal failure. ARF is often described as pre-renal, renal or post-renal, and drugs can be responsible for each of these types of kidney disease.[2]

Pre-renal (or haemodynamic) acute renal failure

In healthy people, autoregulation maintains adequate renal blood flow as blood pressure changes. This homeostatic mechanism serves to protect normal renal blood flow in a number of different disease states that are characterised by hypotension (e.g. congestive heart failure and artherosclerotic renal artery stenosis). There are a number of hormones and autocrine factors acting on renal blood vessels to mediate this

autoregulation (Figure 11.1).[3] Understanding these mechanisms makes it easier to guess which type of drugs of may be responsible for pre-renal ARF.

Drugs that decrease renal perfusion will have an adverse effect on renal function. This is seen as an acute reduction in glomerular filtration rate (GFR), which is usually reversible on

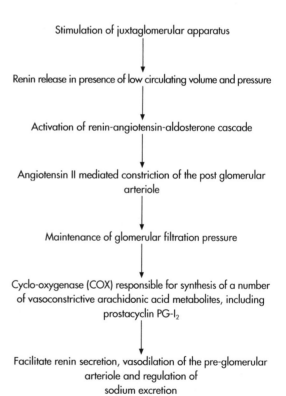

Figure 11.1 Autoregulation of renal blood flow through hormones and autocrine factors acting on renal blood vessels.

restoring blood supply to the kidneys. When not corrected, persistent renal hypoperfusion will ultimately lead to ischaemic acute tubular necrosis. Any drug that compromises circulation may induce ARF. This can include drugs that decrease cardiac output and those that increase peripheral vasoconstriction.

Volume depletion

Volume depletion with water and electrolyte loss can occur with excessive use of laxatives or diuretic therapy, in particular loop diuretics. This can cause particular problems in the elderly, but severe renal failure rarely occurs except in patients with pre-existing renal disease. Lithium in combination with diuretics leads to synergistic toxicity. Non-steroidal anti-inflammatory drugs (NSAIDs) can exacerbate pre-renal effects by further decreasing renal perfusion. They impair the ability of the renal vasculature to adapt to falls in perfusion pressure or to an increase in the vasoconstrictor balance. Hypokalaemia from laxative-induced diarrhoea or overuse of diuretics can produce a chronic nephropathy.

Altered renal haemodynamics

Some drugs have specific effects on renal perfusion. Haemodynamic ARF is a recognised complication of treatment with angiotensin-converting enzyme (ACE) inhibitors and angiotensin II receptor antagonists. These alter renal haemodynamics through their vasodilator effects on the efferent glomerular arterioles. This is particularly evident in patients with pre-existing renal artery stenosis. A sharp rise in a patient's serum creatinine after starting an ACE inhibitor may indicate the presence of bilateral renal artery stenosis. ACE inhibitor use in such patients is contraindicated. Reno-vascular disease has been found in 34% of elderly patients with heart failure. Any renal damage that has occurred is usually reversible if the drug is discontinued promptly. Other risk factors for ACE inhibitor-induced renal disease are hypovolaemia, severe chronic heart failure, polycystic kidney disease and hypertensive nephropathy.

Angiotensin II has a number of intra-renal effects, including:

- Regulation of renal blood flow
- Regulation of GFR
- Regulation of tubular reabsorption of sodium
- Inhibition of renin release.

In patients with severe renal impairment or renal artery stenosis, angiotensin II acts within the kidney to constrict the efferent glomerular arteriole and maintains glomerular filtration. ACE inhibitors block this effect and cause vasodilatation of the efferent arteriole, leading to a sudden decrease in GFR and hence ARF.

The frequency of ACE inhibitor-induced renal failure varies between 6 and 23% in patients with bilateral stenosis and increases to 38% in patients with unilateral stenosis on a single kidney.

NSAIDs inhibit the production of prostaglandins E_2, D_2 and I_2 within the kidney. These are potent vasodilators that are crucial in maintaining renal circulation to the glomerulus and medulla. This is especially important when vasoconstrictor substances such as angiotensin II or antidiuretic hormone (ADH) are increased. This can occur in conditions such as heart failure and severe hypertension. Inhibition of prostaglandin synthesis leads to vasoconstriction and a subsequent decrease in renal blood flow, GFR and urine volume.

Renal function usually recovers if NSAID therapy is withdrawn early enough, although permanent damage can occur. There is little evidence that NSAIDs impair renal function in otherwise healthy individuals.

Other

Some renally toxic drugs affect renal function by more than one mechanism, including vasoconstriction. Renal transplant units have immunosuppressive regimens based on using calcineurin inhibitors (ciclosporin or tacrolimus). High blood levels of ciclosporin and tacrolimus are associated with a negative effect on renal haemodynamics. They cause intense vasoconstriction of the microvasculature within the kidney, resulting in reduced renal perfusion, a fall in GFR and hypertension.

Doses must be adjusted to maximise the therapeutic effect and minimise the renal damage. High blood levels will obviously be associated with renal damage, but low blood levels are associated with increased risk of rejection of the transplanted kidney. Many drugs that affect the cytochrome P450 system will interact with these drugs to alter blood levels.

Intrinsic renal toxicity

This type of renal failure is often described as a 'renal' cause of renal failure, and can be subdivided into four categories: vascular, glomerular, tubular and interstitial.

Vascular

The lumen of the blood vessels may become blocked either by atheroembolic disease or by foreign material that causes an inflammatory reaction that obliterates the lumen. This vasculitis causes inflammation and necrosis in the vessel wall. Drugs are not usually the cause of vascular renal damage.

Glomerular

Drug-induced glomerulonephritis is an immune-mediated disease where antigen–antibody complexes accumulate within the glomerulus. You then get an inflammatory response due to the depositing of immunoglobulins and complement in the base membranes and blood vessels. The result is a reduced GFR, salt and water retention, increased intravascular volume and hypertension. Proteinuria may also be present and the patient can develop nephrotic syndrome. Many drugs are known to cause glomerulonephritis (Table 11.1).

Tubular

Acute tubular necrosis (ATN) can occur due to renal ischaemia or nephrotoxic agents or both. It can arise from the direct toxic affect of drugs or their metabolites on the renal tubules. ATN can occur with normal doses, but more often results from high-dose treatment or accumulation of the drug due to pre-existing renal impairment. ARF may develop after short- or long-term drug exposure. Risk factors include advanced age, pre-existing renal impairment, hypertension, heart disease, peripheral vascular disease and diabetes. Drug-induced ATN is usually associated with oliguria and a significant proportion of patients require renal replacement therapy on a temporary basis.

Nephrotoxic agents should be avoided if at all possible in patients at highest risk of developing ATN. Drugs that are most often associated with ATN are listed in Table 11.2.

Maintenance of adequate hydration and therapeutic drug monitoring where appropriate may minimise the risk of developing ATN.

Interstitial

Acute interstitial nephritis (AIN) is a hypersensitivity reaction that is characterised by a fall in GFR within hours, days or months of exposure to a particular drug. The decrease in GFR is often associated with proteinuria and haematuria. The interstitium is infiltrated with

Table 11.1 Drugs known to cause glomerulonephritis

- Allopurinol
- Dapsone
- Halothane
- NSAIDs
- Penicillins
- Probenecid
- Sulfonamides
- Tolbutamide
- Captopril
- Gold
- Hydralazine
- Penicillamine
- Phenindione
- Rifampicin
- Thiazide diuretics
- Procainamide
- Psoralen
- Levamisole

Table 11.2 Drugs associated with acute tubular necrosis

• Aciclovir	• Furosemide
• Aminoglycosides	• Gold
• Amphotericin	• Ifosfamide
• Cephalosporins	• Lithium
• Cisplatin	• Mannitol
• Contrast media	• NSAIDs
• Ciclosporin	• Paracetamol
• Ethylene glycol	• Tacrolimus
• Foscarnet	• Vancomycin

inflammatory cells, including eosinophils. The other classic clinical signs are low-grade pyrexia, rash and arthralgia.

A large number of different drugs are commonly implicated in causing AIN (Table 11.3).

AIN is thought to account for up to 15% of hospital admissions due to ARF. It is important to identify the causative agent and withdraw this drug from treatment in the patient. Recovery of renal function usually occurs over a period of one month to a year after withdrawal

Table 11.3 Drugs commonly implicated in causing acute interstitial nephritis

• Allopurinol	• Isoniazid
• Aminosalicylates	• Lithium
• Amlodipine	• Mesalazine
• Azathioprine	• NSAIDs
• Bumetanide	• Penicillins
• Carbamazepine	• Phenobarbital
• Cephalosporins	• Phenytoin
• Cimetidine	• Proton pump inhibitors
• Co-trimoxazole	• Quinolones
• Diltiazem	• Ranitidine
• Erythromycin	• Rifampicin
• Furosemide	• Sulfonamides
• Gentamicin	• Thiazides
• Gold	• Vancomycin
• Interferon	

of the offending drug, but permanent impairment may occur.

Chronic interstitial nephritis is also known as analgesic nephropathy. It is often under-diagnosed as patients under-report their use of analgesics. It can cause acute and chronic renal failure. ARF may result from allergic reactions, direct toxic tubule damage or reduction on renal blood flow.[4] Chronic damage is often seen after prolonged use of analgesics. The analgesic combinations containing salicylates, caffeine or paracetamol seem to increase the risk of chronic tubular interstitial disease.

Post-renal damage (obstructive uropathy)

Obstruction to urine flow through the kidneys can be caused by a number of factors. Ureteric fibrosis, renal calculi, blood clots and mechanical blockage can all occur with drug therapy.

Anticoagulants can cause bleeding in patients, which can subsequently lead to blood clot formation and ureteric obstruction. Retroperitoneal haemorrhage following overtreatment with anticoagulants can also cause ureteric obstruction due to external compression of the ureters. Patients with severe renal impairment may be at greater risk of this due to uraemia induced platelet dysfunction, leading to a greater risk of bleeding.

Retroperitoneal fibrosis is overgrowth of fibrous tissue in the peritoneum. The ureters can become embedded in the fibrous tissue, causing unilateral or bilateral obstruction and renal failure. This has been associated with methotrexate, methysergide, beta-blockers, methyldopa, bromocriptine and pergolide. Ureteric fibrosis has been associated with analgesic nephropathy. Symptoms of retroperitoneal fibrosis include malaise, back and flank pain and weight loss. Although the condition usually regresses on discontinuation of the causative drug, this tends to be slow and surgical intervention is often necessary to prevent further deterioration in renal function.

Crystallisation of urate and stone formation within the ureteric lumen predisposes to obstructive nephropathy. Treatment of myelo-proliferative disorders with cytotoxic drugs can cause tumour lysis to occur. This can lead to uric acid crystals being deposited in the renal tubules to such an extent that blockage occurs. This is particularly a problem if the patient has a high tumour burden. The use of prophylactic allopurinol or rasburicase plus adequate fluid intake may decrease this risk.

Crystalluria can also occur with sulfona-mides, acetazolamide, mercaptopurine, metho-trexate, cisplatin, probenecid, naftidofuryl, aciclovir, indinavir, cidofovir and ganciclovir. A high intake of fluid should be maintained in patients to minimise the risk of crystalluria.

Conclusion

There are many factors involved in drug-induced renal failure, with some drugs having more than one mechanism of causing damage. ARF is common in hospitalised patients and is associated with significant morbidity and mor-tality. Pharmacists can play an important role in the management of this patient group. They can identify possible drug causes of renal failure, ensure further nephrotoxic drugs are not pre-scribed during the recovery and treatment of renal failure and advise on appropriate dose adjustments for drugs according to renal func-tion or renal replacement therapy.

 CASE STUDY

Mr NT is a 40-year-old father of two, diagnosed with testicular teratoma. He has normal renal function (EDTA-measured creatinine clearance of 92 mL/min) and is treated with: prednisolone, vincristine 1 mg/m^2, methotrexate 300 mg/m^2, bleomycin 7.5 mg $\times$ 2 doses, cisplatin 120 mg/m^2.

Mr NT is 5 feet 6 inches tall and weighs 101 kg. His body surface area is 2.09 m^2.

One week later, a routine set of blood tests shows:

- Urea 15.1 mmol/L (3.0–6.5 mmol/L)
- Creatinine 200 μmol/L (60–120 μmol/L)
- Sodium 137 mmol/L (135–145 mmol/L)
- Potassium 2.8 mmol/L (3.5–5.0 mmol/L)
- Magnesium 0.35 mmol/L (0.7–1.0 mmol/L)
- Calcium (corrected) 1.87 mmol/L (2.2–2.65 mmol/L).

Q1. What are the metabolic abnormalities?

Q2. What has caused these abnormalities?

Q3. How can you avoid this complication?
On his next admission, Mr NT was given his chemotherapy as per protocol.

Two days later, he was found to be pyrexial with a temperature of 39.80°C, and his full blood count revealed that he was neutropenic, with a WBC count of 1.3 $\times$ 10^9/L (normal range 3.7–11.0 $\times$ 10^9/L), and an absolute neutrophil count of 0.1 $\times$ 10^9/L (normal range 1.5–7.5 $\times$ 10^9/L).

(continued overleaf)

CASE STUDY (continued)

He was prescribed empirically the following drugs:

- Amikacin IV 700 mg twice daily
- Ceftazidime IV 2 g three times daily
- Metronidazole IV 500 mg three times daily.

His biochemistry over the following days was as follows:

	Day 2	Day 3	Day 4	(Normal range)
Sodium (mmol/L)	143	141	144	135–145
Potassium (mmol/L)	5.3	5.5	6.2	3.5–5.0
Calcium (mmol/L)	2.01	1.97	1.93	2.1–2.6
Magnesium (mmol/L)	0.97	0.86	0.73	0.7–1.0
Phosphate (mmol/L)	1.29	1.57	2.01	0.70–1.25
Urea (mmol/L)	7.3	10.6	15.4	3.0–6.5
Creatinine (μmol/L)	155	235	481	60–120

Q4. What has happened now?

Q5. Comment on the antibiotic therapy he has been prescribed. Do you need to intervene?

Q6. What would you recommend?

References

1. Ashley C, Holt S. Renal disease (1): acute renal failure. *Pharm J* 2001; 266: 625–628.
2. Waring S. Features and management of drug-induced renal failure. *Prescriber* 5 Feb 2006: 59–63.
3. Ashley C. Renal failure – how drugs can damage the kidney. *Hosp Pharm* 2004; 11: 48–53.
4. Lameire N, Van Biesen W, Vanholder R. Acute renal failure. *Lancet* 2005; 365: 417–430.

12

Autoimmune kidney disease

Marc Vincent

Autoimmunity is an abnormal condition in which the body reacts with constituents of its own tissues. The normal response of the immune system is to produce antibodies to foreign antigens such as bacteria or viruses. Activated B-cells recognise the foreign antigen and stimulate antibody production. This reaction activates the complement system, which amplifies the B-cell response causing lysis of antigenic cells. Autoimmunity occurs when the immune system produces antibodies to self-antigens in body tissues (autoantibodies). Autoimmune kidney damage usually occurs as a result of autoantibodies directed towards the antigens in the glomerulus, causing glomerulonephritis.

The more common autoimmune kidney diseases are shown in Figure 12.1 and it is these which will be discussed here. There are other kidney diseases which may come under the umbrella of autoimmune kidney disease but they are less common and beyond the scope of this chapter.

The clinical manifestations associated with autoimmune kidney disease can be disease-specific but those associated with glomerular injury are often the same or similar. Definitive diagnosis is based on immunological determination and kidney biopsy. The immunological markers of the different diseases are shown in Figure 12.1.[1]

Pathogenesis

Glomerular injury is caused by type II or type III antibody-mediated reactions, but the cause of antibody formation is often not known or is poorly understood.

Type II reactions describe cytotoxic reactions resulting when an antibody reacts with the antigenic components of a cell or tissue. The antigen–antibody formation may activate cytotoxic cells such as killer T-cells or macrophages which cause cell injury and usually involves complement activation. This antibody-mediated reaction is seen in Goodpasture's syndrome secondary to antiglomerular basement membrane antibodies (anti-GBM) and in systemic vasculitis secondary to antineutrophil cytoplasmic antibodies (ANCA).

Type III reactions involve deposition of antibody–antigen immune complexes in vessels or tissues. The immune complexes may be deposited in various tissues where they activate the complement system, causing the release of lysosomal enzymes and cytokines and cell injury. Kidney damage results when immune complexes localise in the glomerulus. Immune complexes are deposited in the glomerular capillary wall, causing an inflammatory response and glomerulonephritis. Several autoimmune kidney diseases secondary to immune complex formation are shown in Figure 12.1.

Clinical manifestations

Regardless of the pathogenesis, patients usually present with one of six clinical syndromes:

- Microscopic haematuria (seen only on microscopic examination) with or without proteinuria

145

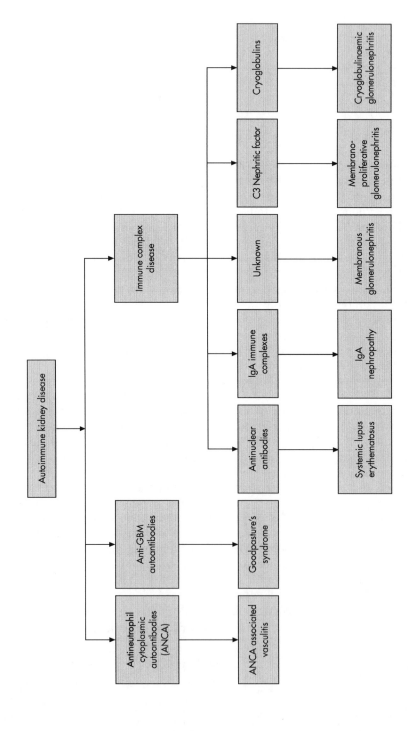

Figure 12.1 Autoimmune kidney diseases and their immunological markers. Adapted from the *Merck Manual*.[1]

- Macroscopic haematuria (visible with the naked eye)
- Nephrotic syndrome
- Nephritic syndrome
- Rapidly progressive glomerulonephritis
- Chronic glomerulonephritis.

Microscopic haematuria

Haematuria is caused by small breaks in the glomerular basement membrane that allow leakage of red blood cells into the urine. Proteinuria may result from alterations in glomerular permeability or tubulointerstitial damage. Microscopic haematuria ($>10 \times 10^6$ red cells/L) and non-nephrotic proteinuria (<3 g/day) may occur in isolation or together but renal function remains normal with no evidence of systemic disease. When haematuria and proteinuria occur together the risk of progressive renal dysfunction is much greater and warrants close monitoring and possibly renal biopsy.

Macroscopic haematuria

In episodic macroscopic haematuria urine is often a smoky brown colour rather than red and clots are unusual. Macroscopic haematuria is typically painless but may be accompanied by loin pain secondary to renal capsular swelling.

Nephrotic syndrome

Nephrotic syndrome is characterised by severe proteinuria (>3 g/day) and oedema. Low serum albumin occurs secondary to protein loss, causing a fall in plasma oncotic pressure and exacerbating oedema. Low serum albumin also causes the liver to increase production of low-density lipoproteins (LDL) with consequent hyperlipidaemia. Platelet aggregation is enhanced, causing a hypercoagulable state which increases the risk of venous thromboembolism. Kidney function may be normal, but may deteriorate if nephrotic syndrome is prolonged. Nephrotic patients are also at increased risk of infection partly due to

fragile water-logged skin and impaired immune function.

Nephritic syndrome

Nephritic syndrome develops as a consequence of glomerular inflammation. This leads to a reduction in glomerular filtration rate (GFR), non-nephrotic proteinuria, haematuria, oedema and hypertension.

Rapidly progressive glomerulonephritis

Rapidly progressive glomerulonephritis (RPGN) is characterised by signs of glomerular inflammation and a rapid decline in renal function over weeks or even days. Patients may present as an emergency requiring dialysis. Many patients with RPGN have a systemic autoimmune disease. The histological hallmark is glomerular crescents, giving rise to the name 'crescentic glomerulonephritis'. Crescents are so-called due to their appearance on histological cross-section and are a poor prognostic sign. They develop from the proliferation of epithelial cells and mononuclear phagocytes in Bowman's capsule.

Chronic glomerulonephritis

Chronic glomerulonephritis is characterised by progressive renal insufficiency, glomerular inflammation, haematuria and frequently, hypertension. This term describes the chronic kidney disease that ensues with long-standing glomerulonephritis, such as that in IgA nephropathy.

Principles of treatment

The treatment of autoimmune kidney disease consists of both supportive and disease specific therapies. Supportive therapies are those used to treat most forms of kidney dysfunction and aim to preserve renal function by reducing proteinuria, controlling oedema, and treating hypertension. Disease-specific therapies include various immunosuppressive therapies and plasma exchange in an attempt to suppress the autoimmune disease itself.

Antineutrophil cytoplasmic autoantibody (ANCA)-associated vasculitis

The vasculitides are a heterogeneous group of uncommon diseases characterised by inflammatory cell infiltration and necrosis of blood vessel walls. Vasculitis affecting the kidneys is largely associated with autoantibodies against components of the cytoplasm of neutrophils known as antineutrophil cytoplasmic autoantibodies (ANCA). ANCA-associated vasculitides include the syndromes Wegener's granulomatosis, Churg–Strauss syndrome and microscopic angitis, all of which can also affect alveolar capillaries causing pulmonary haemorrhage and dermal venules, causing purpura. There are many other types of vasculitis not associated with ANCA, though renal impairment is usually less common and less severe. Vasculitis associated with IgA deposition (Henoch–Schönlein purpura) and cryoglobulinaemia are discussed later under their respective headings. Vasculitis may also occur with the following drug treatment: penicillamine, hydralazine and propylthiouracil. Rarely, leukotriene antagonists such as montelukast can cause a Churg–Strauss-like syndrome, and this usually occurs on reduction or withdrawal of oral steroid therapy.

Pathogenesis and antineutrophil cytoplasmic autoantibodies

Antineutrophil cytoplasmic autoantibodies are thought to have a pathogenic role in the development of necrotising vasculitis. The most common theory is detailed below:

1 A viral infection stimulates cytokine release which 'primes' neutrophils causing migra-

tion of granules containing cytolytic enzymes to the surface of the neutrophils.
2 ANCAs then bind to the enzymes (antigens) on the surface of the neutrophils, most commonly myeloperoxidase (MPO) or proteinase-3 (PR3). The formation of this ANCA–enzyme complex causes activation of neutrophils which then bind to blood vessel walls.
3 Degranulation then occurs, causing release of cytolytic enzymes which in turn causes inflammation and injury to the blood vessel wall. The resultant inflammation results in apoptosis of neutrophils and vessel endothelial cells.

ANCA is a sensitive marker and is raised in 80–90% of patients with ANCA-associated vasculitides but may also be raised in anti-GBM disease, inflammatory bowel disease, rheumatoid arthritis, hepatitis, bacterial endocarditis and cystic fibrosis, though the titre is generally less marked. ANCA may rise and fall with disease activity but must be interpreted together with clinical parameters and treatment should not be initiated purely based on the ANCA titre. A rise in ANCA should, however, prompt clinical evaluation. Immunofluorescence assay produces two major staining patterns: a diffuse cytoplasmic ANCA (c-ANCA) and the more concentrated perinuclear ANCA (p-ANCA). ANCAs are further tested by enzyme immunoassay to determine their specificity for the enzymes PR3 and MPO. Most c-ANCAs have specificity for PR3 and most p-ANCAs for MPO, though this association is not absolute. c-ANCA/PR3-ANCA is more commonly associated with Wegener's granulomatosis, p-ANCA/MPO-ANCA is more commonly associated with Churg–Strauss syndrome, and microscopic angitis is commonly associated with either.

Epidemiology

ANCA-associated vasculitides most frequently present from mid-life onwards though may occur at any age. They have a slight male preponderance and affect people from any race. The incidence is 1–2 per 100 000 population per year. Wegener's granulomatosis may be more frequent in colder climates, with the opposite being true for microscopic angitis.[2]

Clinical manifestations

Renal involvement is common in ANCA-associated vasculitides and usually presents as rapidly progressive glomerulonephritis. Table 12.1 shows the relative organ systems involved in the ANCA-associated vasculitides.[2]

Vasculitis may also present with generalised symptoms secondary to inflammation such as fever, malaise, anorexia, arthralgias and commonly a flu-like syndrome. Skin involvement is usually purpura secondary to dermal venulitis and is most commonly observed on the lower extremities. Nodular lesions are common in Wegener's granulomatosis and Churg–Strauss syndrome but rare in microscopic angitis. Nodules are caused by dermal or subcutaneous arteritis and by necrotising granulomatous inflammation.

Upper and lower respiratory tract symptoms are more common in Wegener's granulomatosis and Churg–Strauss syndrome. These conditions can also have pulmonary haemorrhage secondary to necrotising granulomatous inflammation. By definition, microscopic angitis does not have granulomatous lesions. Upper respiratory manifestations include sinusitis and rhinitis and are more common in Wegener's granulomatosis. Ocular inflammation may also occur. Destruc-tion of bone causing septal deformity requires granuloma so does not occur in microscopic angitis.

Mononeuritis multiplex is the most common neurological manifestation and is more frequent in Churg–Strauss syndrome. Gastrointestinal involvement may present as abdominal pain, blood in the stool, mesenteric ischaemia and rarely perforation. The liver and pancreas may also be affected.

Diagnosis

All ANCA-associated vasculitides are capable of producing clinically indistinguishable symptoms, so thorough clinical evaluation together with immunology screen and renal biopsy are required. Wegener's granulomatosis is characterised by granulomatous inflammation involving the respiratory tract and necrotising glomerulonephritis is common. Churg–Strauss syndrome is characterised by eosinophil-rich and granulomatous inflammation affecting the respiratory tract and is associated with asthma and eosinophilia. Microscopic angitis is characterised by necrotising glomerulonephritis and pulmonary capillaritis but is distinguished from Wegener's granulomatosis and Churg–Strauss syndrome as granulomatous lesions are absent, as is eosinophilia. Glomerulonephritis is less common in patients with Churg–Strauss syndrome.

Table 12.1 The relative organ involvement in ANCA-associated vasculitides

Organ	% Incidence		
	Microscopic angitis	Wegener's granulomatosis	Churg–Strauss syndrome
Kidney	90	80	45
Skin	40	40	60
Lungs	50	90	70
Musculoskeletal	60	60	50
CNS	30	50	70
Gastrointestinal	50	50	50
ENT	35	90	50

Adapted from ref. 2.

Prognosis of ANCA-associated vasculitides

Without treatment, the majority of patients would die within a year but with the advent of immunosuppressive regimens 84% now survive a year and 76% survive for 5 years. End stage renal failure (ESRF) develops in up to a third of patients, but the most life-threatening complication remains pulmonary haemorrhage. The higher the serum creatinine at initiation of treatment, the more likely it is that treatment will fail. Other poor prognostic signs include age over 60 years and rapidly progressive glomerulonephritis.[3]

Treatment of ANCA-associated vasculitides

Due to the high relapse rates in ANCA-associated vasculitides, long courses of immunosuppressive therapy are required which have associated complications. This toxicity is an added burden on the already immunocompromised patient with renal impairment. Treatment consists of three phases: induction, maintenance and treatment of relapses. A summary of immunosuppressive regimens is shown in Table 12.2.

Induction

Induction treatment is given for several months to patients with severe acute disease which needs to be aggressively treated to prevent rapid progression of the disease. Treatment aims to induce remission using relatively high doses of cyclophosphamide and prednisolone and usually takes 3–6 months. Induction therapy may be continued for a further three months post remission to prevent early relapse. Prednisolone dosages may be tapered during induction to reduce adverse effects. Although this combination is very effective, it is limited by long-term toxic effects, requiring alternative approaches for maintenance therapy.

Corticosteroids

In rapidly progressive disease pulsed IV methylprednisolone is given at a dose of 1 g daily for 3 days then converted to oral prednisolone 1 mg/kg/day. Pulsed methylprednisolone may be omitted in less severe disease. Efficacy relates to the suppression of the acute and chronic inflammatory processes and immune cell function. Reversible short-term adverse effects include sodium and water retention, hypertension, hyperglycaemia, CNS stimulation, peptic

---

Table 12.2   Immunosuppressive regimens in autoimmune kidney disease

Disease	Induction therapy	Maintenance therapy
ANCA-associated vasculitis	IV cyclophosphamide 15 mg/kg every 2 weeks for three doses then monthly for six months PLUS IV methylprednisolone 1 g/day for 3 days then oral prednisolone 1 mg/kg/day	Azathioprine 2 mg/kg/day PLUS low-dose prednisolone 5–10 mg/day
Goodpasture's syndrome	Plasma exchange PLUS oral cyclophosphamide 2 mg/kg/day PLUS IV methylprednisolone 1 g/day for 3 days then oral prednisolone 1 mg/kg/day	Continue oral cyclophosphamide PLUS low-dose prednisolone 5–10 mg/day
Lupus nephritis	IV cyclophosphamide 500 mg every 2 weeks for 3 months PLUS oral prednisolone 0.5–1 mg/kg/day	Azathioprine 2 mg/kg/day OR mycophenolate mofetil 1 g twice daily

ulceration and immunosuppression. Prolonged administration can lead to other adverse effects including osteoporosis, cataracts, skin fragility, myopathy, Cushingoid facies, hirsutism, alopecia and fat redistribution. The incidence of any adverse events increases with cumulative corticosteroid dose.

Gastroprotection with a proton pump inhibitor should be considered for all patients on corticosteroid therapy but particularly for those with additional risk factors such as advancing age and concomitant NSAID therapy. Osteoporosis prophylaxis should also be considered using calcium and vitamin D supplements and bisphosphonates. Bisphosphonates have been shown to reduce both bone loss and fracture rates in patients on corticosteroid therapy.[4] Although bisphosphonates are unlicensed in patients with a creatinine clearance less than 30–35 mL/min, they are used in practice, with weekly alendronate or risedronate being the agents of choice. HRT including tibolone may be considered in postmenopausal females.

Cyclophosphamide

Cyclophosphamide is a prodrug converted by hepatic microsomal enzymes to the alkylating agents 4-hydroxy-cyclophosphamide and phosphoramide mustard, which alkylate guanidine nucleotides thus blocking cell division. Significant dose reductions are required in renal impairment as 5–25% is excreted unchanged in the urine.

Intravenous therapy is the treatment of choice in most units although there is no consensus on a specific dosing regimen. A meta-analysis compared pulsed IV cyclophosphamide to daily oral cyclophosphamide and concluded that there was no difference in mortality or progression to ESRF. There was, however, a higher relapse rate following IV therapy and more adverse events following daily oral therapy.[5] Oral treatment tends only to be used when IV therapy is not possible or there has been good response to IV therapy and oral therapy is more convenient for the patient.

Bladder toxicity is caused by renal excretion of the metabolite acrolein which can cause haemorrhagic cystitis and an increased risk of bladder cancer. Mesna is used prophylactically

with IV cyclophosphamide therapy as it inactivates acrolein, thus preventing urothelial toxicity. The dose of oral mesna is 40% of the cyclophosphamide dose and is given at 2 hours before, 2 hours after and 6 hours after the cyclophosphamide infusion.

Cyclophosphamide can also lead to nausea and vomiting, myelosuppression with neutropenia, infections due to immunosuppression, alopecia and infertility. Prophylactic therapies should be used where appropriate as discussed below. The incidence of leukaemia and lymphoma is increased with prolonged administration. Sperm banking should be offered to adult male patients, where appropriate, before any exposure to cyclophosphamide. Egg retrieval and preservation methods in female patients are still under investigation and are currently not routine practice. One major drawback of egg retrieval is the time required to promote egg proliferation, which is often not compatible with the urgent clinical need for immunosuppressive treatment.

A suggested regimen is IV cyclophosphamide 15 mg/kg every two weeks for three doses then monthly for six months. The cyclophosphamide dose is generally reduced by about 25% in moderate renal impairment (creatinine clearance 10–20 mL/min) and 50% in severe renal impairment (<10 mL/min). Some units further reduce doses in elderly patients as they are more likely to suffer neutropenia and other adverse events. A full blood count should be checked 10 days after the pulse is given as this is the nadir for bone marrow suppression. Subsequent doses should be reduced or withheld if the white cell count drops below 4×10^9/L or platelet count drops below 100×10^9/L. Concomitant allopurinol should be avoided as it can increase cyclophosphamide levels and the risk of myelosuppression.

Methotrexate

The NORAM trial compared daily oral cyclophosphamide with weekly methotrexate and adjunctive prednisolone in patients with Wegener's granulomatosis and renal involvement. There was no difference between groups in achieving remission, but patients with multiorgan involvement and those with pulmonary disease took longer to achieve remission with methotrexate.[6] Overall relapse rate was also higher in the methotrexate group. In practice, methotrexate is little used in patients with renal impairment due to its high renal excretion (80–90%), which increases the risk of severe toxicity.

Infliximab and rituximab

Infliximab, a monoclonal antibody that binds to tumour necrosis factor alpha, and rituximab, a monoclonal antibody directed against the CD20 antigen on the surface of B-lymphocytes, have shown some promise as induction therapy in the treatment of ANCA-associated vasculitides where therapy with cyclophosphamide and steroids has failed. Evidence so far is limited to small studies and case reports for both agents. Further evidence is required to define the role of these new agents in clinical practice and to determine their safety profiles in this patient group.

Maintenance and relapse

The maintenance phase usually starts at least 3–6 months after initial treatment at which point cyclophosphamide therapy is usually converted to azathioprine to reduce long-term toxic effects. Azathioprine therapy may be tapered gradually and it may be possible to stop prednisolone therapy altogether. If the patient's condition relapses, treatment may be stepped back up and induction therapies added depending on the severity of the relapse. Additional therapies such as plasma exchange or IV immunoglobulins may also be required.

Azathioprine and mycophenolate

In the CYCAZAREM trial, patients received daily oral cyclophosphamide to induce remission, then one group continued cyclophosphamide therapy while the other group was converted to azathioprine. There was no difference in relapse rate and adverse effects were comparable.[7]

Azathioprine is converted in the liver to 6-mercaptopurine, which inhibits purine biosynthesis. Azathioprine also suppresses inflammatory response and lymphocyte function. Adverse effects include nausea and vomiting, dose-dependent myelosuppression and reversible cholestatic hepatotoxicity. There is an increased incidence of skin cancers and lymphomas following administration with prolonged use. Patients being treated with azathioprine should limit their sun exposure and use high-factor sun block when out in the sun. Elimination of azathioprine requires hepatic metabolism by xanthine oxidase, leading to a significant interaction with the xanthine oxidase inhibitor allopurinol. Concomitant therapy with allopurinol results in an increase in azathioprine levels of up to two-thirds, increasing the risk of toxicity unless the azathioprine dose is reduced significantly. Mycophenolate may be a useful alternative when azathioprine is not tolerated or when concomitant allopurinol is required.

Plasma exchange

The MEPEX trial involved patients with Wegener's granulomatosis or microscopic angitis presenting with rapidly progressive glomerulonephritis and investigated whether adjunctive plasma exchange was superior to methylprednisolone pulses. All patients were treated with daily oral cyclophosphamide and prednisolone and received maintenance therapy with azathioprine for a further six months. Recovery of renal function was more frequent with plasma exchange (67%) compared with the methylprednisolone group (49%).[6] The mechanism of plasma exchange may relate to the removal of ANCA. It is still unknown whether plasma exchange is helpful in other groups of patients such as those with pulmonary haemorrhage or less severe disease. In practice plasma exchange tends to be used in combination with methylprednisolone.

Immunoglobulins

Intravenous immunoglobulins may occasionally be used as an additional agent for patients with relapsing or refractory disease. Immunomodulatory doses of immunoglobulins used to treat autoimmune conditions are considerably larger than those used to treat immunodeficiency states. The usual dose is 400 mg/kg/day for 5 days. Some preparations contain sucrose, which can rarely induce osmotic injury to renal tubules and acute renal failure. Patients who may be at increased risk are those with pre-existing renal impairment, diabetes, volume depletion, sepsis, paraproteinaemia, those over 65 years and those receiving concomitant nephrotoxic drugs.

Adjunctive treatments

Anti-infectives are often used prophylactically in patients receiving cyclophosphamide therapy, and although evidence is lacking, most units use prophylactic antibiotics to some extent. The most commonly used is co-trimoxazole for prophylaxis against *Pneumocystis jiroveci* (previously known as *P. carinii*) pneumonia (PCP). If co-trimoxazole is contraindicated then dapsone may be used and both of these require dose adjustment dependent on renal function. Co-trimoxazole may reduce upper respiratory symptoms in Wegener's granulomatosis but does not affect relapse rate.[8] Fungal prophylaxis is used in some units and varies from nystatin mouthwash to oral fluconazole.

Goodpasture's syndrome

Goodpasture's syndrome is a rare hypersensitivity disorder of unknown cause, characterised by circulating anti-GBM antibodies, pulmonary haemorrhage and rapidly progressive glomerulonephritis. Goodpasture's syndrome is caused by antibodies against specific types of collagen in the glomerular and alveolar basement membranes (anti-GBM antibodies). The antibody binds to these membranes, triggering destructive inflammation which causes rapidly progressive glomerulonephritis, often with pulmonary haemorrhage. Cigarette smoking and inhalation injury are thought to prime capillaries, increasing their susceptibility to damage by anti-GBM antibodies.

Epidemiology

Goodpasture's syndrome is rare, with an estimated incidence of 1 per 2 million in white European populations. It accounts for 5% of all cases of glomerulonephritis and 10–20% of rapidly progressive glomerulonephritis cases. Patients with Goodpasture's syndrome are usually young men in their 30s or elderly

women in their 70s. Mortality without treatment is 90–95% but with aggressive treatment this falls to 10–20%. The disease occurs in any race but is most common in white Europeans.[9]

Clinical manifestations

The diagnosis of Goodpasture's syndrome is dependent on clinical symptoms, the presence of anti-GBM antibodies and the absence of other antibodies such as ANCA. It usually presents with haemoptysis, dyspnoea and rapidly progressive renal failure. Pulmonary haemorrhage may precede renal failure by months or years and almost exclusively occurs in smokers. Pulmonary haemorrhage is usually precipitated by infection and varies from mild haemoptysis to profound haemorrhage, leading to respiratory failure. Haemoglobin should be monitored as a fall may indicate active bleeding. Pulmonary haemorrhage can also occur in systemic lupus erythematosus, rheumatoid arthritis, microscopic polyarteritis and Wegener's granulomatosis, but these can usually be distinguished by specific antibody tests and renal biopsy.

As with pulmonary haemorrhage, renal failure may also occur in isolation. Renal biopsy shows rapidly progressive glomerulonephritis with crescent formation (crescentic glomerulonephritis). Immunofluorescent staining shows linear deposition of immunoglobulins and complement in the GBM and sometimes in the alveolar–capillary basement membrane. Patients presenting with severe renal injury with crescents on biopsy may not respond to treatment.

Treatment

If Goodpasture's syndrome is treated early, most patients recover and relapse is uncommon. If left untreated, however, most patients die rapidly from pulmonary haemorrhage or renal failure. Assisted ventilation and haemodialysis are often required in the acute stage. Subsequent management requires pulsed methylprednisolone with oral cyclophosphamide and repeated plasma exchange to remove circulating anti-GBM antibodies. Platelet count should be monitored as plasma exchange can lead to consumption of platelets. Fresh frozen plasma should be administered at the end of plasma exchange if the patient is at risk of bleeding. Intensive daily plasma exchange is required to adequately reduce circulating antibodies and restore renal function. Improvement is usually evident within a few days of treatment.

Maintenance immunosuppressive therapy usually continues in the form of oral cyclophosphamide 2 mg/kg/day and prednisolone 1 mg/kg/day (Table 12.2). Prednisolone therapy is maintained for at least four weeks then slowly tapered to 5–10 mg daily, which should be continued until treatment is withdrawn. Oral cyclophosphamide may be tapered by 25 mg every 2–3 months according to disease activity. Duration of treatment varies considerably and may be required for up to 18 months in some patients. Some patients progress to ESRF and require dialysis or transplantation. Recurrence of Goodpasture's syndrome after kidney transplantation is rare.[9]

Systemic lupus erythematosus

Systemic lupus erythematosus (SLE) is a chronic inflammatory connective tissue disorder of unknown cause that can affect almost any organ or system in the body. When SLE affects the kidneys it is termed lupus nephritis. SLE follows a relapsing–remitting course which varies widely from rapidly progressive to relatively benign, often with long periods of remission, interspersed with relapses termed 'flares'. SLE affects at least 12 in 100 000 people in the UK, and 90% of cases occur in women. It usually presents between the ages of 15 and 40 and is more prevalent in Afro-Caribbean and Asian populations than in the white population. Prognosis is usually good provided acute episodes are treated aggressively.[11]

Pathogenesis

The cause and pathogenesis of SLE is not completely understood but genetic, environmental and hormonal factors may be implicated in producing immunological defects. These defects give rise to antibodies to nuclear components of cells, termed antinuclear antibodies (ANAs). In contrast to Goodpasture's syndrome, ANAs are less specific and result in the deposition of immune complexes throughout the body, including the glomeruli, vasculature and skin tissue. The deposition of immune complexes causes an inflammatory response in the affected tissue.

Diagnosis

The fluorescent test for ANA is positive and high in titre in the vast majority of SLE patients, though the presence of ANA is not limited to SLE. Anti-double-stranded DNA antibodies (anti-dsDNA) are a specific diagnostic marker for SLE and are present in most patients. Disease activity may be affected by hormonal mechanisms, with flares very rare after the menopause and hormone replacement therapy (HRT) increasing flares in some patients. Drug-induced causes of SLE flares such as hydralazine should be borne in mind.

About a third of patients with lupus have antiphospholipid antibodies (APAs) in their circulation, which may increase the coagulability of blood. This increases the risk of arterial and venous thrombosis, low platelet count, miscarriages and a skin rash called livedo reticularis.

Clinical manifestations

Systemic lupus erythematosus may present abruptly with fever or develop insidiously over months or years with episodes of fever and malaise. It is a multisystem disease which can affect almost any part of the body. The American College of Rheumatology suggests that a diagnosis of SLE is likely when four or more of the following clinical features are present:[2]

- Malar rash ('butterfly' rash across the cheeks)
- Discoid rash
- Skin photosensitivity
- Oral ulcers

- Non-erosive arthritis
- Serositis
- Renal involvement (proteinuria or haematuria)
- Neurological disorder (seizures, psychosis)
- Haematological disease (leucopenia, thrombocytopenia, lymphopenia)
- Immunological disorder (anti-dsDNA antibodies, APAs)
- Raised antinuclear antibodies (ANAs).

Lupus nephritis

Around 50% of patients with SLE develop clinically evident renal disease, though this is largely benign with only a small minority of patients developing ESRF.[11] The World Health Organization has classified lupus nephritis based on the nature of glomerular lesion (Table 12.3[2]). Glomerular lesions may change over time and usually more than one type of lesion is present.

Classes I and II lupus nephritis have an excellent prognosis and are monitored but not specifically treated. Classes III and IV or proliferative lupus nephritis are more fulminant, requiring aggressive treatment to induce remission and prevent significant renal morbidity and mortality. Class IV has the worst prognosis without treatment though most patients survive with aggressive treatment. Class V, or membranous lupus, is characterised by nephrotic syndrome but treatment regimens are less well defined than classes III and IV.

Lupus nephritis flares may present as nephrotic or nephritic syndrome. Nephritic syndrome is often accompanied by low complement levels and rising anti-dsDNA antibodies. Lupus nephritis flares are common despite treatment and occur in up to two-thirds of patients. They are more common if steroids are used alone compared with when immunosupression with cyclophosphamide or mycophenolate is used. Other risk factors for lupus nephritis flares include young age, male gender, black race, severe SLE, delay in initiating treatment, delay in achieving remission, partial response to treatment and rising anti-dsDNA antibodies. Renal function can be preserved if additional immunosuppressive therapy is started early on relapse, though some patients will progress to ESRF requiring dialysis or transplantation.

Treatment

Treatment varies depending on the severity of disease. Mild lupus nephritis associated with classes I, III and V usually only requires symptomatic therapy and occasionally moderate doses of corticosteroids, for example 10–15 mg of prednisolone. More severe lupus nephritis associated with class III or IV nephritis usually requires immunosuppressive therapy. The goal of long-term immunosuppressive therapy is to suppress lupus with minimum side-effects. It is usually possible to stop treatment after several years provided the patient has stable renal function, normal immunology and no proteinuria.

Treatment of extrarenal manifestations

The most common symptoms of SLE are fatigue and pain in the joints and muscles which can be managed with NSAIDs and paracetamol. The risks and benefits of NSAIDs in patients with renal impairment should be carefully assessed and if considered essential then renal function should be closely monitored. Gastroprotection should be considered, especially if the patient is taking NSAIDs regularly or with concomitant steroids. Hydroxychloroquine is often used for cutaneous SLE or arthralgias not controlled by

Table 12.3 WHO classification of lupus nephritis

Category	Histological picture	Incidence
Class I	Normal glomeruli	<10%
Class II	Mesangial glomerulonephritis	10–20%
Class III	Focal proliferative glomerulonephritis	15–20%
Class IV	Diffuse proliferative glomerulonephritis	50%
Class V	Membranous glomerulonephritis	15%

From ref. 2.

NSAIDs and paracetamol. The dose is 200–400 mg daily which may then be reduced once control is achieved. Hydroxychloroquine is relatively safe and well tolerated. Though retinal toxicity is rare, affecting 1 in 1800 patients, patients should have annual eye tests and be referred to an ophthalmologist if there is any change in visual acuity.[12] Patients with high levels of APAs should be prescribed aspirin 75–150 mg daily as thromboprophylaxis. Patients with cerebral lupus and patients with APA who have already suffered thromboses or miscarriages should be considered for warfarin therapy as they are at risk of further thromboses.

Immunosuppression

Immunosuppressive therapy for SLE is dependent on disease severity. In lupus nephritis, treatment is similar to that for systemic vasculitis but regimens differ slightly based on evidence (see Table 12.2). As in vasculitis, studies involving infliximab and rituximab are limited, with therapy being reserved for patients with disease resistant to standard therapies. Concerns have been raised that infliximab may not be suitable in SLE due to an increased risk of developing ANA and worsening disease activity.

Corticosteroids

Mild SLE flares can be controlled with 'one-off' doses of intramuscular methylprednisolone which may avoid long-term steroid use. More acute flares may require a course of daily oral prednisolone starting at 20–30 mg daily, reducing slowly dependent on disease activity. Higher doses of steroids are reserved for more severe disease such as lupus nephritis and cerebral lupus, which require IV pulses of methylprednisolone followed by oral prednisolone 1 mg/kg/day. Hirsutism and weight gain may be particularly troublesome given that most patients are younger females.

Cyclophosphamide

Cyclophosphamide is used in combination with steroids to treat the most severe forms of SLE including lupus nephritis. Most protocols in UK

units use IV pulsed cyclophosphamide of varying frequency and dose. The Euro-Lupus Nephritis Trial compared a high-dose to a low-dose cyclophosphamide regimen and found comparable results in treatment failure, renal remission, renal flares and side-effect profiles. All patients received three pulses of methylprednisolone followed by oral prednisolone therapy. The low-dose cyclophosphamide protocol was 500 mg every two weeks for six doses compared with the high-dose regimen of 500 mg/m^2 monthly for six months then quarterly for two pulses. Azathioprine 2 mg/kg/day was started in all patients two weeks after the last cyclophosphamide pulse.[13]

Azathioprine and mycophenolate

Azathioprine is usually used to replace cyclophosphamide as maintenance therapy as in the protocol above but it may also be used to allow reduction of steroid dose in patients who have recurrent flares when the prednisolone dose is reduced. Mycophenolate mofetil may be an alternative to azathioprine and has been used in recent studies to induce remission. Mycophenolate acts by inhibiting lymphocyte proliferation, antibody formation and generation of cytotoxic T-cells. Several trials investigating its use in lupus nephritis have shown that mycophenolate may be at least as effective as oral cyclophosphamide and possibly more effective than IV pulsed cyclophosphamide therapy.[14] Although mycophenolate may cause more nausea and diarrhoea, this is usually self-limiting and is appealing, considering the more serious adverse effects with cyclophosphamide. Limitations of the above studies include variations in type and extent of renal injury amongst patients and the limited follow-up time, so further studies are warranted to confirm these findings.

IgA nephropathy

IgA nephropathy is a form of glomerulonephritis characterised by deposition of immunoglobulin A (IgA) in the GBM. IgA nephropathy is highly variable and its clinical course may vary from slow progression to rapidly progressive glomerulonephritis. Although IgA nephropathy is a non-systemic disease only affecting the kidney, IgA deposition may also be associated with systemic illnesses, most commonly Henoch–Schönlein purpura and SLE. Henoch–Schönlein purpura is a small-vessel vasculitis affecting the skin, joints, gut and kidney. It has the same renal features of IgA nephropathy but is differentiated by extrarenal features caused by tissue deposition of IgA.

Pathophysiology

Kidney biopsy shows deposition of IgA and complement in the GBM indicating that this is the result of deposition of immune complexes leading to the activation of the complement cascade. On biopsy, glomeruli may be normal, but with long standing disease there are varying degrees of glomerular sclerosis and tubulo-interstitial scarring which represent chronic kidney damage. Acute renal failure shows as necrotising glomerulonephritis with crescent formation and renal tubular occlusion with red cell casts.

Epidemiology

Distribution of IgA nephropathy varies with geographic area throughout the world and is more common in Asia than in Europe and the USA. IgA nephropathy is more common in white and Asian populations and is rare in Afro-Caribbean populations. It has a male predominance of at least 2:1 and can affect all ages, but is most common in the second and third decade of life.[15] Henoch–Schönlein purpura is most common in the first decade of life, though it may occur at any age.

Clinical features

IgA nephropathy follows a benign course in most patients, but many still progress to end stage renal disease, which develops in about 15% of patients by 10 years and 20% by 20 years.[15] IgA nephropathy may be picked up on routine blood or urine analysis as raised plasma creatinine or proteinuria but usually presents with either episodic macroscopic haematuria or persistent microscopic haematuria.

Acute renal failure with oedema, hypertension and oliguria occurs in less than 5% of patients. It can present as rapidly progressive glomerulonephritis or mild glomerular injury with macroscopic haematuria secondary to tubular damage. Chronic renal failure is usually slowly progressive, taking many years to develop to ESRF.

In IgA nephropathy, macroscopic haematuria is largely associated with upper respiratory tract infections and usually presents within 48–72 hours after the infection begins. Macroscopic haematuria may also follow tonsillectomy, vaccination, strenuous physical exercise and trauma. Between episodes of gross haematuria many patients have persistent microhaematuria, proteinuria or both. Microscopic haematuria is usually associated with proteinuria and occasionally nephrotic syndrome. Patients with microscopic haematuria have a higher risk of progressive renal failure than those with macroscopic haematuria, possibly because they are identified later. Sustained hypertension, impaired renal function and proteinuria above 1 g/day are poor prognostic signs. The symptoms and course of IgA nephropathy is influenced by the susceptibility of the glomeruli to injury which is likely to have a genetic component.

Henoch–Schönlein purpura usually begins with a palpable purpuric skin rash involving the feet, legs and arms. Most patients have a fever accompanied with polyarthralgia with associated tenderness and swelling of the ankles, knees, hips, wrists and elbows. Abdominal pain and melaena may also be present secondary to gut vasculitis. Up to half of patients will develop haematuria and proteinuria. Henoch–Schönlein purpura usually remits within four weeks of onset, but frequently recurs after a disease-free period of several weeks. In most patients the disorder subsides without serious complications; however, some patients go on to develop chronic renal failure.

Supportive treatment

Supportive treatment aims to prevent worsening of renal function and concentrates on aggressive management of hypertension and proteinuria. ACE inhibitors are the agent of choice to treat hypertension as they also have beneficial effects on proteinuria. Proteinuria should also be treated with ACE inhibitors in normotensive patients if tolerated as, in addition to their effect on blood pressure, they may decrease proteinuria by decreasing intraglomerular pressure. ACE inhibitors have been shown to preserve renal function in patients with proteinuric IgA nephropathy.[16] Angiotensin II receptor blockers can be used for patients who cannot tolerate ACE inhibitors due to persistent cough. They can also be added to maximal ACE inhibitor therapy (unlicensed), which may have an additive effect on reducing proteinuria, but whether this has further beneficial effects on renal function is not yet known.

Immunosupressive treatment

The risk benefit for immunosuppressive regimens is often unfavourable due to the slowly progressive nature of IgA nephropathy, but may be beneficial in the small minority of patients with rapidly progressive disease. Prednisolone may reduce proteinuria and preserve renal function in those patients with preserved renal function and minimal glomerular injury, though the benefit of prednisolone over aggressive supportive therapy has not yet been proven.[17] The immunosuppressive regimen of choice is usually prednisolone monotherapy, as no clear benefit has been shown with other agents. Daily oral cyclophosphamide in addition to prednisolone should be reserved for those with rapidly progressive disease.[18] Even with immunosuppression, up to half of these patient will progress to ESRF within 12 months. Patients may be switched to azathioprine once in remission, as in vasculitis and SLE, though caution should be exercised as there have been rare reports of anaemia and leucopenia with concomitant ACE inhibitor therapy and

azathioprine. Renal transplantation is effective but IgA nephropathy recurs in 20–60% of patients and usually progresses slowly, with graft loss occurring in less than 10% of patients.[15]

Treatment of Henoch–Schönlein purpura

Treatment of Henoch–Schönlein purpura is somewhat different, requiring only symptomatic management. Prednisolone may be used to treat arthralgias, abdominal pain and oedema but has no effect on the course of renal disease. Immunosuppressive regimens with cyclophosphamide with prednisolone may be beneficial in severe nephritis. Plasma exchange may also be beneficial in severe nephritis but there is little evidence to confirm this.

Membranous glomerulonephritis

Membranous glomerulonephritis is a condition that mainly affects adults and is characterised by the insidious onset of nephrotic syndrome. Patients usually have normal renal function and normal or elevated blood pressure. Membranous glomerulonephritis is usually idiopathic but may be secondary to other diseases such as SLE, hepatitis, malaria and malignancies. Drugs may also precipitate membranous glomerulonephritis, including gold, penicillamine, captopril and lithium. Membranous glomerulonephritis is thought to be due to the deposition of immune complexes in the GBM, though antigens associated with idiopathic disease have not been identified.

About a third of patients remit spontaneously without further relapses. Another third develop chronic renal impairment and a further third progress to ESRF. Patients usually present with oedema, proteinuria (>3 g/day) and occasionally haematuria and hypertension. Hypertension may be secondary to deteriorating renal function. Patients may also present with nonspecific symptoms such as anorexia, malaise and fatigue.

Supportive treatment

Asymptomatic patients should be monitored for deterioration in renal function but are not actively treated as their long-term prognosis is good. Patients with oedema are treated symptomatically with diuretics. Supportive therapies such as ACE inhibitors should be prescribed initially, adding in an angiotensin II receptor blocker if required, as in IgA nephropathy.

Immunosuppressive treatment

Immunosuppressive therapies are reserved for patients with severe symptomatic disease who are at most risk from disease progression. This includes patients with severe nephrotic syndrome (proteinuria >10 g/day) and renal impairment which cannot be controlled with supportive therapies.

Prednisolone monotherapy is not generally used as it has no effect on remission or preservation of renal function. Monotherapy with daily oral cyclophosphamide has been shown to reduce proteinuria and preserve renal function and is given at a dose of 1.5–2 mg/kg/day. Chlorambucil is an alkylating agent which can be used in an alternative regimen as below:

- Days 1–3: intravenous methylprednisolone 1 g/day
- Days 1–28: chlorambucil (0.2 mg/kg/day)
- Days 29–56: prednisolone (0.5 mg/kg/day).

This cycle is repeated for three cycles (six months in total).

For patients intolerant of cytotoxic therapy, ciclosporin may be used at 4–6 mg/kg/day but patients frequently relapse following withdrawal. There is currently no consensus on a specific immunosuppressive regimen.[19]

Membranoproliferative glomerulonephritis

Membranoproliferative glomerulonephritis is an uncommon cause of chronic glomerulonephritis mainly affecting children and young adults.

Although it can be idiopathic, it more often occurs secondary to other diseases such as SLE, cryoglobulinaemia, hepatitis and some malignancies. Membranoproliferative glomerulonephritis is characterised by chronic immune complex deposition in the glomerulus causing glomerulosclerosis. The antibodies thought to be involved in its pathogenesis are known as nephritic factors, most commonly C3 nephritic factor.

Clinical manifestations

Membranoproliferative glomerulonephritis presents with nephrotic syndrome in the vast majority of patients and is usually accompanied by microscopic haematuria. Occasionally macroscopic haematuria, acute renal failure and hypertension occur. Kidney biopsy is required to confirm diagnosis and differentiate the disease from membranous nephropathy. In general the long-term prognosis is poor, with ESRF occurring in 50% of patients by 3–5 years and 75% by 10 years.

Treatment

Treatment strategies are variable due to the scarcity of randomised controlled trials. Supportive treatment is the same as that for membranous nephropathy, though there is little evidence to support prednisolone or other immunosuppressive therapy in these patients. Antiplatelet therapy is the only intervention shown to be of benefit in adult patients with membranoproliferative glomerulonephritis. The probable mechanism for antiplatelet therapy is platelet inhibition and altered renal haemodynamics. Combination therapy with aspirin and dipyridamole is usually the drug regimen of choice.[20]

Cryoglobulinaemic glomerulonephritis

Cryoglobulins are immunoglobulins that undergo reversible precipitation when plasma is cooled while flowing through small blood vessels. Cryoglobulin immune complexes may deposit in any part of the body, resulting in inflammation and vasculitis. Cryoglobulinaemic glomerulonephritis occurs when cryoglobulin immune complexes deposit in the glomerular capillaries. The survival rate for patients with renal impairment is around 60% at 5 years from diagnosis. The occurrence of cryoglobulins may be idiopathic but is strongly associated with hepatitis C infection, and may also be seen in other autoimmune diseases including SLE.

Clinical manifestations

Skin involvement is very common, including purpura and Raynaud's phenomenon, and is due to the precipitation of immune complexes in the small blood vessels of the skin. Ischaemic necrosis of the skin may also occur. Arthralgia and myalgia are common but progressive arthritis is very rare. Pulmonary involvement may result in dyspnoea and cough. Abdominal pain may be present secondary to vasculitis affecting the gut. Arterial thrombosis, though rare, can occur secondary to increased serum viscosity. Renal failure may present with isolated haematuria, proteinuria or nephrotic syndrome and is a serious complication, following a progressive course similar to that of membranoproliferative glomerulonephritis.

Treatment

Patients with myalgia or arthralgia may be treated with paracetamol or, if necessary, NSAIDs, though these must be used with caution in renal impairment. Patients with mild to moderate arthritis may respond to low doses of steroids with or without hydroxychloroquine. If there is evidence of renal disease or vasculitis immunosuppressive therapy may be required. Combination therapy with oral cyclophosphamide and prednisolone are the agents of choice as discussed under ANCA-associated vasculitis. Life-threatening disease requires plasma exchange in addition to immunosuppression.

If there is a secondary cause then the main focus of therapy is to treat the underlying disease. SLE should be treated as discussed earlier. Cryoglobulinaemic glomerulonephritis is associated with hepatitis C infection in the vast majority of patients and should be treated with pegylated interferon and ribavirin, though expert opinion should be sought.[21]

Conclusions

Autoimmune kidney disease covers a wide range of diseases which cause varying degrees of renal dysfunction from mild renal impairment to life-threatening rapidly progressive glomerulonephritis. Rapidly progressive disease always requires immunosuppressive therapies which carry their own risks and managing the toxic effects of these agents may be just as challenging as managing the disease itself. Less severe disease may not require immunosuppressants at all, so the risks and benefits of treatment should be weighed carefully against the severity of disease.

CASE STUDIES

Case 1

Mrs X is 74 years old and is admitted to the nephrology ward with acute renal failure (GFR <10 mL/min) and haemoptysis. A full immunology screen is positive for c-ANCA in high titre and the chest X-ray shows evidence of granulomatous lesions.

Q1. What diagnosis is most likely to be made?

Q2. What initial treatment would you recommend?

Q3. How would you monitor this therapy?

Q4. What adjunctive therapies would you consider for this patient?

Q5. What advice would you give to the patient regarding their new treatment regimen?

Case 2

Mr Y, aged 22 years, is admitted to the nephrology ward for control of hypertension. Urinalysis is positive for microscopic haematuria and proteinuria. On routine blood chemistry serum creatinine is raised at 167 μmol/L.

Q1. What drug therapy would you suggest?

Q2. What is the target blood pressure for this patient?

Six months later Mr Y is readmitted with persistent hypertension despite supportive therapy. A 24-hour urine collection is performed showing a protein excretion of 2 g/day and a creatinine clearance of 36 mL/min. The consultant advises a kidney biopsy which shows IgA and complement deposition in the GBM.

Q3. What is the prognosis for Mr Y?

Q4. What further drug therapy would you recommend?

References

1. *The Merck Manual*, 17th edn. 1999, Section 17, Chapter 224, p. 1857.
2. Feehally J, Johnson K. *Comprehensive Clinical Nephrology*, 2nd edn. London: Harcourt, 2003, Section 5 Chapters 26 and 27.
3. Booth A, Almond MK, Burns A *et al.* Outcome of ANCA-associated renal vasculitis: a 5-year retrospective study. *Am J Kidney Dis* 2003; 41: 776–784.
4. Royal College of Physicians. *Glucocorticoid-induced Osteoporosis*. London: Royal College of Physicians, December 2002.
5. de Groot K, Dwomoa A, Savage C. The value of pulse cyclophosphamide in ANCA associated vasculitis: meta analysis and critical review. *Nephrol Dial Transplant* 2001; 16: 2018–2027.
6. de Groot K, Jayne D. What is new in the therapy of ANCA-associated vasculitides? *Clin Nephrol* 2005; 64: 480–484.
7. Jayne D, Rasmussen N, Andrassy K *et al.* A randomized trial of maintenance therapy for

vasculitis associated with antineutrophil cytoplasmic autoantibodies. *N Engl J Med* 2003; 349: 36–44.

8. Stegeman C, Cohen Tervaert JW, de Jong PE, Kallenberg CGM and the Dutch Co-trimoxazole Wegener Study Group. Co-trimoxazole for the prevention of relapses of Wegener's granulomatosis. *N Engl J Med* 1996; 335: 16–20.

9. Kluth D, Rees A. Anti-glomerular basement membrane disease. *J Am Soc Nephrol* 1999; 10: 2446–2453.

10. *The Merck Manual of Diagnosis and Therapy*, 18th edn. 2007, Chapter 5 Section 50.

11. Hildebrand J. Systemic lupus erythematosus. *E-Medicine* 2005; updated 21 November.

12. Rahman A. Drug treatment of systemic lupus erythematosus. *Hosp Pharm* 2001; 8: 69–73.

13. Houssiau FA, Vasconcelos C, D'Cruz D *et al*. Immunosuppressive therapy in lupus nephritis: the Euro-Lupus Nephritis Trial, a randomized control trial of low-dose versus high dose intravenous cyclophosphamide. *Arthritis Rheum* 2002; 46: 2121–2131.

14. Ginzler E, Aranow C. Mycophenolate mofetil in lupus nephritis. *Lupus* 2005; 14: 59–64.

15. Brake M, Somers D. IgA Nephropathy. *eMedicine* 2006, updated 23 August.

16. Praga M, Gutiérrez E, González E *et al*. Treatment of IgA nephropathy with ACE inhibitors: a randomized controlled trial. *J Am Soc Nephrol* 2003; 14: 1578–1583.

17. Pozzi C, Andrulli S, Del Vecchio L *et al*. Corticosteroid effectiveness in IgA nephropathy: long-term results of a randomized controlled trial. *J Am Soc Nephrol* 2004; 15: 157–163.

18. Samuels J. Immunosuppressive agents for treating IgA nephropathy (review). *The Cochrane Library*, 2006 Issue 3.

19. Ponticelli C, Passerini P. Treatment of membranous nephropathy. *Nephrol Dial Transplant* 2001; 16 (Suppl 5): 8–10.

20. Kathuria P. Membranoproliferative glomerulonephritis. *eMedicine* 2006; updated 11 April.

21. Edgerton C. Cryoglobulinaemia. *eMedicine* 2006; updated 26 January.

13

Paediatric kidney disease

Susan Patey

This chapter provides a guide to the particular challenges that face the paediatric renal pharmacist from the initial calculation of glomerular filtration rate to dosing and administration of medicines. It will deal with chronic renal failure and its progression to end stage, dialysis and transplantation.

Many medicines are not approved for paediatrics either because explicit approval has not been obtained by the manufacturers as studies have not been performed in children or because of toxic effects on development as observed in animal experiments (e.g. quinolones). Some of these medicines, however, are used in vital indications by paediatricians, thus licensed preparations may be used 'off label' and some preparations suitable for paediatrics may be made by specials manufacturers (unlicensed).

The issue of licensing of medicines for children is being addressed by the European Commission. In its section on medicines, the National Service Framework for Children published in October 2004,[1] envisages that all children and young people will receive medicines that are safe and effective in formulations that can be easily administered, are appropriate to their age and have minimum impact on their education and lifestyle. Children, young people and their parents or carers need to be well-informed and supported to make choices about their medicines and to become competent in the administration of medicines. Children with chronic renal failure are often required to take a large number of different medicines, which are then replaced by another set of medicines following a renal transplant.

The causes of chronic kidney disease in children are very different to those in adults, as most children with renal failure have been born with abnormal kidneys (e.g. polycystic or dysplastic kidneys). Less commonly, an illness can cause damage to the kidneys during childhood (e.g. lupus nephritis, haemolytic uraemic syndrome, Henoch–Schönlein purpura nephropathy). Occasionally, there may be a genetic cause such as cystinosis, a metabolic disease or congenital nephrotic syndrome, which often requires bilateral nephrectomy.

As in adults, the markers for renal function are creatinine and glomerular filtration rate (GFR).

Creatinine and glomerular filtration rate

Creatinine is a very good marker of kidney function, but because it comes from muscle, the blood level is dependent on the size of the child in addition to how well the kidneys are working. Therefore, the creatinine level in an adult would be higher compared with that in a child and, similarly, a higher level would be found in a child than in a baby. One would expect the creatinine to rise throughout childhood until adulthood is reached. For this reason the Cockroft and Gault equation for calculating GFR is unsuitable for use in paediatric patients. An alternative formula which provides a good approximation of GFR in children is that derived by Morris *et al.* in 1982 using height/serum creatinine:[2]

$$\text{GFR (mL/min)} \text{ (corrected to } 1.73 \text{ m}^2) = \frac{40 \times \text{height (cm)}}{\text{Serum creatinine (µmol/L)}}$$

163

(Creatinine level of 1 mg/mL = 88.5 μmol/L)
This equation cannot be applied to infants and neonates.

As the Morris equation is corrected for body surface area, the resultant GFR in mL/min does not require further manipulation when making dosage decisions based on references that utilise GFRs that have been normalised to 1.73 m² (e.g. Guy's and St Thomas' Paediatric Formulary, *British National Formulary for Children*, Daschner's paediatric dosing tables).[3]

Others have identified methods of estimating GFR in children without the use of height or weight.[4]

The normal range of GFR is 80–120 mL/min/1.73 m². A GFR between 60 to 80 is usually considered to indicate mild chronic renal failure (CRF), 30–60 moderate, and below 30 severe CRF. When the GFR falls below 15 mL/min/1.73 m², dialysis or transplantation is usually necessary.

GFR is low at birth, averaging 3 mL/min/1.73 m² in the term baby, rapidly increases during the first six months of life and then increases gradually to adult values by 1–2 years. In the neonatal period the GFR may be standardised to body weight as this correction produces less variability (Table 13.1).

Usually when both kidneys are affected and the GFR is below normal, the kidney function gets progressively worse, although this does not always happen and it may remain stable for many years, or even improve, especially in the first year of life. Abnormal kidneys may not be able to grow as the child grows, and therefore become progressively smaller relative to the child's body size. This may be particularly the case during puberty, when the child is growing very fast, so this may be a time when kidney function declines more rapidly. Many children with abnormal kidneys are unable to concentrate their urine so pass very large volumes. They therefore need to drink a lot to compensate, particularly if they have extra fluid losses such as with diarrhoea, vomiting or fever.

Monitoring and treatment of children with chronic renal failure

Nutrition and growth

Chronic renal failure can affect growth, mainly due to poor nutrition, which may be because of reduced appetite or vomiting. All infants and children CRF should be referred to a dietician. The aim is produce a diet that will control symptoms and prevent complications, particularly uraemia and renal bone disease, and will promote optimum growth but will preserve residual renal function. Tube feeding or a gastrostomy is often required to supplement oral intake. Height, weight and head circumference

---

Table 13.1 Approximate GFR based on age, weight and body surface area

	Weight (kg)	BSA (m²)	GFR	
			mL/min	mL/min/1.73 m²
Premature infants	1.0	0.1	0.2	3.5
Newborns	2.0	0.15	0.5	6.0
	3.2	0.2	1.5	13.0
1 month	4.0	0.25	7.5	52.0
3 months	6.0	0.35	11.0	54.0
1 year	9.2	0.45	30.0	115.0
10 years	30.0	1.0	70.0	120.0
Adults	70.0	1.73	120.0	120.0

BSA, body surface area; GFR, glomerular filtration rate.
From ref. 5.

must be plotted on a growth chart to monitor growth and development. If vomiting is a problem, domperidone may be prescribed at a dose of 200–400 µg/kg three to four times a day, although this should be used with caution in infants under one month of age due to the possibility of extrapyramidal side-effects (this indication is unlicensed for use in children). Very rarely, if growth is poor despite optimum nutrition, growth hormone may be prescribed.

Blood pressure

Blood pressure varies with age. It can be low in some children with CRF as their kidneys 'leak' salt and water. These children usually need to drink a lot and may need sodium chloride supplements. A 1 mmol in 1 mL solution is available as a 'special' and should be given orally, initially at a dose of 1–2 mmol sodium/kg/day in 3–4 divided doses and adjusted as necessary.

Children who are salt losers or able to deal with salt normally may develop problems as their renal function declines.

Some children are unable to lose salt and water as they should and consequently will need to reduce their salt intake. These children are likely to develop high blood pressure and will need appropriate treatment (diuretic, calcium channel blocker, angiotensin-converting enzyme (ACE) inhibitor etc.).

The measurement of blood pressure in children, particularly the younger age group, requires practice and specialist paediatric skills and knowledge. The US Task Force report on blood pressure is a good reference source, which takes into consideration the child's gender, age and height percentiles.[6]

The focus here is to use medicines that preferably can be used once daily, maximising treatment dosage before adding a further medicine. Compliance in infants and children can be a particular problem as they are often on multiple medicines. The agent(s) used will be from the following groups: ACE inhibitor; beta-blocker; calcium channel blocker; diuretic. A beta-blocker should not be used alone as first-line therapy (Table 13.2).

The clinical situation, including the presence of any proteinuria, will determine which group is used initially. If the GFR is <10 mL/min/1.73 m^2 always start with the lowest dose.

For infants (less than 1 year old) use shorter acting agents for flexibility of dosage: propranolol instead of atenolol; captopril instead of enalapril (Table 13.3). Once stable, the patient may be changed to the longer acting antihypertensive agent.

Proteinuria

The presence of protein in the urine has been shown to increase the rate of decline of renal function. An ACE inhibitor or angiotensin II receptor blocker may be prescribed.

Bicarbonate

The kidneys are responsible for regulating the acidity of the blood. Sodium bicarbonate may need to be prescribed. For chronic replacement a 1 mmol in 1 mL solution is available as a 'special'. The initial oral dose is 1–2 mmol/kg/day for infants and 70 mmol/m^2/day for older children, given in 2–4 divided doses and adjusted according to plasma levels.

Urea

Urea is produced when protein in the diet is broken down so that it can be used in the body for growth. The urea level will therefore depend upon the protein and calorie intake in the diet. It will rise if the protein intake is very high or the calorie intake is very low, as this reflects the breakdown of protein from muscle as a source of energy. A high urea level can make a child feel very ill. The dietitian will provide advice on controlling the urea level. The aim is to keep plasma levels below 20 mmol/L or below 30 mmol/L in children over 10 years of age.

Calcium, phosphate and parathyroid hormone

The kidneys are responsible for maintaining a healthy balance of calcium, phosphate and vita-

Table 13.2 Long-term treatment of hypertension in children and adolescents as used at Great Ormond Street Hospital, London

Drug	Route	Normal starting dose	Normal and maximum dose range	Divided doses in a day	Preparations and comments
Amlodipine	Oral	100–200 µg/kg per dose	1.25 mg (body weight 6–15 kg) 2.5 mg (body weight 15–25 kg) 5 mg (body weight >25 kg)	1	Tablets 5 mg, 10 mg Tablets may be dispersed in water and still maintain long acting effect
Atenolol[a]	Oral	1 mg/kg per dose	1–2 mg/kg/day Maximum 100 mg/day or 50 mg/day when GFR <10 mL/min/1.73 m^2	1	Tablets 25, 50, 100 mg Syrup 25 mg in 5 mL Caution in asthma although cardioselective
Enalapril	Oral	100 µg/kg per dose	200–500 µg/kg in a day Maximum 600 µg/kg in a day or 40 mg/day	1	Tablets 2.5 mg, 5 mg, 10 mg Commencing treatment in pregnancy and hyperkalaemia contraindicated Caution in renal artery stenosis and when GFR <30 mL/min/1.73 m^2 Avoid in neonates – especially premature
Furosemide	Oral	500 µg/kg per dose	1–4 mg/kg/day	1–4	Tablets 20 mg, 40 mg Syrup 50 mg in 5 mL

[a] Recent studies in adults[8,9] and NICE recommend that atenolol should not be used alone as first-line therapy.

min D in the body to ensure strong and healthy bones. The kidneys are responsible for getting rid of the phosphate from food. Phosphate is present in protein-containing food, particularly dairy products. In CRF the level of phosphate in the blood rises, which causes increased production of the parathyroid hormone (PTH). An excessive level of PTH causes damage to the bones, the bone marrow and the lining of the blood vessels. The amount of phosphate in the diet should therefore be controlled. Treatment is started if the plasma phosphate is above 1.7 mmol/L or above 2 mmol/L in neonates. A phosphate binder such as calcium carbonate, (licensed as Calcichew, Adcal, unlicensed as dispersible tablets and suspension), calcium acetate ('off label') or, if the calcium level is high, magnesium carbonate (unlicensed) or sevelamer ('off label') is given with food to bind the dietary phosphate in the gut and stop its absorption.

In infants the phosphate binder may be added to the feed but must be mixed well to avoid precipitation. The dose is tailored to the child's phosphate level and can appear to be a very large dose. If the child is receiving an overnight feed a proportionately larger dose of the phosphate binder may be added to that feed.

In kidney failure calcium is lost from the bones and thus the body so the calcium level needs to be maintained. Some calcium may be derived from the calcium in the phosphate binder but often a vitamin D preparation such as alfacalcidol will also be prescribed and this will raise the serum calcium by increasing gastrointestinal calcium absorption. Alfacalcidol which is available as a liquid in addition to capsules should only be prescribed in nanograms or micrograms, not millilitres.

Even if blood calcium and phosphate levels are brought under control, high PTH levels can

Table 13.3 Antihypertensive agents for infants less than 1 year old

Drug	Route	Normal starting dose	Normal and maximum dose range	Divided doses in a day	Preparations and comments
Captopril	Oral	50 µg/kg per dose	0.5–3 mg/kg/day Maximum 6 mg/kg/day	3	Tablets 2 mg, 12.5 mg, 25 mg Very soluble in water Caution in renal artery stenosis, hyperkalaemia and when GFR <30 mL/min/1.73 m^2 Test dose required
Propranolol	Oral	1 mg/kg per dose	1–4 mg/kg/day Maximum 8 mg/kg/day	3	Syrup 50 mg in 5 mL Contraindicated in asthma and heart failure When GFR <20 mL/min/1.73 m^2 start at lower dose

Various reference sources used: Great Ormond Street Hospital, Guy's and St.Thomas' Formulary etc.

also be caused by the lack of the active form of vitamin D. Vitamin D from food (and sunlight) needs to be activated by the kidney, so the more usable form alfacalcidol is given.

Renal bone disease begins very early in kidney failure so it is important that the blood PTH is measured regularly, in addition to the frequent monitoring of calcium and phosphate. The PTH should be in the range 0.7–5.6 pmol/L.

Anaemia (haemoglobin and iron levels)

The kidney is responsible for making the hormone erythropoietin, necessary for making red blood cells. Children with CRF often become anaemic and the level of haemoglobin in the blood falls. Erythropoietin is usually given as a subcutaneous injection once a week, or intravenously three times a week if on haemodialysis. Iron also needs to be given, either orally or intravenously.

The National Institute for Health and Clinical Excellence (NICE) has produced a clinical practice guideline on 'Anaemia management in people with chronic kidney disease'.[7] The guidance states that for children aged 2 years and older, haemoglobin range should be maintained at the target range for adults (i.e. between 10.5 and 12.5 g/dL), and for children aged under 2 years treatment should maintain stable haemoglobin levels between 10 and 12 g/dL (Table 13.4).

Use intravenous iron if persistently low ferritin levels are recorded (<100 µg/L) despite

Table 13.4 Evaluation of anaemia as used at Great Ormond Street Hospital, London

Age	Normal (standard deviation) range for haemoglobin (g/dL)	Evaluate for anaemia when the haemoglobin falls to (g/dL)
< 6 months	11.5 (9.5–13.5)	<10
6–24 months	12.0 (10.5–13.5)	<11
By 12 years of age	13.5 (11.5–15.5)	<12

Table 13.5 Target haemoglobin levels	
Age	Target haemoglobin (g/dL)
<6 months	> 9.5
6–24 months	>10
>2 years	>10.5

oral iron. Haemoglobin should be measured once or twice a month and iron status every three months.

Children should achieve their target haemo-globin within six months of being seen by a paediatric nephrologist, unless there is a specific reason (Table 13.5).

All children should achieve a serum ferritin of >100 and <800 µg/L whether or not they are receiving epoetin. The NICE clinical guideline contains an overview outlining the key stages of managing anaemia in chronic kidney disease (CKD).[7]

Figure 13.1 describes the management of renal anaemia in children at Great Ormond Street Hospital, including commencement of erythropoietin therapy.

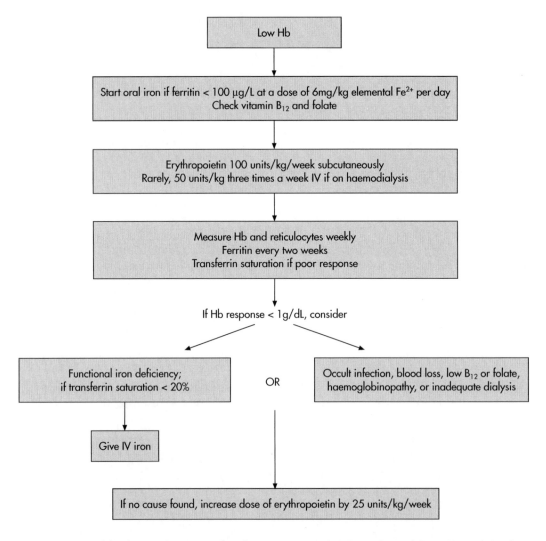

Figure 13.1   Protocol for the commencement of erythropoietin as used at Great Ormond Street Hospital, London.

Table 13.6 Dose of folic acid

Age	Dose
Infants	250 µg/kg once daily
Children 1–5 years	2.5 mg daily
Children >5years	5 mg daily

Folic acid

Folic acid is also needed to make red blood cells but also seems to have a protective effect on the heart and blood vessels. The dosage used in children is shown in Table 13.6.

Potassium

Progressive renal failure can be associated with potassium retention. Hyperkalaemia generally does not occur until GFR is <10% of normal, however regular biochemical assessment must be carried out in all patients. Possible causes of hyperkalaemia include: inadequate energy intake; medicines such as the ACE inhibitors or the potassium-sparing diuretic spironolactone; a high dietary intake of potassium; constipation.

Transplantation

Ideally transplantation should be carried out before dialysis for the following reasons:

- A successful transplant is the best treatment for children as it makes their lives as normal as possible.
- Long-term mortality is lower with a transplant than on dialysis.
- The risk of calcium deposits in blood vessels with long-term blood vessel damage is high on dialysis.
- It is important to preserve access points for dialysis (arm and leg veins for haemodialysis, peritoneum for peritoneal dialysis) for future use.

Transplantation without dialysis may not always be possible in some conditions that require bilateral nephrectomies and/or a period of dialysis (e.g. in focal and segmental glomerulosclerosis). Transplantation in the child is often live-related (i.e. the kidney is taken from a living relative) so can be pre-emptive.

Pre-transplantation all vaccines must be up to date (including BCG, hepatitis B, varicella). Glandular fever (EBV) vaccine may be available soon. An accelerated immunisation procedure may be carried out so that the child is ready for transplantation by the age of 19–24 months (Tables 13.7 and 13.8).

At Great Ormond Street Hospital, the following guidelines on immunisation for infants and children with CRF are used:

- All children must complete all routine childhood vaccines.
- BCG, varicella, pneumococcal and hepatitis B vaccines must be added in children approaching dialysis and transplantation.
- Immunisations must begin as soon as possible in the child born with severe CRF (including infants with congenital nephrotic syndrome) as the schedule can rarely be completed before 18 months of age.
- Only in exceptional circumstances can transplantation occur without completing the full schedule.

Important general points:

- Routine immunisation in the first year of life is with the following vaccines: diphtheria, tetanus, acellular pertussis (DTaP), inactivated polio, *Haemophilus influenzae* type b conjugate (Hib) (Pediacel), pneumococcal vaccine (Prevenar) and meningococcal group C conjugate.
- Before school or nursery school entrance (but preferably one year after completing the primary course) a booster of diphtheria, tetanus, acellular pertussis and inactivated polio should be given.
- Measles, mumps and rubella (MMR) vaccination may be given at 13 and 16 months in the infant in or approaching end stage renal failure (ESRF).
- Over 10 years of age give a booster dose of low-dose diphtheria, tetanus and inactivated polio and MMR.

Table 13.7 Immunisation schedule for infants and children with chronic renal failure (GFR <60 mL/min/1.73 m²) as used at Great Ormond Street Hospital, London

Age (months) (Can be varied)	BCG SSI (Statens Serum Institut)[a]	Diphtheria, tetanus, acellular pertussus (DTaP), Haemophilus influenzae type b (Hib) and inactivated polio (IPV) (Pediacel) Deep SC or IM	7-valent Pneumococcal conjugated vaccine (Prevenar) IM	Meningococcal group C conjugate Deep SC or IM	Hepatitis B[b] IM	MMR (measles, mumps and rubella) Deep SC or IM	Varicella-zoster vaccine SC	Influenza vaccine IM
0	✓ Or at any time up to 6 years of age with no skin test (Mantoux) required, unless born in or visited a high-incidence country							
2		✓	✓					
3		✓		✓				
4		✓	✓	✓				
6					✓ (0.5 mL)			Given each autumn for at-risk patients >6 months old.
7					✓ (0.5 mL)			
12		✓ (Hib no DTaP/IPV)		✓	✓ (0.5 mL)			
13	Over the age of 6 years only if negative tuberculin skin test (Mantoux); delay transplant for 3 months	If not previously immunised: 1–10 years give 1 dose of Hib (but for full cover should have had 3 doses of Pediacel)	✓ If not previously immunised: 12 months–5 years: 2 doses separated by 2 months interval >5 years: conjugate vaccine is NOT given		Booster doses may be required	✓ If not predicted for ESRF can have 2nd dose with pre-school booster		
16						✓		
18							✓ if booster required	

[a] For notes on intradermal dose see Table 13.8.

[b] For notes on accelerated immunisation schedule see Table 13.8.

After second birthday, single dose of 23-valent pneumococcal polysaccharide vaccine (Pneumovax II).

Before school or nursery school entry if not 'on call': Booster doses of diphtheria, tetanus, acellular pertussis, inactivated polio (Infanrix-IPV, Repevax).

Over 10 years of age: Booster dose of low-dose diphtheria, tetanus and inactivated polio (Revaxis). If schedule followed at 19 months proceed to transplant.

Table 13.8   Notes on immunisation schedule for infants and children with chronic renal failure

Vaccine	Comments
BCG SSI (Statens Serum Institut)	May be given to some newborns routinely
	Can be given up to the age of 6 years without a prior Mantoux test, unless born in or visited (>1 month) a high-incidence country. Over the age of 6 years give only if tuberculin skin test (Mantoux) negative (NB Tuberculin testing should not be carried out within 3 weeks of receiving a live vaccine as response may be falsely negative)
Age <12 months	BCG dose 0.05 mL by intradermal injection
Age >12 months	BCG dose 0.1 mL by intradermal injection
	May be given simultaneously with another live vaccine but if not given at the same time, allow an interval of at least 3 weeks
	In neonates the vaccine must be given intradermally into the upper arm only (preferably the left deltoid region). Do not use the same arm for further immunisation for 3 months
	Delay transplantation for 3 months after BCG
Hepatitis B	All patients who will need ESRF management should be immunised against hepatitis B, preferably pre-emptively while the GFR remains relatively high
	Can be given at any age at intervals of 0, 1 and 6 months
	An accelerated course can be used so that the third dose is given 2 months after the first dose (i.e. doses at 0, 1 and 3 months and a booster dose at 12 months)
	For IM administration: The anterolateral thigh (IM) is the preferred site in infants and young children. The deltoid muscle is the preferred site in older children. It should not be injected into the buttock as vaccine efficacy is reduced
Dose for pre-dialysis patients: Engerix B (GlaxoSmithKline) by IM injection	
Birth to 10 years	3 doses of 0.5 mL (10 µg)
Age 10–15 years	3 doses of 1 mL (20 µg)
HB-Vax Pro (Aventis Pasteur) by IM injection	
Under 10 years	3 doses of 0.5 mL (5 µg)
Age 10–15 years	increase dose to 1 mL (10 µg)
	These doses should be doubled for patients on dialysis and 4 doses given at 0, 1, 2 and 6 months
	Check anti HBsAg antibodies 2–3 months after the third dose
	Dialysis patients should be monitored annually and revaccinated if necessary
Antibodies	
100 iu/L	Protective – give booster every 5 years
10–100 iu/L	Poor responder – give booster at 1 and 5 years
<10 iu/L	Non-responder – repeat course of vaccine
MMR	Give at 13 months (0.5 mL by deep SC or by IM injection). If ESRF not imminent, 2nd MMR can be given with pre-school booster. If in ESRF, 2nd MMR can be given at 16 months of age (interval of at least 3 months after 1st vaccine)

(continued overleaf)

Table 13.8   (continued)

Vaccine	Comments
MMR (continued)	Children <4 years old with a GFR <30 mL/min/1.73 m² should have their pre-school/nursery school booster (2nd MMR) brought forward. Older children – a 2nd MMR is advised unless there is definite serological evidence of immunity. If administering at the same time as other injections, use a separate syringe and needle; give MMR first as it is less painful, and use a different limb. Alternatively, a second appointment can be made. Other live vaccines may either be given on the same day or at least 3 weeks later
	Check measles antibody response 2–4 weeks after completing MMR course
	An initial negative or equivocal antibody result should be repeated. In vaccinated children who have had a previously positive measles IgG but are found to be negative/equivocal on retesting, the conventional wisdom is that primed memory cells will respond to a measles challenge. However, if blood or blood products have been given 3 months prior to the test, the measles IgG may be transiently positive and a retest will be required
	Delay transplantation for 1 month after MMR course
Varicella vaccine (Varilrix or Varivax)	Can be given with, or 4 weeks after MMR vaccine if non-immune (check titres). Ensure lymphocyte count >1.2 × 10⁹/L
	Delay for 3 months if patient has received immunoglobulin or a blood transfusion because of likelihood of vaccine failure due to passively acquired varicella antibodies
	Salicylates should be avoided for 6 weeks after varicella vaccination as Reye's syndrome has been reported following the use of salicylates during natural varicella infection
	In 'healthy' patients if a measles containing vaccine is not given at the same time as the varicella vaccine an interval of at least one month must elapse between vaccines. Measles vaccination may lead to short-lived suppression of the cell mediated response
Dose:	
Age >12 months–12 years	1 dose (0.5 mL) SC (upper arm-deltoid region). May need a booster dose after an interval of 2 months
Age >13 years	2 doses with an interval between doses of 4–8 weeks
	In high-risk patients additional doses might be required
	Check titres (ELISA) after 2–3 months. If no seroconversion a second dose is given
	Delay transplantation for 1 month after vaccination course if seroconversion demonstrated
Pneumococcal vaccines	
Saccharide conjugated vaccine-7-valent (Prevenar)	Previously recommended for immunosuppressed children aged 2 months to 5 years or who have CRF and/or nephrotic syndrome, although now routine in the UK at 2 and 4 months (with DTP/IPV and Hib) and at 13 months (with MMR)
For previously unvaccinated older infants and children:	
Age 6 months–12 months	2 doses (0.5 mL) at least a month apart. A third dose is recommended after the 1st birthday
Age 12 months to 5 years	2 doses (0.5 mL) with an interval of at least 2 months between doses
	The vaccine is not necessary in children over 5 years of age

→

Table 13.8 (continued)

Vaccine	Comments
Pneumococcal vaccines (continued) Pneumococcal polysaccharide vaccine-23-valent (Pneumovax II)	
All children between 2 and 5 years	who have received the pneumococcal saccharide vaccine need a single dose (0.5 mL) to provide protection against the serotypes of *Str. pneumoniae* not covered in the conjugate vaccine
	Leave an interval of at least 2 months between the two vaccines
Children >5 years	need a single dose
Children >10 years	can be revaccinated if high risk (e.g. nephrotic syndrome)
Influenza vaccine	Annual vaccination is recommended from the age of 6 months

For up to date information refer to the Department of Health website at www.doh.gov. uk and to the vaccine manufacturer's literature.

NICE has recently published its final appraisal determination on immunosuppressive therapy for renal transplantation in children and adolescents.[10] Between April 2003 and March 2004 approximately 130 patients (7% of those who underwent renal transplantation) were under 18 years of age. The document recognises that organ transplantation is not considered fully successful for children and adolescents unless they grow and develop as normal after transplantation. Concordance due to complex medication regimens and/or associated side-effects may be a problem. The document considers the use of: the induction agents basiliximab and daclizumab; the calcineurin inhibitors ciclosporin and tacrolimus; and azathioprine and corticosteroids. The use of mycophenolate mofetil in corticosteroid reduction or withdrawal strategies is recommended only within the context of randomised clinical trials, mycophenolate sodium is currently not recommended and sirolimus is only recommended when proven intolerance to calcineurin inhibitors (including nephrotoxicity) necessitates the complete withdrawal of these treatments.

The document also recognises that some medicines may be prescribed outside the terms of their UK marketing authorisation. 'Health-care professionals prescribing these medicines should ensure that children and adolescents receiving renal transplants and/or their legal guardians are aware of this, and that they consent to the use of these medicines in these circumstances.'[10]

Each paediatric unit will have its own renal transplant protocol, which will be continually subject to trials of combinations of drugs to optimise the preservation of the graft with minimal side-effects. In children the use of steroids and their effect on linear growth is a major factor in considering the rapid reduction of steroids or steroid-free immunosuppressant regimens. As the regimens are complex they will not be discussed here.

Patients are continually monitored for infection, including viral infections and opportunistic protozoal, fungal and bacterial infections, post-transplant lymphoproliferative disorders, de novo post-transplant diabetes mellitus and evidence of rejection.

Dialysis

Waste products are cleared from the blood by diffusion. The strong solution, blood containing creatinine and urea, passes to the weaker solution, the dialysate. Excess water is removed by ultrafiltration. In peritoneal dialysis glucose from the dialysate draws water from the blood; in haemodialysis the machine draws water from the blood. Waste and water pass into the dialysis fluid (dialysate) for removal from the body. The dialysis membrane keeps the dialysis fluid and blood apart. In peritoneal dialysis the peritoneum (layer of cells that lines the abdomen and covers the guts) is the membrane; in haemodialysis a filter is used.

Peritoneal dialysis

This can be undertaken at home so that the child can go to school. A soft catheter (Tenckhoff) is tunnelled under the skin into the abdomen, the tip being in the pelvis. To allow the incision to heal properly and prevent any risks of infection dialysis is not usually started for 3–4 weeks if possible. Constipation may displace the tube so to avoid this lactulose is given.

Continuous ambulatory peritoneal dialysis

In continuous ambulatory peritoneal dialysis (CAPD), the bag is hung and allowed to run into the abdomen. The fluid is then left in the abdomen until the next time when the old fluid will be drained out and replaced with fresh fluid. This is done four times a day: morning, lunchtime, late afternoon and before bed. It may be better for older children who want to be able to go out in the evenings.

Continuous cycling peritoneal dialysis

Also called automated peritoneal dialysis (APD), in continuous cycling peritoneal dialysis (CCPD) a machine, rather than gravity, is used to push the fluid in and out of the abdomen. Dialysis takes place at night whilst the child is asleep. Usually 10–12 hours on the machine is needed so this is better for younger children. Sometimes an extra cycle can be put in during the day so that the length of time overnight can be shortened in the older children. Usually some fluid is left in during the day. Initial dialysis fluid volumes are 10 mL/kg gradually increasing up to 45–50 mL/kg (or 1100–1400 mL/m^2).

Peritonitis associated with dialysis

If infection enters into the abdomen, peritonitis will develop. The dialysate, which is usually clear becomes cloudy and the child develops abdominal pain and may have a temperature. Peritonitis may be treated by giving antibiotics intravenously or added to the dialysate. The protocol used at Great Ormond Street Hospital is shown in Table 13.9.

Review after 24–48 hours with blood culture and peritoneal dialysis fluid (PDF) results. If blood culture is negative, change to intraperitoneal (IP) treatment as above. If blood culture is positive, continue IV antibiotics according to sensitivities, and consider adding IP antibiotics.

Continuing antibiotic therapy will be modified according to the identity and sensitivity of the organisms cultured. It is essential to liaise with medical microbiology. It may be helpful to consider substituting flucloxacillin 50 mg/L for sensitive Gram-positive organisms if there is concern about the development of resistance to vancomycin, and changing to the use of gentamicin 5 mg/L or amikacin 25 mg/L for sensitive Gram-negative organisms if ciprofloxacin resistance is a concern. When no bacteria are isolated both antibiotics are continued.

Dialysis regimen for peritonitis

- All children should initially be treated with CCPD (home choice) using usual TTV (total therapy volume) but with a TTT (total therapy time) of 24 hours. This will give the same number of cycles per day but with increased dwell times and should be continued for 2 days (48 hours). Antibiotics and heparin should be added to all of the dialysis fluid bags if applicable (heparin only if on IV antibiotics).
- Close observations of fluid balance and plasma potassium levels should be performed.
- If the white blood cell count (WBC) is $<100 \times 10^6$/L after 48 hours, continue on usual dialysis regimen adding antibiotics to the PDF as above (including last fill if on CCPD). If the WBC is $>100 \times 10^6$/L after 48 hours continue cycling regimen.

Table 13.9 Protocol for treatment and prevention of peritonitis in children on peritoneal dialysis as used at Great Ormond Street Hospital, London

Clinical presentation	Cloudy dialysate fluid	±
	Abdominal pain	±
	Fever	±
	History of line break/contamination	
Assessment	Either local infection with minor systemic signs or associated severe systemic illness. Send sample of PDF effluent for cell count and differential, Gram stain & culture (MC&S). PDF sample should be 50–100 mL, with the dwell time and fill volume indicated on the form Perform a CRP, WBC and differential blood cultures if clinically indicated	
Diagnosis	WBC >100 × 10^6/L	±
	Organisms on Gram stain (Gram positive / negative or yeasts)	±
	Positive culture	
Note:	If WBC 50–100 × 10^6/L and patient's symptoms/signs suggestive of peritonitis, initiate treatment If WBC 50–100 × 10^6/L and patient asymptomatic, hold dialysis and repeat specimen in 4–6 hours	
Treatment with antibiotics		
If local signs/minor systemic illness:	Initially use both IP vancomycin and ciprofloxacin until Gram stain/culture of PDF available. Then modify treatment accordingly	
Gram-positive organisms		
Gram-negative organisms	Vancomycin (15 mg/L) IP	
No organisms seen but WBC >100 × 10^6/L	Ciprofloxacin (20 mg/L) IP Vancomycin (15 mg/L) IP + ciprofloxacin (20 mg/L) IP + heparin 200 units/L (for 48 hours cycling and continue as clinically indicated) + nystatin oral suspension 100 000 units **four** times a day whilst on antibiotics	
If severe systemic illness:	Initially use both IV vancomycin and ciprofloxacin until Gram stain/culture of PDF available. Then modify treatment accordingly	
Consider this approach with immunocompromised patient		
Gram-positive organisms	Vancomycin 10 mg/kg stat IV (if 24-hour level <10 mg/L give further dose)	
Gram-negative organisms	Ciprofloxacin 5 mg/kg IV 12 hourly (max 400 mg 12 hourly)	
No organisms seen but WBC >100 × 10^6/L	Vancomycin 10 mg/kg stat IV (if 24-hour level <10 mg/L give further dose) + ciprofloxacin 5 mg/kg dose 12 hourly IV (max dose 400 mg 12 hourly) + heparin 200 units/L IP (for 48 hours cycling and continue as clinically indicated) + nystatin oral suspension 100 000 units four times a day whilst on antibiotics	

- Duration of treatment: 14 days (may require up to four weeks for *Staph. aureus*).
- Send daily PDF samples to microbiology to monitor treatment response.
- Send sample for eosinophil count to haematology if culture-negative peritonitis and persistent cloudy effluent. If >10% leucocytes are eosinophils this is suggestive of eosinophilic peritonitis. May also have a peripheral blood eosinophilia. No extra treatment indicated.
- In most cases the patient can go home after

48 hours to continue treatment. The community team is involved if parents cannot add antibiotics to bags.

- Remove catheter if the following develop: fungal peritonitis; severe intra-abdominal sepsis and septicaemic shock; exit site or tunnel infection due to the same organism as the peritonitis (recurrence within four weeks with the same organism); no decline or increase in dialysate white cell count after 3–4 days if infection severe or 7 days if infection mild.
- Consider removal of catheter if child remains symptomatic after 3–4 days.

Post-surgical peritonitis (within two weeks of procedure)

A raised PDF white cell count is often found following an intraperitoneal procedure (i.e. placement of peritoneal dialysis catheter) but symptomatic peritonitis is uncommon. The operative procedure is covered with IV antibiotics (amikacin 10 mg/kg and teicoplanin 10 mg/kg stat) and the catheter is capped off following frequent flushes until the dialysate is clear. The catheter is flushed weekly but a PDF sample should only be sent to microbiology if the child is symptomatic. Treatment will be indicated in a symptomatic child with a rising WBC on serial PDF samples.

Line break/contamination

If a line break/contamination occurs when peritoneal dialysis has commenced:

- Perform a line change and obtain PDF sample as before.
- If WBC is <100 × 10⁶/L add vancomycin and ciprofloxacin (as above) to dialysis bags for 48 hours but continue usual dialysis regimen.
- If WBC is >100 × 10⁶/L then treat as peritonitis (as above).

If line break/contamination occurs before peritoneal dialysis has commenced:

- Perform a line change. Give IV antibiotics for 48 hours and continue as clinically indicated.

A summary of the treatment of peritonitis in peritoneal dialysis is given in Table 13.10.

Frequent episodes of peritonitis can damage the peritoneum and reduce the length of time that peritoneal dialysis can be given. On average, peritoneal dialysis can be used for 5 years before it ceases to work properly.

Haemodialysis

For haemodialysis there needs to be access to the blood vessels so that blood can be taken out of the body, passed through a filter to clean it, and then returned to the body. Access is via a catheter or by a fistula. Haemodialysis takes place for 4 hours on 3 days per week. Schooling is arranged whilst the child is on haemodialysis.

The catheter used for haemodialysis needs to be relatively large to allow high blood flow speeds – a Permcath consisting of two lumens (one for blood to leave the body and one for return) is placed in the vessels in the neck. Permcaths are only used in an emergency or if haemodialysis is short term or in young children as they easily become infected and may damage the blood vessel. If the catheter becomes infected, vancomycin or teicoplanin 'line-locks' may be used according to the sensitivities of the infecting organism.

Older children are dialysed via a fistula. An artery is joined to a vein in the arm; this makes the vein increase in size and become tougher so that needles can be placed into the vein and high blood speeds through the filter can be obtained. A local anaesthetic cream is used before the needles are put in. The vessels in the neck are preserved and the infection risk is reduced. After creation the fistula will take 4–6 weeks before it is usable.

Paediatric haemodialysis brings another set of challenges and requires specialist knowledge and expertise.

Fluid restriction on dialysis

This is dependent upon how much urine is passed (a small amount is lost in stools and sweat) and restriction will depend upon how well fluid is removed with peritoneal dialysis,

Table 13.10 Treatment of peritonitis

	Treatment
Recurrent peritonitis Consider risk factors: Revisit exchange technique	
Tenckhoff catheter exit site or tunnel infection	Swab exit site and obtain ultrasound scan of tunnel. May need further course of oral antibiotics (up to 6 weeks) according to sensitivities. Infected superficial cuff can be exteriorised and shaved. If inner cuff of catheter involved will need catheter replacement
Staph. aureus infection	Check if child or carers are nasal carriers. If positive nasal swabs, apply topical nasal mupirocin twice a day
Gastrostomy exit site	If appears infected obtain swab and treat appropriately

Note: Replace peritoneal dialysis catheter if refractory peritonitis (i.e. relapsing or >2 recurrent infections) as possible biofilm formation

Fungal peritonitis Children at risk: Frequent broad-spectrum antibiotic usage	Start treatment with liposomal amphotericin – 1 mg/kg as a daily dose IV, changing if possible after 48 hours (following fluconazole sensitivity testing and identification) to fluconazole 12 mg/kg IV as a single daily dose for 48 hours decreasing to 6 mg/kg/ day (max dose 200 mg daily) for a total of at least 2 weeks If functioning renal transplant, adjust dose based on renal function Then continue with oral fluconazole for further 4 weeks. Most *Candida albicans* (germ tube-positive yeast) is sensitive to fluconazole
Immunosuppressed post transplant with peritoneal dialysis catheter in situ Gastrostomy (but no significant relationship)[2]	Catheter removal as soon as possible.

Note: Re-initiation of peritoneal dialysis is common following successful treatment of fungal peritonitis.[11,12]

and how much fluid the child can tolerate being taken off with haemodialysis in a relatively short time.

On peritoneal dialysis, what is taken in must equal what comes out if the child is not to retain fluid and gain weight (oedema). Higher concentrations of dialysate will pull off more fluid. In the infant and young child a lot of adjustment is required with dialysis concentrations, types of fluid and fill volumes to optimise growth (not oedema) and development. The amount of protein in the diet is increased as protein is lost in the dialysate. Some sugar will be absorbed from the dialysate.

On haemodialysis, if too much is drunk between dialysis sessions the blood pressure goes up and the child can become very unwell, particularly during the process of fluid removal. The child will also need to stay on the machine longer. On haemodialysis, potassium must be monitored carefully.

Neither type of dialysis is good at removing phosphate so a phosphate binder is essential. High levels of phosphate and PTH are important

Table 13.11 Intravenous iron dose in haemodialysis

	Maintenance dose
Ferritin <100 µg/L and T$_{SAT}$ <20%	A 7 mg/kg (max 200 mg) IV stat dose is given, followed by 2 mg/kg/dose IV every 2 weeks (max single dose 100 mg)
Ferritin >100 and <800 µg/L, T$_{SAT}$ 20%	2 mg/kg/dose IV every 2 weeks (max single dose 100 mg)
Ferritin >800 µg/L, T$_{SAT}$ >50%	No treatment required

The serum ferritin (µg/L), iron (µmol/L) and transferrin (µmol/L) should be measured monthly.
Transferrin saturation (T$_{SAT}$) can be calculated as follows: T$_{SAT}$ = iron/2 × transferrin (%).
From ref. 13.

causes of cardiovascular disease. The mortality is about 700 times higher in young adult patients on long-term dialysis than in the normal population.

Erythropoietin and iron needed before dialysis will need to be continued, but iron is usually given intravenously during haemodialysis as iron sucrose (off-label) at the doses shown in Table 13.11.

The risk of death in children on dialysis is about 1% per year.

Drug prescribing in renal disease

Compared with adult patients there are few published studies on drug dosing for children with renal impairment. Age, weight or body surface area needs to be considered in addition to renal function. Dosage based on body weight is often inappropriate and may result in underdosing in small infants. Adjusting the dose to body surface area gives a better estimate of the dose for an infant or child. Surface area increases at a lower rate than body weight during a child's growth and many physiological parameters that are important for drug distribution and elimination are closely correlated to surface area. Immature liver and kidney functions in newborns markedly improve during the first months of life, altering drug metabolism. Changes in gastrointestinal motility, gastric pH, nausea and vomiting all alter drug absorption. Gut motility and gastric emptying time are delayed in neonates.

The gastric pH is alkaline at birth. Gastric acid secretion begins within a day or two and adult levels are reached at age 5–12 years. Intestinal enzyme activities affecting drug absorption may be subject to age-dependent alterations. Protein binding is altered by acidosis, malnutrition and inflammation. The extent to which drugs are cleared by haemodialysis or peritoneal dialysis is also important.

Drug action can also interfere with a child's development (e.g. long-term corticosteroids can inhibit growth and cause osteoporosis).

To date it is impossible to accurately determine all factors that may influence drug metabolism in children in every paediatric age group. Thus continual observation and wherever possible careful monitoring of drug levels is essential, particularly in those with a narrow therapeutic range.

References such as the *British National Formulary for Children*, Guys & St Thomas Paediatric Formulary or Daschner's dosing tables[3] may be used.

The Great Ormond Street protocols listed in this chapter are those in current use but are regularly subject to review and may change.

Acknowledgements

To all the staff in the nephrology unit at Great Ormond Street Hospital, London and to Kuan Ooi, pharmacy department, for assistance in proofreading and formatting.

CASE STUDY

A 1-day-old term baby (weight 3 kg) is admitted in chronic renal failure with a diagnosis of bilateral dysplastic kidneys.

Urea and electrolytes are as follows (normal ranges within parentheses):

- Sodium 136 mmol/L (133–146 mmol/L)
- Potassium 3.9 mmol/L (3.2–6.0 mmol/L)
- Total CO_2 23 mmol/L (17–27 mmol/L)
- Urea 5.0 mmol/L (0.7–5.0 mmol/L)
- Creatinine 234 μmol/L (53–97 μmol/L)
- Calcium 2.27 mmol/L (1.96–2.66 mmol/L)
- Magnesium 0.78 mmol/L (0.66–1.0 mmol/L)
- Phosphate 2.38 mmol/L (1.5–2.6 mmol/L)
- Albumin 29 g/L (26–36 g/L)
- PTH 10.0 pmol/L (0.7–5.6 pmol/L)
- Liver function tests within normal range
- Haemoglobin 12 g/dL (13.5–19.5 g/dL).

Q1. How would you determine the baby's GFR?

Q2. Describe the therapy that should be initiated and why.

Q3. How would you ensure that the child maintains optimum growth and development?

Q4. The parents are told that the baby will need to start dialysis in the very near future, and will ultimately require a transplant. The parents are very keen to donate a kidney as soon as possible. They are aware of the work up required, but what is the earliest age that a transplant could go ahead and why?

A peritoneal dialysis catheter is inserted and peritoneal dialysis started. Once dialysis is stabilised and after extensive training, mum feels confident to perform the dialysis at home. The baby is discharged. However 2 days later mum phones the unit to say that her baby was screaming and had a temperature. She had also noticed that the effluent dialysis bag was cloudy.

Q5. What is the likely diagnosis and what would you therefore recommend that mum should do?

References

1. Department of Health. *Medicines standard: National Service Framework for Children, Young People and Maternity Services.* October 2004. http://www.dh.gov.uk
2. Morris MC, Allanby CW, Toseland P, Haycock GB, Chantler C. Evaluation of a height/plasma creatinine formula in the measurement of glomerular filtration rate. *Arch Dis Child* 1982; 57: 611–615.
3. Daschner M. Drug dosage in children with reduced renal function. *Pediatr Nephrol* 2005; 20: 1675–1686.
4. Mattman A, Eintracht S, Mock T *et al.* Estimating pediatric glomerular filtration rates in the era of chronic kidney disease staging. *J Am Soc Nephrol* 2006; 17: 487–496.

5. Fawer CL, Torrado A, Guignard JP. Maturation of renal function in full term and premature neonates. *Helv Paediatr Acta* 1979; 34: 11–21.

6. National High Blood Pressure Education Program. Working Group on high blood pressure in children and adolescents. *Pediatrics*. 2004; 114 (Suppl 4th report): 555–576. http://pediatrics.aappublications.org/cgi/reprint/114/2/S2/555

7. National Institute for Health and Clinical Excellence (NICE). Clinical guideline 39: Anaemia management in chronic kidney disease: Understanding NICE guidance. September 2006. http://guidance.nice.org.uk/cg39/publicinfo/pdf/English

8. Carlberg B, Samuelsson O, Lindholm LH. Atenolol in hypertension: is it a wise choice? *Lancet* 2004; 364: 1684–1689.

9. Anglo Scandinavian Cardiac Outcomes Trial (ASCOT) study aiming to evaluate different treatment strategies to prevent cardiovascular disease in hypertensive patients. http://www.ascotstudy.org

10. National Institute for Health and Clinical Excellence (NICE). Final appraisal determination: Immunosuppressive therapy for renal transplantation in children and adolescents. 2006. http://www.nice.org.uk

11. The Mupirocin Study Group. Nasal mupirocin prevents *Staphylococcus aureus* exit site infection during peritoneal dialysis. *J Am Soc Nephrol* 1996; 7: 2403–2408.

12. Warady B, Bashir M, Donaldson L. Fungal peritonitis in children receiving PD: A report of the NAPRTCS. *Kidney Int* 2000; 58: 384–389.

13. Morgan HEG, Gautam M, Geary DF. Maintenance intravenous iron therapy in pediatric haemodialysis patients. *Pediatr Nephrol* 2001; 16: 779–784.

Further reading

Stein A, Wild J. *Kidney Failure Explained*, 2nd edn. London: Class Publishing, 2002. [Although this book is about adults living with kidney disease it is very well written and presented.]

Rees L, Brogan P, Webb N. *Handbook of Paediatric Nephrology*. Oxford: Oxford University Press, 2006.

14

Renal pharmacy in critical care

John Dade

A large proportion of patients admitted to an intensive care unit (ICU) will experience some reversible changes in their renal function during the course of their admission as a consequence of their critical illness. A smaller and significant number will develop acute renal failure (ARF). This chapter will concentrate on the pharmaceutical needs of patients who develop ARF and require an ICU admission. It will also briefly review the use of drug therapies, specific to the critical care, in patients with renal dysfunction.

Acute renal failure is a common problem in the intensive care unit and affects approximately 10 000 patients in the UK annually.[1] This equates to 5–20% of ICU admissions, depending on the individual ICU's patient mix. Lower rates are seen in single speciality units (e.g. cardiothoracic ICUs), and higher rates in general ICUs.

Acute renal failure is a serious medical condition. Even if you allow for the severity of their concurrent illness, patients with ARF have a significantly worse outcome; patients receiving ventilation and renal replacement have an ICU mortality rate in excess of 50%, whereas on average 20–25% of all patients fail to survive their ICU admission. Worse still, a significant number of individuals that recover to leave ICU will die before leaving hospital, resulting in a total hospital mortality rate of approximately 70% in ARF patients, compared with 35–40% for all ICU admissions. The outlook for those patients who survive ARF, however, is good, with less than 10% remaining dialysis-dependent in the longer term.[1]

Pharmacists who work with critically ill patients will spend a significant part of their time managing the causes and consequences of renal failure. Consequently they will require an understanding of the following issues amongst others:

- The causes of renal impairment in critically ill patients and how this can be prevented. This is a key role bearing in mind the mortality rates once ARF occurs.
- How renal replacement techniques are performed, particularly continuous haemofiltration and continuous haemodialysis.
- How to adjust drug therapy to allow for the effects of renal impairment and replacement (e.g. dosage, fluid allowance, adverse events and contraindications).

Preventing acute renal failure

Acute renal impairment and ARF most commonly occurs following a period of underperfusion of the kidney (pre-renal failure), typically as a result of hypotension and/or hypovolaemia. The causes for underfilling and low blood pressure can vary, but the management is almost always the same (i.e. administer fluids, and where necessary support the blood pressure). Pharmacists can play a key role in encouraging these treatments, and crucially reversing any drug-induced causes of hypovolaemia and hypotension. Common causes for hypovolaemia that should be considered include excessive diuretic therapy, unnecessary fluid restrictions, and high gastrointestinal losses. Causes of hypotension include administration of hypotensive medications (e.g. antihypertensive drugs and many other cardiovascular agents) and sedative agents (e.g. propofol – a very common cause of low BP), and opioids. See also Chapter 11.

Pharmacists should also be aware that sicker patients are at a higher risk of developing ARF and be vigilant to ensure that the use of nephrotoxic medications is kept to the absolute minimum, particularly in the acutest phase of the illness. Drugs to consider include non-steroidal anti-inflammatory drugs (NSAIDs), radiological contrast agents, aminoglycosides, amphotericin, ciclosporin, and tacrolimus.

Finally the role of drug therapy in the prevention of renal failure is currently very limited. The use of low-dose dopamine infusions, loop diuretics and mannitol has declined significantly as evidence of their lack of efficacy has been published. The only possible exception is the use of alkaline diuresis in the prevention of ARF due to high myoglobin levels. This can occur following significant tissue injury (e.g. trauma), pressure areas or drug-induced rhabdomyolysis (e.g. statins). This treatment involves the maintenance of a high output of alkalinised urine (pH >6–6.5), which is achieved by administering a combination of sodium chloride 0.9%, sodium bicarbonate (1.4–8.4% according to protocol and urinary pH), and other fluids.

Renal replacement therapy in the intensive care unit

Up until 5–10 years ago the majority of ICUs in district general hospitals did not have facilities for renal replacement and patients were usually transferred to tertiary ICUs for management. In the last 5 years the picture has changed considerably as haemofiltration equipment has become more widely available. A survey published in 2003 found that 90% of ICUs in the UK provided renal replacement therapy in house, and this figure has increased to close to 100% in the intervening years.[1] This change has had a number of knock-on effects, the principal being that in most ICUs renal replacement is nowadays solely provided by the critical care team, with varying back-up support from nephrology teams. Only one-third of ICUs providing haemofiltration are based in hospitals with renal units, nephrologists and renal pharmacy specialists on site.

Renal replacement therapies used in UK intensive care units

There is a considerable difference between the techniques used for long-term renal support in the dialysis-dependent population and those used in the ICU. A survey published in 2003 demonstrated that the following techniques were used in UK ICUs:[1]

- Continuous veno-venous haemofiltration (CVVHF) 88%
- Continuous veno-venous haemodiafiltration (CVVHDF) 70%
- Intermittent haemodialysis 30%
- Intermittent haemofiltration 16%
- None 11%.

These findings reflect the fact that CVVHF and to a lesser extent CVVHDF, are the mainstay methods used for renal replacement in ICU, particularly in the earlier more critically ill phase of a patient's admission. The remaining discussion will concentrate on these techniques as they are rarely used outside of critical care areas, such as ICU high dependency units (HDUs). Intermittent techniques are used in some ICUs but usually when the ICU patient is recovering from their acute illness, as their treatment becomes less invasive. See Chapter 8.

Continuous renal replacement therapies

The procedures of haemofiltration and haemodialysis are physiologically disruptive, and regularly induce acute changes in blood pressure, fluid balance and many other parameters. Critically ill patients are particularly sensitive to these effects, and many cannot tolerate intermittent courses of renal replacement. As a result, continuous modes of haemofiltration and haemodialysis have been developed. Put simply, continuous renal replacement techniques are what you get if you run intermittent techniques at lower rates of clearance and blood flow, and over a longer, unspecified period of time. The physical processes occurring, including those that control drug clearance, are identical to those occurring in intermittent techniques. Refer to Chapter 8 for a fuller description.

Medications required during renal replacement therapy

A number of medicines are necessary to perform haemodialysis or haemofiltration. These are the renal replacement fluid, anticoagulants and, in some ICUs, electrolytes, as these may be added to the replacement fluid.

Renal replacement fluid

Renal replacement fluids are water-based mixtures of a buffer and basic electrolytes, formulated to be close to the components of an ideal extracellular fluid. They can be presented in a number of ways but in most ICUs haemofiltration fluid will be used as a dialysis fluid in haemodialysis, and a haemofiltration fluid in haemofiltration. This fluid is the major product for controlling blood chemistry.

During the process of renal replacement a patient's electrolyte and solute levels will gradually move closer to the components of the replacement fluid (i.e. waste products and drugs removed, electrolytes equilibrated and buffers replaced). A range of haemofiltration fluids are available, most of which have similar formulations. The major differences are in the choice of buffer, and the level of electrolytes, principally potassium.

Potassium

The optimum blood potassium for the majority of ICU patients will be within the range of 4–5 mmol/L. In patients with renal failure this can be maintained in a number of ways:

- Some units will use a potassium-free haemofiltration as the standard fluid, and once the initial high potassium is controlled they will maintain the serum potassium by a combination of intravenous potassium and/or adding potassium to the haemofiltration fluid to a defined concentration.
- Other units will use a potassium-containing haemofiltration fluid containing 2 or 4 mmol/L potassium. This is used alongside a potassium infusion if it is necessary to increase blood potassium levels. A potassium-free haemofiltration fluid is used if there is an urgent requirement to reduce blood potassium.

Both methods have their advantages and disadvantages, but the latter method is more widely used as it is simpler to operate, and uses smaller quantities of concentrated potassium injection, a product whose use is increasingly being restricted in UK hospitals.

Buffers – lactate vs. bicarbonate

Until recently, the choice of renal replacement buffer in critically ill patients was limited to precursor substances, principally lactate, and less commonly acetate, that are metabolised to the natural physiological buffer bicarbonate by the liver. These products were used for practical reasons as bicarbonate haemofiltration fluids are unstable and cannot be supplied as a ready mixed solution. For the majority of ICU patients, lactate-based fluids are well tolerated, as they are able to metabolise the precursors to bicarbonate and buffer their acidotic blood.

A small minority of patients are unable to metabolise lactate to an adequate degree. This results in worsening acidosis as there is insufficient buffer generated, and because of accumulation of the lactate, which is an acid in its own right. Patients at risk of this 'lactate intolerance' include those with significant hepatic impairment, and poor perfusion states secondary to severe sepsis, severe cardiac failure and systemic inflammatory response syndrome. Lactate intolerance becomes apparent if the acidosis fails to respond or worsens, and there are significant rises in blood lactate following the initiation of CVVHF/HDF. Until recently, managing acidosis in these patients was very challenging, but this has been improved with the availability of bicarbonate-based haemofiltration fluids. These are mixed at the point of use and therefore have a much better shelf life.

Anticoagulation

Both haemodialysis and haemofiltration require the use of an extracorporeal blood circuit to deliver blood to the artificial kidney. As a result, some method of anticoagulation is necessary to both maintain blood flow and to prevent the build-up of micro-thrombi that reduce the efficiency of the artificial kidney. This latter process is very important for continuous renal replacement techniques, as filter lives need to be optimised to achieve effective control of blood chemistry.[3]

The commonest anticoagulant used in this context is unfractionated heparin. This is typically infused to achieve a clotting time of 2 times normal (each hospital will use a different assay, e.g. APTT, KCTT, ACT). Unlike in most areas of medicine, unfractionated heparin is generally favoured over low-molecular-weight heparins, because the latter is less easily monitored at the bedside.

If heparin is not effective, there are concerns about bleeding, or there are side-effects or contraindications (e.g. thrombocytopenia), some units will use epoprostenol (prostacyclin 5 ng/kg/min) as an alternative agent. However this agent is very expensive and many units restrict its use as much as possible. Other approaches include pre-dilution of blood with haemofiltration fluid, or using no anticoagulation if the patient's clotting is very deranged. Newer techniques include the use of citrate, heparinoid or hirudins, but these are rarely used in the UK.

Drug dosing in patients receiving continuous renal replacement therapy

A variety of strategies can be adopted when making dosage decisions in patients receiving continuous renal replacement therapy. The key information that you require is the urea clearance rate of the technique in use. This can be obtained from a number of sources but is largely dependent on the filtration rate (for haemofiltration devices), or the dialysis fluid rate (for a haemodialysis device). In practice, the haemofiltration fluid flow rate will be roughly equivalent to the filtration rate of a haemofiltration device. In most ICUs the clearance rate for either device will be in the region of 25–40 mL/min, but you should check for the exact figure for accuracy and also because as a small number of units may use significantly higher flow rates.

Once you have this figure you can start to make dosing decisions. Strictly speaking, you may wish to review literature to obtain details on drug clearance but in practice pharmacists look up the dosage recommended for this creatinine clearance rate in the drug's summary of product characteristics (SPC) and recommend this dosage. This method will give a reasonable dosage decision in most situations. If you have inadequate information to calculate dosage your best option is to seek guidance from a more experienced colleague. Finally, for drugs such as aminoglycosides and vancomycin the best option is to adjust dosages according to blood levels.

Drug therapies specific to critical care areas

Analgesia and sedation

A large majority of ICU patients will receive a combination of an analgesic and sedative drug(s) during their admission. The indications for these drugs are principally to control postoperative or procedural pain, to facilitate ventilation, and to manage delirium and agitation.

Mechanical ventilation is an uncomfortable process commonly associated with agitation. Strong opioids are administered to control the pain of the process, and where necessary to depress respiratory drive as this makes ventilation easier. Sedative drugs are prescribed to manage agitation, to prevent the patient from pulling out their endotracheal tube and lines, and to induce anaesthesia. Opioids can provide some useful sedative effects, and on occasion it maybe possible to manage patients, particularly the elderly, using an opioid alone. In the majority of cases, however, the doses of opioid required to maintain adequate sedation would be excessive and result in adverse effects and accumulation. As a consequence, sedative anaesthetic agents are co-prescribed to manage agitation and to facilitate the ventilation process. Finally in the rarer more serious cases it may also be necessary to use muscle relaxants to paralyse the patient if they fail to synchronise with the ventilator, or if paralysis is required to control symptoms.

Because most of the drugs used undergo renal excretion or hepatic metabolism, oversedation due to accumulation of the parent drug and/or active metabolites is a risk in ICU patients as kidney or liver impairment is relatively commonplace. To some extent this accumulation is unavoidable (e.g. where a patient's clinical condition requires high dosages or if a prolonged period of sedation is necessary), but oversedation can be minimised by a number of strategies, such as use of drugs that are less likely to accumulate, regular review of dosages, sedation scoring and daily sedation holds.

The characteristics of individual sedative agents will be discussed below but as a generality those that are the least prone to accumulation (e.g. alfentanil, remifentanil, propofol) are also the most expensive. This means that financial considerations inevitably come into play when deciding the optimal regimen for sedation, as these drugs form the major component of many ICUs' expenditure. On a more practical level, the majority of ICUs prefer to use a limited range of agents to manage patients as this reduces the likelihood of staff being unfamiliar with the drugs in use and consequently being more likely to use them inefficiently. As a result, in practice the choice of drug is affected by factors other than duration of action and tendency to accumulate.

Strategies to reduce oversedation

Sedation scoring is a numerical system of recording how sedated a patient is. There are many scoring systems in use, but they are only useful if clinical staff use the data to tailor dosages on a regular basis. On many occasions this does not happen as well as it should, and consequently sedation scoring is not universally popular. A more recent innovation, daily sedation hold, has been more enthusiastically received. In this method, sedation is stopped each morning and only reinstated once the patient recovers, and if there is an ongoing clinical need. Because of its simplicity this system is very efficient at preventing oversedation, however it cannot be used in patients whose clinical management is likely to be compromised if sedation is removed (e.g. head injuries, high ventilation requirements). In these cases the adjustment of dosing reverts to traditional methods (e.g. sedation scoring), observing physiological markers (e.g. raised heart rate/ blood pressure), and the experience of the clinical team.

Opioids

Strong opioids are the foundation for any sedation and analgesia used in ICU. The agents in most common use are morphine, fentanyl, alfentanil and, more recently, remifentanil.

Morphine is the most popularly used opioid in ICUs in the UK because it is inexpensive and provides excellent analgesia in patents with good renal and liver function. The parent drug undergoes hepatic metabolism to a series of pharmacologically very active metabolites: morphine-3-glucuronide (M3G) and morphine-6-glucuronide (M6G). These metabolites are excreted by the kidney, and accumulate in renal impairment, but are both significantly cleared during haemofiltration or haemodialysis. Because of this profile, morphine needs careful prescribing and administration in patients with renal impairment to prevent significant accumulation. On occasion this can delay awakening for many days. Regular dosage review, daily sedation holds and, where appropriate, renal replacement therapy are essential to prevent significant accumulation.

Fentanyl duration of effect is affected as much by the duration of use as by any other factors. In the early phase of treatment the duration is short because the agent redistributes extensively throughout the body and the drug itself is metabolised by hepatic metabolism (half-life ~2–12 hours). Used for short periods, fentanyl does not accumulate clinically, but if longer term infusions are used, redistribution from central compartments and its slow excretion may result in delayed recovery. This effect is seen in all patients and is not significantly affected by renal function.

Alfentanil has a short duration of action, a small volume of distribution, is hepatically metabolised to inactive metabolites, but is expensive compared with morphine and fentanyl. Recovery from alfentanil is unlikely to be delayed due to renal impairment, but can be delayed in hepatic impairment. It is probably the agent of choice in renal impairment but many units choose to use other agents for economic reasons.

Remifentanil is metabolised by serum esterases, and does not accumulate in renal or liver impairment. It has a very short duration of action but is expensive compared with all of the other opioids. To date there is limited experience with the use of this agent, and it is principally being used because of the quality of its sedation in difficult to manage patients rather than its duration of action and the reduced risk of accumulation, which is most likely to be most advantageous in patients with significant liver dysfunction.

The pharmacokinetics of the main medications used in the ICU are summarised in Table 14.1.

Sedative anaesthetic agents

In the UK the commonest sedative agents used are the benzodiazepines (midazolam, and less commonly lorazepam) and propofol. A range of other sedatives may also be used in specific cases or where sedation is difficult to achieve. Discussion of these agents (ketamine, haloperidol, clonidine, isoflurane) is beyond the scope of this text.

Midazolam is the most widely used sedative agent in the UK. When used for short-term sedation and in patients with good renal and liver function it provides excellent quality sedation and is not associated with delayed awakening. Midazolam undergoes hepatic metabolism to a series of metabolites, principally 1-hydroxymidazolam glucuronide. This has weak sedative effects but accumulates significantly in renal impairment and has been demon-strated to be responsible for significantly delayed awakening. As a result, this agent should be used with caution in patients with renal impairment, particularly for long durations of sedation.

Lorazepam has a longer duration of action than midazolam but its metabolites are pharmacologically inactive. Because of its long half-life there is a significant propensity for accumulation in any patient, but this is unlikely to be aggravated by renal impairment. As a result, lorazepam is increasingly been seen as an alternative sedative agent to midazolam. However there have been concerns about adverse effects secondary to its excipient agent propylene glycol causing hyperlactaemia and other metabolic effects.

Propofol is the shortest acting anaesthetic available and it provides an excellent quality of sedation that is rapidly reversible in the majority of patients. It rarely accumulates in patients, including those with renal impairment, because it undergoes metabolism, predominantly by the liver to inactive substances. Until recently propofol was an expensive agent and its use was limited because of cost, however since the expiry of its patent this agent is now relatively cheap and its use is increasing. It is probably the agent of choice in patients with renal dysfunction. The major concerns with propofol are its hypotensive effect and the so called 'propofol infusion syndrome' that has been reported in patients receiving very high doses over a prolonged period of time.

Muscle relaxants

A range of non-depolarising muscle relaxants are available for use in the ICU, most units using atracurium, vecuronium, or less commonly cisatracurium and rocuronium.

Atracurium is a short-acting agent with a duration of action of 20 minutes. It undergoes systemic metabolism by Hofmann elimination to largely inactive metabolites, and it does not accumulate in renal or liver dysfunction. One of its metabolites, laudanosine, does accumulate markedly in renal failure but there is little evidence that this causes any clinically relevant side-effects.

Vecuronium has a slightly longer duration of action than atracurium. It is metabolised in the

Table 14.1   Pharmacokinetics of intensive care unit medications

Drug	Pharmacokinetics	Duration of action	Effect of renal failure
Alfentanil	Hepatic, inactive metabolites	Half-life 1–4 hours	Minimal. Small increased in free fraction, therefore doses slightly reduced
Fentanyl	Redistribution, hepatic metabolism	Half-life 2 hours. Duration increases with time due to redistribution	Minimal
Morphine	Hepatic, active metabolites (morphine glucuronides) excreted renally	Half-life morphine is 1–4 hours. Half-life morphine glucuronides is 4–50 hours	Significant risk of accumulation of active metabolites
Remifentanil	Systemic metabolism by serum esterases	3–10 minutes. Metabolites essentially inactive	Minimal
Lorazepam	Hepatic metabolism, glucuronide metabolite is inactive	Half-life 5–10 hours	Small increase in duration
Midazolam	Hepatic metabolism, active metabolite (1-OH midazolam)	1.5–12 hours	Significant risk of accumulation of active metabolite
Propofol	Predominantly hepatic metabolism	30–60 min	Minimal
Atracurium	Systemic metabolism – Hofmann elimination	20–30 min	Minimal Metabolite laudanosine not muscle relaxant
Vecuronium	Hepatic metabolism to active metabolites	Half-life 0.5–1.2 hours	Accumulation of active metabolites

liver to a series of metabolites, including 3-hydroxy-vecuronium, which has approximately 50% the activity of the parent drug. These metabolites are excreted renally and can cause delayed recovery in patients with kidney impairment. As a result, vecuronium is probably not the first choice muscle relaxant in renal failure, but it maybe used if patients start to develop resistance to atracurium, a phenomenon that is fairly common.

Prevention of stress ulceration

ICU patients, particularly those receiving mechanical ventilation, have an increased risk of developing gastric and duodenal ulcers due to the physiological stress of their illness. A num-

ber of strategies are used to minimise this risk, including prophylactic H_2-antagonists, proton pump inhibitors, sucralfate, and early establishment of enteral feeding.

The best evidence is for the use of H_2-antagonists or sucralfate. Both treatments reduce the incidence of stress ulceration to similar degrees, but there is a tendency towards higher rates of hospital-acquired pneumonia in patients receiving H_2-antagonists. Despite this evidence most ICUs use intravenous H_2-blockers because they are easier to administer than enteral sucralfate which can cause complications with prolonged use in conjunction with enteral feeding. Also, because it contains aluminium there have been concerns expressed about the use of sucralfate in patients with ARF because of the known association of aluminium-containing medicines with renal bone disease and dialysis dementia in patients with ESRD. The H_2-antagonist most commonly used is ranitidine 50 mg three times daily (reduced to twice daily in severe renal impairment). Sucralfate is given enterally at a dose of 1 g every 4–6 hours.

Of the other treatments, enteral feeding is widely used, and is probably effective once the patient has started to absorb food, as this indicates a working and adequately perfused gastrointestinal tract. There is, however, surprisingly little published evidence on its use. Proton pump inhibitors are increasingly being used, but with little evidence, and until proven otherwise there will remain concerns about the incidence of pneumonia as this is probably related to changes in gastric pH.

Thromboprophylaxis

Intensive care unit patients typically have a higher risk of thromboembolic complications because of their pre-existing or presenting conditions (e.g. pneumonia, cardiac disease). As a result, most units will give the higher doses of thromboprophylaxis (i.e. enoxaparin 40 mg daily, dalteparin 4000 units daily) to all patients with 'normal' clotting function. Patients with ARF may, however, require either a lower dose of prophylactic agent because of the increased half-life of some heparin products in renal impairment (e.g. enoxaparin). Alternatively, treatment may be omitted because they are receiving concurrent anticoagulant medication as part of their renal replacement therapy.

'Inotropic' therapy

A wide range of agents are used to optimise cardiovascular function in critically ill patients. These range from vasopressor agents such as norepinephrine (noradrenaline), phenylephrine and argipressin that are used to increase vascular tone and blood pressure, through inotropic/vasodilator agents such as dobutamine, enoximone, milrinone that are used in cardiogenic shock, to mixed agents that have intropic, vasodilating and vasopressor effects

depending on dosage (e.g. epinephrine (adrenaline), dopamine). Readers should refer to other sources for a more detailed insight into the clinical use of these agents, but as most of these agents have extremely short half-lives and are metabolised systemically, general renal impairment has little effect on their duration of action. The only exception is the phosphodiesterase inhibitors milrinone and enoximone that have a longer duration of action and do accumulate in renal failure. These agents should therefore be used at lower than average doses. However, as dosing is generally titrated to effect, clinically significant accumulation rarely occurs.

General comments on administering drugs to patients with renal impairment

The rules for prescribing drugs in renal impairment are the same as you would apply in any other clinical area, but a few specific points of guidance are worth considering.

A large number of drugs are administered by intravenous injection, and this can impose a significant fluid input particularly in sicker patients receiving multiple infusions. It may therefore be necessary to try to restrict fluid intake. A number of options should be considered. First you should attempt to give medicines by enteral routes if this is feasible, and does risk impaired absorption for medicines that are critical for recovery. If you need to fluid restrict you should consult the SPC and where necessary minimum infusion guides (e.g. UKCPA Critical Care Group Minimum infusion volumes for fluid restricted critically ill patients[4]). This latter document gives largely anecdotal advice but is invaluable.

Finally, when managing patients who are extremely sick and have immediately life-threatening infections etc., if dosage reductions are necessary, it is worth delaying these to ensure that the patient receives sufficient dose of a drug to give them a chance of responding. In practice, most pharmacists will delay dosage reductions until the following day as this period of 'overdosing' is highly unlikely to be harmful to the patient.

CASE STUDY

MF is a 19-year-old man weighing 70 kg who was admitted to the ICU with severe sepsis secondary to presumed meningococcal meninigitis. On admission he is severely hypotensive, and anuric. He is prescribed cefotaxime and benzylpenicillin, is sedated for ventilation, and is commenced on norepinephrine (noradrenaline) to increase his blood pressure.

His blood results on admission give a creatinine of 123 µmol/L and a urea of 7.3 mmol/L.

Q1. Assess his renal function, and decide whether it will be necessary to adjust the dosage of his antibiotics and any other medications.

Q2. The standard protocol for sedating patients on the ICU uses a combination of morphine and midazolam. The clinical staff are concerned about drug accumulation with these agents. What are the options to prevent accumulation?

Twelve hours following admission, MF remains anuric, has a significant metabolic acidosis (pH 7.21, lactate 5.3 mmol/L), requires norepinephrine (noradrenaline) to maintain adequate blood pressure, and ventilatory support. Continuous veno-venous haemofiltration is commenced.

Q3. The CVVHF system is configured to an ultrafiltration rate of 30 mL/kg/h. Are any dosage modifications required for the drugs mentioned above and for the following additional agents – enoxaparin SC 40 mg once daily, ranitidine IV 50 mg three times daily, and IV insulin infusion to maintain a blood glucose of 5–8 mmol/L?

The consultant prescribes drotrecogin alfa (activated protein C) as treatment for severe sepsis, at a dose of 24 µg/kg/h.

Q4. Are any dosage modifications required for this agent, and are any additional precautions necessary?

Q5. What options are available to manage MF's metabolic acidosis?

References

1. Wright SE, Bodenham A, Short AIK, Turney JH. The provision and practice of renal replacement therapy on adult intensive care units in the United Kingdom. *Anaesthesia* 2003; 58: 1063–1069.
2. Pruchnicki MC, Dasta JF. Acute renal failure in hospitalised patients: Part II. *Ann Pharmacother* 2002(July/August); 36: 1261–1267.
3. Oudemans-van-Straaten HM, Wester JPJ, dePont ACJM, Schetz MRC. Anticoagulation strategies in continuous renal replacement therapy: can the choice be evidence based? *Intensive Care Med* 2006; 32: 188–202.
4. UK Clinical Pharmacy Association, Critical Care Group. Minimum infusion volumes for fluid restricted critically ill patients, 3rd edn. May 2006. Available from www.ukcpa.org.uk

15

Pain control in renal impairment

Stephen Ashmore

The clinical efficacy of most analgesic drugs is altered by impaired renal function, not simply because of altered clearance of the parent drug, but also through accumulation of toxic or therapeutically active metabolites. Some analgesic agents can aggravate pre-existing renal disease, causing direct damage and thus altering their excretion.

This chapter will cover the basic rules for prescribing analgesics in patient with varying degrees of renal impairment. Published evidence of efficacy is quoted for a wide range of agents which have been employed to treat different types of pain. Specific renal doses for individual agents can be found in *The Renal Drug Handbook*,[1] or in the relevant summary of product characteristics (SPC).

Assessing pain

The assessment and ongoing measurement of pain are essential to diagnosing and treating painful conditions. A visual analogue scale from 0 to 10 is often used to assess pain in adults. Patients are asked to mark on a 10-cm scale the point which best represents their pain, where 0 represents no pain and 10 the worst pain imaginable (scores above 7 cm are considered to represent severe pain). Pictorial representations of pain (smiling/sad faces) are often used for children. Advice on recording pain scores should be obtained from acute pain specialists.

A description of the type of pain is also important to aid prescribing. Neuropathic pain requires a different treatment approach to other types of pain, and will be described as burning, stabbing or shooting in nature.

The analgesic ladder

Analgesic prescribing for both acute and chronic pain should always follow a stepwise approach, with ongoing monitoring of pain severity and adjustment of doses and agents. In the acute setting it is important to monitor the patient regularly for signs of toxicity or lack of efficacy. This is particularly important in cases of acute renal failure, where renal function can change rapidly, resulting in increased risk of side-effects or underdosing.

The first step on the analgesic ladder is to use non-opioids such as paracetamol and non-steroidal anti-inflammatory drugs (NSAIDs) (if appropriate for the renal patient); if pain persists mild opioids can be added or substituted. Finally, in severe pain a strong opioid should be used, in combination with an NSAID if necessary.

Analgesics and renal impairment

Analgesics that exhibit the safest pharmacological profile in patients with renal impairment are alfentanil, buprenorphine, fentanyl, ketamine and paracetamol. None of these drugs deliver a high active metabolite load or have a significantly prolonged clearance.

Oxycodone can usually be used without any dose adjustment in patients with renal impairment as the main metabolite, oxymorphone, is only weakly active, and contributes minimally to any clinical effect. However, as hepatic blood flow can be altered in uraemia the half-life of oxycodone can be increased as hepatic clearance is reduced. The manufacturer of oxycodone

191

Table 15.1   Recommendations for drug dosing in renal impairment

Drug	Comments	Recommendations	References
NSAIDs and COX-2 inhibitors	Can affect renal function	Use with caution in mild renal impairment. Avoid in severe renal impairment	4
Gabapentin	Half-life increased and plasma levels raised in renal impairment	Dose adjustment recommended on basis of creatinine clearance	5
Tricyclic antidepressants	Amitriptyline metabolised to active agent in liver	Limited data; metabolite accumulation may increase risk of side-effects	6
Ketamine	Metabolite level increased, but has little activity	Limited data; probably no dose adjustment required	7
Local anaesthetics	Increase in free fraction may result from alterations in protein binding	Risk of toxicity may be affected by acid–base disturbances or serum potassium levels	8–10

Adapted from ref. 2.

therefore recommends cautious use of the drug in chronic renal and hepatic disease, with a low starting dose.[2]

Analgesics that have been used in patients with renal impairment, but may require a reduction in dose include amitriptyline, clonidine, codeine, gabapentin, hydromorphone, lidocaine, methadone, morphine and tramadol.

NSAIDs, dextropropoxyphene (found in co-proxamol) and pethidine are not recommended in patients with significant renal impairment.[3]

Table 15.1 summarises some recent published recommendations for various analgesics in patients with renal impairment. Practice in individual renal units may differ from these recommendations.

Individual agents

Paracetamol

Paracetamol is an effective analgesic and antipyretic. It is absorbed rapidly and well from the small intestine after oral administration and can be given rectally and intravenously.

The mechanism of action of paracetamol remains unclear. It has no known endogenous binding sites, and apparently does not inhibit peripheral cyclo-oxygenase activity. There is increasing evidence of a central antinociceptive effect. Potential mechanisms for this include inhibition of a COX-2 in the CNS, or inhibition of a central cyclo-oxygenase 'COX-3' that is selectively susceptible to paracetamol, and modulation of inhibitory descending serotonergic pathways. Paracetamol has also been shown to prevent prostaglandin production, independent of cyclo-oxygenase activity.[11]

Paracetamol is an effective adjunct to opioid analgesia, opioid requirements being reduced by 20–30% when combined with a regular regimen of oral or rectal paracetamol. The combination of paracetamol 1000 mg plus codeine 60 mg has a number-needed-to-treat (NNT) of 2.2. The addition of an NSAID to paracetamol further improves efficacy.[12]

Intravenous (IV) paracetamol is an effective analgesic after surgery, is as effective as ketorolac, and is equivalent to morphine and better tolerated after dental surgery, although there is evidence of a ceiling effect.[3]

Paracetamol has fewer side-effects than NSAIDs and can be used when the latter are contraindicated (e.g. patients with a history of asthma, renal impairment or peptic ulcers). It should be used with caution or in reduced doses in patients with active liver disease, alcohol-related liver disease and glucose-6-phosphate dehydrogenase deficiency. In these situations, as well as in overdose, the rate of reactive metabolite production can result in liver damage, occasionally with acute renal tubular necrosis.

In cases of severe renal impairment, the elimination of paracetamol is slightly delayed and metabolites may accumulate. It has been suggested that the maximum daily dose of paracetamol for chronic use in patients with end stage renal failure (ESRF) should be reduced to 3 g.[13] However, in practice, few renal units adopt this strategy.

Non-steroidal anti-inflammatory drugs

NSAIDs have analgesic, anti-inflammatory and antipyretic effects and are effective analgesics in a variety of acute pain states. Unfortunately, significant contraindications and adverse effects limit the use of NSAIDs in many patients, including those with renal impairment.

Prostaglandins have many physiological functions including gastric mucosal protection, and renal tubular function which are mainly regulated by COX-1 and are the basis for many of the adverse effects associated with NSAID use. Tissue damage induces COX-2 production, leading to synthesis of prostaglandins that result in pain and inflammation. COX-2 may be 'constitutive' in some tissues, including the kidney. NSAIDs inhibit both COX-1 and COX-2. Aspirin acetylates and inhibits cyclo-oxygenase irreversibly but NSAIDs are reversible inhibitors of the enzymes. The COX-2 inhibitors have been developed to inhibit selectively the inducible form.

When given in combination with opioids after surgery, NSAIDs result in better analgesia and reduce opioid consumption. The addition of an oral NSAID to paracetamol also improves analgesia.[3]

Side-effects

NSAID side-effects are more common with long-term use. In general, the risk and severity of NSAID-associated side-effects is increased in the elderly.

Renal function
Renal prostaglandins regulate tubular electrolyte handling, modulate the actions of renal hormones, and maintain renal blood flow and glomerular filtration rate in the presence of circulating vasoconstrictors. In some clinical conditions, including hypovolaemia and dehydration, high circulating concentrations of vasoconstrictors increase production of intrarenal vasodilators including prostacyclin – maintenance of renal function may then depend on prostaglandin synthesis and thus can be sensitive to brief NSAID administration.

Diclofenac has been shown to affect renal function in the immediate post-operative period after major surgery and administration of other potential nephrotoxins, such as gentamicin, can increase the renal effects of ketorolac.

The risk of adverse renal effects of NSAIDs and COX-2 inhibitors is increased in the presence of factors such as pre-existing renal impairment, hypovolaemia, hypotension, use of other nephrotoxic agents and angiotensin-converting enzyme (ACE) inhibitors.[3]

Platelet function
NSAIDs inhibit platelet function by their effect on COX-1. In patients with bleeding problems or receiving anticoagulants, there is an increased risk of significant surgical blood loss after NSAID administration. See also Cardiovascular risks of NSAIDs and COX-2 inhibitors below.

Gastrointestinal side-effects
Acute gastroduodenal damage and bleeding can occur with short-term NSAID use. The risk is increased with higher doses, a history of peptic ulceration, use for more than 5 days and in the elderly. After 5 days of naproxen and ketorolac use in healthy elderly subjects, ulcers were found on gastroscopy in 20% and 31% of cases respectively.[14]

The gastric and duodenal epithelia have various protective mechanisms against acid and enzyme attack and many of these involve prostaglandin production. Chronic NSAID use is associated with peptic ulceration and bleeding and the latter may be exacerbated by the antiplatelet effect. It has been estimated that the relative risk of perforations, ulcers and bleeds associated with NSAIDs is 2.7 compared with people not consuming NSAIDs.[15]

Bronchospasm
Aspirin-exacerbated respiratory disease (AERD) is a recognised problem in individuals with asthma, chronic rhinitis and nasal polyps. AERD affects 10–15% of people with asthma, can be severe and there is a cross-sensitivity with NSAIDs but not selective COX-2 inhibitors.[16] A history of AERD is a contraindication to NSAID use, although there is no reason to avoid NSAIDs in other people with asthma.

Cyclo-oxygenase-2 selective inhibitors (COX-2 inhibitors)

These agents selectively inhibit the inducible cyclo-oxygenase enzyme COX-2, and spare COX-1. They offer the potential for effective analgesia with fewer side-effects than NSAIDs. At the time of writing there are two COX-2 inhibitors, or coxibs, on the UK market – celecoxib and etoricoxib.

Side-effects

Renal function
COX-2 is continuously produced in the kidney and is increased in response to alterations in intravascular volume. COX-2 has been implicated in maintenance of renal blood flow, mediation of renin release and regulation of sodium excretion. COX-2 inhibitors and NSAIDs have similar adverse effects on renal function.[17]

Platelet function
Platelets produce only COX-1, and hence COX-2 selective inhibitors do not impair platelet function. The use of COX-2 inhibitors reduces surgical blood loss in comparison with

NSAIDs.[18] The lack of antiplatelet effects may be an advantage for the patient with bleeding problems, or when anticoagulants are given.

Significant research has been undertaken into whether COX-2 inhibitors can produce a tendency to thrombosis because they inhibit endothelial prostacyclin production but spare platelet thromboxane synthesis and aggregation.

The VIGOR study, in which patients on low-dose aspirin were excluded, found an increased risk of myocardial infarction for patients given rofecoxib compared with naproxen.[19] Rofecoxib was withdrawn from clinical practice in 2004 because of further concerns about the risks of cardiovascular events including myocardial infarction and stroke.[20] See also Cardiovascular risks of NSAIDs and COX-2 inhibitors below.

Gastrointestinal side-effects
Large outcome studies have demonstrated that COX-2 inhibitors produce less clinically significant peptic ulceration than NSAIDs. Both rofecoxib and celecoxib have been associated with a substantial reduction in endoscopic ulcers compared with NSAID comparators.[3] In the VIGOR study all upper gastrointestinal events were reduced with rofecoxib compared with naproxen.

Bronchospasm
Studies in patients with AERD have shown that analgesic doses of COX-2 inhibitors do not produce bronchospasm in these patients.[16]

Cardiovascular risks of COX-2 inhibitors

Following the results from studies such as VIGOR and the Adenoma Prevention with Celecoxib (APC) Trial[21] the Medicines and Healthcare Products Regulatory Agency (MHRA) reported on the safety of COX-2 inhibitors in February 2005. The conclusions are set out below:

The evidence suggests that selective COX-2 inhibitors, as a class, may cause an increased risk of thrombotic events (e.g. myocardial infarction and stroke) compared with placebo and some NSAIDs, and the risk may increase with dose and duration of exposure. It is not possible to quantify the risk precisely, but it is considered unlikely to exceed one extra serious thrombotic event per 100 patient years, over the rate for no treatment.

It was advised that:

- Patients with established ischaemic heart disease or cerebrovascular disease should be switched to alternative treatment: in addition, the existing contraindication for severe heart failure has been extended to include moderate heart failure (New York Heart Association (NYHA) class II–IV).
- For all patients the balance of gastrointestinal and cardiovascular risk should be considered before prescribing a COX-2 inhibitor, particularly for those with risk factors for heart disease and those taking low-dose aspirin, for whom gastrointestinal benefit has not been clearly demonstrated.
- The lowest effective dose of COX-2 inhibitor should be used for the shortest necessary period. Periodic re-evaluation is recommended, especially for osteoarthritis patients who may only require intermittent treatment.
- Gastroprotective agents should be considered for patients switched to non-selective NSAIDs.[22]

A systematic review and meta-analysis of randomised double-blind trials of celecoxib has shown an increased risk of myocardial infarction with celecoxib therapy, which confirms the advice given above.[23]

Considering the high prevalence of cardiovascular disease in patients with established renal disease it would seem appropriate to avoid the use of COX-2 inhibitors in such patients.

Cardiovascular risks of non-steroidal anti-inflammatory drugs

In August 2005 the MHRA reported on the safety of NSAIDs. The conclusions are set out below:

As NSAIDs exhibit a broad range of COX-2/COX-1 selectivity, it would be important to know if differing degrees of selectivity correlate with differing biological effects. The three most widely used standard NSAIDs have differing levels of COX1/2 selectivity: diclofenac is COX-2 'preferential', whereas ibuprofen and particularly naproxen preferentially inhibit COX-1.

COX-1 must be inhibited by at least 95% before platelet function is affected *in vivo*. Therefore only drugs that are highly selective for COX-1, such as naproxen are likely to be cardioprotective. Whether COX-2 'preferential' drugs such as etodolac and meloxicam share the same pro-thrombotic effects as the highly selective 'coxibs' is uncertain, but from the perspective of platelet aggregation there appears little evidence to suggest that they would differ.

The association between exposure to NSAIDs and coxibs and subsequent risk of myocardial infarction has been investigated in a large number of epidemiological studies. The tentative observation from the epidemiological data alone is that:

- In relation to non- or 'remote' use of NSAIDs, naproxen usage was associated with a slightly protective or null effect with regard to myocardial infarction.
- In relation to non- or 'remote' use of NSAIDs, ibuprofen usage was associated with a slightly increased or null effect with regard to myocardial infarction.
- In relation to non- or 'remote' use of NSAIDs, diclofenac usage was associated with an elevated risk with regard to myocardial infarction.

The evidence of an increased thrombotic risk associated with NSAIDs is much less clear than for coxibs. Based on the available evidence, any increased risk is likely to be small and associated with continuous longer term treatment and high doses.

Most of the available data relate to naproxen, ibuprofen and diclofenac. Some trials have shown naproxen to have a lower thrombotic risk than selective COX-2 inhibitors. However, data on the risk for ibuprofen and diclofenac, relative to COX-2 inhibitors, are less clear. The absence of useful data for other NSAIDs should not be taken to imply a lower risk for these products.

The MHRA concluded that overall, the data on thrombotic risk with traditional NSAIDs are insufficient to warrant changes in current prescribing practice. Any prescribing decision should be based on the overall safety profile of

NSAIDs (particularly gastrointestinal safety profile), and the individual risk factors of the patient. For all NSAIDs, the lowest effective dose should be used for the shortest period of time necessary in order to control symptoms.

Although platelet aggregation studies have demonstrated an interaction between aspirin and ibuprofen, a clinically important effect has not been clearly demonstrated in epidemiological studies or clinical trials. There is less evidence for such an interaction between naproxen and aspirin.[24]

Opioids

Opioids remain the mainstay of systemic analgesia for the treatment of moderate to severe acute pain. Interpatient opioid requirements vary greatly, and opioid doses therefore need to be titrated to suit each patient. In adult patients, age rather than weight is the better predictor of opioid requirements (Table 15.2).[25]

All full opioid agonists given in equi-analgesic doses produce the same analgesic effect, although such equi-analgesic doses are difficult to determine due to interindividual variabilities in kinetics and dynamics.[34]

Most available data do not suggest that any one opioid is superior to another, either in terms of better pain relief, differences in side-effects or patient satisfaction, but rather that some opioids may be better in some patients; although pethidine has been reported to have a higher incidence of nausea and vomiting compared with morphine.[3]

Codeine and dihydrocodeine

Codeine is classified as a weak opioid but the molecule itself is devoid of analgesic activity. The main metabolite of codeine is codeine-6-glucuronide, which has a similar potency to the parent drug and is renally excreted; 2–10% of a dose is metabolised to morphine, which accounts for most of the analgesic effect of codeine.

Dihydrocodeine is a semi-synthetic derivative of codeine, with an analgesic effect independent of its metabolism to dihydromorphine.

Despite the lack of published safety data for dihydrocodeine in patients with renal impairment, and the reported side-effects of codeine in this population, both drugs are widely used in renal units. Codeine is particularly popular, often combined with paracetamol. Patients receiving regular co-codamol 30/500 should be monitored for side-effects.

Dextropropoxyphene

Dextropropoxyphene is a weak opioid with an NNT of 7.7. In the UK it has been used in combination with paracetamol (co-proxamol) but this combination improves pain relief by only 7.3% compared with paracetamol alone and increases the incidence of dizziness.[3]

The major metabolite of dextropropoxyphene is nordextropropoxyphene which is renally excreted; accumulation of nordextropropoxyphene can lead to CNS, respiratory and cardiac depression.

At the time of writing co-proxamol has been withdrawn from the UK market.

Morphine

Morphine remains the most widely used opioid for the management of pain and the standard against which other opioids are compared. Morphine-6-glucuronide (M6G) and morphine-3-glucuronide (M3G), the main metabolites of morphine, are formed by morphine glucuronidation, primarily in the liver. M6G is a mu-opioid agonist and may be more potent than morphine with morphine-like effects, including analgesia. M3G has very low affinity for opioid receptors, has no analgesic activity and animal studies have shown that it may antagonise the analgesic effects of morphine and be responsible for neurotoxic symptoms sometimes associated with high doses of morphine.

Both M6G and M3G are dependent on the kidney for excretion. Impaired renal function, the oral route of administration (first-pass metabolism), higher doses and increased patient age are predictors of higher M3G and M6G concentrations.[35]

Table 15.2 Recommendations for opioid dosing in renal impairment

Drug	Comments	Recommendations	References
Alfentanil	No active metabolites. Alterations in protein binding may lead to increased free drug	No dose adjustment required	26, 27
Buprenorphine	Inactive and weakly active metabolites. Mainly biliary excretion	No dose adjustment required	26, 27
Codeine	Prolonged sedation and respiratory arrest reported. Neuro-excitation with normal doses	Dose adjustment recommended. Use an alternative if possible	26, 27
Dextropropoxyphene	Accumulation of active metabolite can lead to CNS and CVS toxicity	Dose adjustment recommended. Use an alternative if possible	27, 28
Dihydrocodeine	Metabolism probably similar to codeine	Insufficient evidence: use not recommended	26
Fentanyl	No active metabolites	No dose adjustment required	27
Hydromorphone	Neurotoxicity from accumulation of metabolite possible	Dose adjustment recommended. Use an alternative agent if high doses needed	27, 29
Methadone	Mainly inactive metabolites, but 20% excreted unchanged via kidneys	Dose adjustment recommended in severe renal impairment	26, 27
Morphine	Major metabolites excreted via kidneys. Delayed sedation and neurotoxicity from accumulation of metabolites	Dose adjustment recommended. Use an alternative agent if high doses needed	26, 27, 30
Oxycodone	Oxymorphone metabolite has little clinical effect	No dose adjustment required	28
Pethidine	Accumulation of norpethidine can lead to seizures	Dose adjustment required. Use of alternative recommended	26, 27, 31, 32
Tramadol	Increased effects from active metabolite	Dose adjustment recommended. Use an alternative agent in significant renal impairment	27, 33

Adapted from ref. 2.

Diamorphine

Diamorphine (diacetylmorphine) is rapidly hydrolysed to monoacetylmorphine (MAM) and morphine; diamorphine and MAM are more lipid soluble than morphine and penetrate the CNS more rapidly, although it is MAM and morphine that are thought to be responsible for the analgesic effects of diamorphine. There is no difference between parenteral diamorphine and morphine in terms of analgesia and side-effects.[36]

Fentanyl

Fentanyl is increasingly used in the treatment of acute pain because of its lack of active metabolites and fast onset of action. The development of fentanyl patches for the treatment of chronic pain has increased the use of this drug, and is a useful addition to the analgesic formulary for patients with all degrees of renal impairment.

Hydromorphone

Hydromorphone is a derivative of morphine and is between five and ten times as potent as morphine. There is little difference between hydromorphone and other opioids in terms of analgesic efficacy or adverse effects. The main metabolite of hydromorphone is hydromorphone-3-glucuronide, a structural analogue of M3G and, like M3G, it is dependent on the kidney for excretion, has no analgesic action and can lead to dose-dependent neurotoxic effects.[3]

Methadone

Methadone is commonly used for the maintenance treatment of patients with an addiction to opioids because of its good oral bioavailability (60–95%), high potency and long duration of action. In addition, its lack of active metabolites, low cost and additional effects as an N-methyl-D-aspartate (NMDA) receptor antagonist and selective serotonin reuptake inhibitor (SSRI) have led to its increasing use in the treatment of cancer and chronic non-cancer pain. Its use in acute pain treatment is limited by its long and unpredictable duration of action and the risk of accumulation.

Oxycodone

Oxycodone is a potent opioid agonist, with approximately 2–3 times the potency of morphine. Oxycodone is metabolised in the liver primarily to noroxycodone and oxymorphone; oxymorphone is weakly active but contributes minimally to any clinical effect. Despite the minimal activity of oxymorphone the manufacturers of oxycodone caution its use in patients with mild to moderate renal impairment, and contraindicate its use in dialysis patients due to an increase in the elimination half-life of oxycodone.

Pethidine

Pethidine is a synthetic opioid still widely used even though it has multiple disadvantages. Despite a common belief that it is the most effective opioid in the treatment of renal colic, it is no better than morphine. Similarly, pethidine and morphine have similar effects on the sphincter of Oddi and biliary tract and there is no evidence that pethidine is better in the treatment of biliary colic.[3]

Accumulation of the active metabolite norpethidine is associated with neuroexcitatory effects that range from nervousness to tremors, twitches and seizures. As impaired renal function increases the half-life of norpethidine, patients in renal failure are at increased risk of norpethidine toxicity. Naloxone does not reverse and may increase the problems related to norpethidine toxicity.

Tramadol

Tramadol is an atypical centrally acting analgesic because of its combined effects as an opioid agonist and a serotonin and noradrenaline reuptake inhibitor. It is listed as a weak opioid by the World Health Organization.

Tramadol is effective in the treatment of neuropathic pain with an NNT of 3.5. Its adverse effect profile is different from other opioids. The risk of respiratory depression is significantly lower at equianalgesic doses. Significant respiratory depression has been described in patients with severe renal failure, most likely due to accumulation of the metabolite O-desmethyltramadol (M1), which has higher affinity for the opioid receptor.

In addition, tramadol has limited effects on gastrointestinal motor function and causes less constipation than morphine. Nausea and vomiting are the most common adverse effects and occur at rates similar to other opioids. Tramadol does not increase the incidence of seizures compared with other analgesic agents.[3]

Adverse effects of opioids

Common adverse effects of opioids are sedation, pruritus, nausea, vomiting, slowing of gastro-intestinal function and urinary retention. Clinically meaningful adverse effects of opioids are dose-related; once a threshold dose is reached, every 3–4 mg increase of morphine-equivalent dose per day is associated with one additional adverse event or patient-day with such an event.[37]

Respiratory depression can usually be avoided by careful titration of the dose against effect. As respiratory depression is almost always preceded by sedation, the best early clinical indicator is increasing sedation.[38]

Those opioids that are dependent on renal elimination should be used with caution in patients with renal impairment, and the possibility of drug-related side-effects should always be borne in mind. The idea of 'small doses not very often' with titration to effect should form the basis of opioid dosing for many of these drugs in a population at risk of opioid accumulation.

Adjuvant drugs

N-Methyl-D-aspartate receptor antagonists

N-Methyl-D-aspartate (NMDA) receptors are present in peripheral and central nerves. Activation of NMDA receptors is linked to learning and memory, neural development and acute and chronic pain states.

The NMDA receptor antagonist ketamine is used clinically. In chronic pain states such as central pain, complex regional pain syndrome, fibromyalgia and ischaemic and neuropathic pain, there is moderate to weak evidence that ketamine, either as the sole agent or in combination with other analgesics, improves pain and/or decreases the requirement for other analgesic agents.[39]

In patients with severe pain that was incompletely relieved by morphine, the addition of ketamine to the morphine regimen provided rapid, effective and prolonged analgesia.[40]

Most of a dose appears in the urine as hydroxylated and conjugated metabolites; 4% is excreted unchanged or as norketamine. Due to the low amounts of active drug that are excreted via the kidneys, no dose reduction is required for ketamine in patients with renal impairment.

Antidepressant drugs

Antidepressants are effective in the treatment of a variety of chronic neuropathic pain states (Table 15.3). There is also good evidence for the effect of antidepressants in chronic headaches with an NNT of 3.2 and for pain relief, but not improved function, in chronic back pain.[3]

Currently the use of antidepressants for acute neuropathic pain is mainly based on extrapolation of the above data. However, amitriptyline and venlafaxine are effective in the treatment of established neuropathic pain following breast surgery. In addition there is a possible preventive effect – given before and continued after surgery, venlafaxine significantly reduced the incidence of chronic pain at six months, and amitriptyline given to patients with acute herpes zoster reduced the incidence of postherpetic neuralgia at six months.[3]

Clinical experience in chronic pain suggests that tricyclic antidepressants (TCAs) should be

Table 15.3 Antidepressants for the treatment of diabetic neuropathy and postherpetic neuralgia (placebo-controlled trials)

Efficacy	NNT (95% CI)
Diabetic neuropathy	
TCAs	2.4 (2.0–3.0)
SSRIs	6.7 (3.4–435)
Postherpetic neuralgia	
TCAs	2.1 (1.7–3.0)
Minor adverse effects	NNH (95% CI)
Pooled diagnoses	
TCAs	2.8 (2.0–4.7)
SSRIs	No data available
Major adverse effects	NNH (95% CI)
Pooled diagnoses	
TCAs	17.0 (10–43)
SSRIs	Not different from placebo

NNT, number-needed-to-treat; NNH, number-needed-to-harm; TCA, tricyclic antidepressant; SSRI, selective serotonin reuptake inhibitor; CI, confidence interval.

Adapted from refs 41 and 42.

started at low doses, in contrast to the treatment of depression (e.g. amitriptyline 5–10 mg at night). Subsequent doses can be increased slowly if needed, in order to minimise the incidence of adverse effects.

TCAs are mainly hepatically metabolised, and there is little indication for dose reduction in renal failure, although metabolite accumulation at higher doses may increase the incidence of side-effects. The cardiovascular side-effects of these agents may limit their use in certain patients.

Evidence for the use of SSRIs in pain, consists of a number of small studies and anecdotal reports including:

- Slight but significant improvement of diabetic neuropathy symptoms was reported with citalopram 40 mg daily in a small placebo-controlled study.[43]
- Duloxetine is licensed for the treatment of diabetic neuropathy. Duloxetine treatment effectively reduced neuropathic pain in patients with diabetic neuropathy in two randomised, double-blind, placebo-controlled studies.[44] Duloxetine is contraindicated in patients with severe renal impairment (creatinine clearance <30 mL/min).
- The case of a 31-year-old woman with autonomic and peripheral neuropathy secondary to insulin-dependent diabetes mellitus and major depression is reported. Fluoxetine therapy was titrated up to 40 mg per day. After seven months without pain the patient's pain and depression returned, accompanying deterioration in her disease state. A dosage increase to 60 mg/day was quickly followed by pain relief, and later followed by improvement of her depression.[45]
- A 47-year-old man with back pain and depression due to injuries to his neck and back during a fall, benefited from mirtazapine therapy.[46] Mirtazapine 15 mg at bedtime was initiated and after one month his mood improved. His back pain also decreased from a 10 to a 3 on a 10-point scale. He was able to walk greater lengths with less difficulty and without his legs becoming 'weak'.
- Paroxetine 10–60 mg/day (median 40 mg/day) was effective in relieving symptoms of diabetic neuropathy in a single-blind, dose-

escalation study in 19 diabetic patients. The most commonly reported adverse effects were fatigue, sweating and nausea.[47]
- Venlafaxine relieved the unremitting pain of diabetic peripheral neuropathy in eight patients who found no relief from a variety of other treatments. NSAIDs, paracetamol, carbamazepine, capsaicin and amitriptyline were not successful, either due to lack of efficacy or to intolerable side-effects. Within 2–8 days of beginning treatment, all eight patients responded to venlafaxine 37.5 mg twice daily with dramatic relief in symptoms associated with painful peripheral neuropathy. No serious side-effects were observed.[48] Eleven patients with type II diabetes mellitus and painful diabetic neuropathy had a 75–100% reduction in pain within a few days after beginning venlafaxine.[49] All patients had been treated unsuccessfully with other medications known to alleviate the pain associated with diabetic peripheral neuropathy. No adverse effects were reported. Two patients who were pain-free stopped taking venlafaxine and had a recurrence of pain 2–3 days later. When venlafaxine was restarted, the pain was relieved promptly.

The disposition of venlafaxine and its active metabolite, o-desmethylvenlafaxine, is altered in renal disease. Venlafaxine clearance is decreased by approximately 30 to 35% in patients with renal dysfunction. Total daily dose should be reduced by 25% in patients with mild to moderate renal impairment. The total daily dose should be reduced by 50% in patients with creatinine clearance values less than 30 mL/min. The reduced dose could be given once a day because of the prolonged half-life in this population.[50]

Anticonvulsant drugs

Anticonvulsants have been used to treat chronic neuropathic pain and various systematic reviews have shown their efficacy in a variety of neuropathic pain states (Table 15.4).

In acute pain after surgery, sodium valproate is of no benefit, whereas peri-operative gabapentin leads to substantial reductions in both post-operative analgesic requirements and pain.[3]

Table 15.4 Anticonvulsants for the treatment of diabetic neuropathy and postherpetic neuralgia (placebo-controlled trials)

Efficacy	NNT (95% CI)
Diabetic neuropathy	2.7 (2.2–3.8)
Postherpetic neuralgia	3.2 (2.4–5.0)
Minor adverse effects	NNH (95% CI)
Pooled diagnoses	2.7 (2.2–3.4)
Major adverse effects	NNH (95% CI)
Pooled diagnoses	Not different from placebo

NNT, number-needed-to-treat; NNH, number-needed-to-harm; CI, confidence interval.
Adapted from ref. 42.

Carbamazepine

In a systematic review, carbamazepine was found to have an NNT of 2.6 in trigeminal neuralgia and 3.3 in diabetic neuropathy.[51] The number-needed-to-harm (NNH) was 3.4 for minor adverse effects and 24 for severe adverse effects.

Only 1% of a dose is excreted renally. Carbamazepine has been reported as causing reversible acute renal failure, although this is rare.[52]

Gabapentin

In the same review the NNTs for gabapentin ranged between 3.2 and 3.8 in the treatment of chronic neuropathic pain states. The NNH for a minor adverse effect compared with a placebo was 2.6 (2.1–3.3). Gabapentin is also effective in the treatment of post-amputation phantom pain.[53] It should be used with caution in patients with renal impairment, and doses reduced to avoid accumulation.[54]

Lamotrigine

The NNT of lamotrigine, based on a limited number of studies in trigeminal neuralgia, is 2.1 (1.3–6.1).[51] In single-dose studies in subjects with end stage renal failure, plasma concentrations of lamotrigine were not significantly altered. However, accumulation of the glucuronide metabolite is to be expected; caution should therefore be exercised in treating patients with renal failure.[55]

Pregabalin

Pregabalin is structurally related to gabapentin and is licensed for the treatment of peripheral neuropathic pain. Like gabapentin it requires significant dosage reduction in renal impairment.[56] It has been shown to be an effective analgesic agent in placebo-controlled trials, but trials comparing it with other agents are awaited.

Sodium valproate

Sodium valproate has an NNT of 3.5 for at least a 50% reduction in migraine frequency.[57] The NNHs for nausea, tremor, dizziness and drowsiness were 3.3, 6.2, 6.5 and 6.3 respectively. The NNH for withdrawals due to adverse effects with sodium valproate was 9.4.

In patients with renal insufficiency, it may be necessary to decrease the dosage due to reduced albumin levels and associated increased free drug levels. As monitoring of plasma concentrations may be misleading, dosage should be adjusted according to clinical monitoring.[58]

Membrane stabilisers

Intravenous lidocaine infusions are effective in reducing pain in chronic neuropathic pain conditions.[3] Overall, the strongest evidence is for use of membrane stabilisers in pain due to peripheral nerve trauma.[59]

Mexiletine has been used in the treatment of refractory neuropathic pain in patients who have responded to IV lidocaine, with which it has structural similarities. Oral mexiletine showed limited efficacy with an NNT of 10 for diabetic neuropathy. It has been shown to have normal clearance in patients with creatinine clearances >10 mL/min, with up to 15% of a dose excreted unchanged in the urine.[60]

References

1. Ashley C, Currie A. *The Renal Drug Handbook*, 2nd edn. Oxford: Radcliffe Medical Press, 2004.
2. Oxycontin summary of product characteristics. Napp Pharmaceuticals Ltd, 2005.
3. Australian and New Zealand College of Anaesthetists and Faculty of Pain Medicine. *Acute*

CASE STUDY

A 33-year-old female haemodialysis patient has a 2-year history of left hand pain following a fractured metacarpel after falling off a horse. The pain worsens in cold weather. Her hand is stiff on movement which causes pain and restricts her activities. Her hand swells intermittently and becomes blue and cold. She has been told that the pain has no physical cause and that she must be imagining it. She feels that no one believes her and is concerned she may be going mad.

Previous medical history:

- IgA nephropathy
- Low mood
- Gastric ulcer three months ago.

Drug history:

- Fluoxetine 20 mg once daily
- Bisoprolol 2.5 mg once daily
- Calcichew 2 three times daily
- Alfacalcidol 0.25 µg once daily
- Vitamin B Co Forte 2 once daily
- Lansoprazole 30 mg once daily.

Presenting complaint:
Seems drowsy, withdrawn and low in mood. Says she sleeps very poorly. Diagnosis of complex regional pain syndrome.

Doctor prescribes:

- Amitriptyline 50 mg every night
- Tramadol MR 100 mg twice daily
- Guanethidine blocks.

Q1.   Comment on this prescription. What interventions might you make?

Pain Management: Scientific Evidence. Australian and New Zealand College of Anaesthetists, 2005.

4. Royal College of Anaesthetists. *Guidelines for the Use of Non-steroidal Anti-inflammatory Drugs in the Perioperative Period.* Oxford: Royal College of Anaesthetists, 1999.

5. Blum RA, Comstock TJ, Sica DA *et al.* Pharmacokinetics of gabapentin in subjects with various degrees of renal function. *Clin Pharmacol Ther* 1994; 56: 154–159.

6. Liebermann JA, Cooper TB, Suckow RF *et al.* Tricyclic antidepressant and metabolite levels in chronic renal failure. *Clin Pharmacol Ther* 1985; 37: 301–307.

7. Koppel C, Arndt I, Ibe K. Effects of enzyme induction, renal and cardiac function on ketamine plasma kinetics in patients with ketamine long-term analgesosedation. *Eur J Drug Metab Pharmacokinet* 1990; 15: 259–263.

8. Crews JC, Weller RS, Moss J *et al.* Levobupivacaine for axillary brachial plexus block: a pharmacokinetic and clinical comparison in patients with normal renal function or renal disease. *Anesth Analg* 2002; 95: 219–223.

9. Rice AS, Pither CE, Tucker GT. Plasma concentrations of bupivacaine after supraclavicular brachial plexus blockade in patients with chronic renal failure. *Anaesthesia* 1991; 46: 354–357.

10. McEllistrem RF, Schell J, O'Malley K *et al.* Interscalene brachial plexus blockade with lidocaine in chronic renal failure – a pharmacokinetic study. *Can J Anaesth* 1989; 36: 59–63.

11. Mancini F, Landolfi C, Muzio M *et al.* Acetaminophen down-regulates interleukin-1 beta-induced nuclear factor-kappa B nuclear translocation in a human astrocytic cell line. *Neurosci Lett* 2003; 353: 79–82.

12. Rømsing J, Møiniche S, Dahl JB. Rectal and parenteral paracetamol, and paracetamol in combination with NSAIDs, for postoperative analgesia. *Br J Anaesth* 2002; 88: 215–226.

13. Bennett WM, Aronoff GR, Golper TA *et al. Drug Prescribing in Renal Failure*, Philadelphia, PA: American College of Physicians, 1994.

14. Goldstein JL, Kivitz AJ, Verburg KM *et al.* A comparison of the upper gastrointestinal mucosal effects of valdecoxib, naproxen and placebo in healthy elderly subjects. *Aliment Pharmacol Ther* 2003; 18: 125–132.

15. Ofman JJ, MacLean CH, Straus WL *et al.* A meta-analysis of severe upper gastrointestinal complications of nonsteroidal antiinflammatory drugs. *J Rheumatol* 2002; 29: 804–812.

16. West PM, Fernandez C. Safety of COX-2 inhibitors in asthma patients with aspirin hypersensitivity. *Ann Pharmacother* 2003; 37: 1497–1501.

17. Curtis SP, Ng J, Yu QF *et al.* Renal effects of etoricoxib and comparator nonsteroidal anti-inflammatory drugs in controlled clinical trials. *Clin Ther* 2004; 26: 70–83.

18. Hegi TR, Bombeli T, Seifert B *et al.* Effect of rofecoxib on platelet aggregation and blood loss in gynaecological and breast surgery compared with diclofenac. *Br J Anaesth* 2004; 92: 523–531.

19. Bombardier C, Laine L, Reicin A *et al.* Comparison of upper gastrointestinal toxicity of rofecoxib and naproxen in patients with rheumatoid arthritis. VIGOR Study Group. *N Engl J Med* 2000; 343: 1520–1528.

20. US Food and Drug Administration (FDA). *FDA Public Health Advisory: Safety of Vioxx*. US Food and Drug Administration, 2004.

21. Solomon SD, McMurray JJV, Pfeffer MA *et al.* the Adenoma Prevention with Celecoxib (APC) Study Investigators. Cardiovascular risk associated with celecoxib in a clinical trial for colorectal adenoma prevention. *N Engl J Med* 2005; 352: 1071–1080.

22. Medicines and Healthcare Products Regulatory Agency. Updated advice on the safety of selective COX-2 inhibitors. February 2005.

23. Caldwell B, Aldington S, Weatherall M *et al.* Risk of cardiovascular events and celecoxib: a systematic review and meta-analysis. *J R Soc Med* 2006; 99: 132–240.

24. Medicines and Healthcare Products Regulatory Agency. Cardiovascular safety of non-steroidal anti-inflammatory drugs. Overview of key data. August 2005.

25. Macintyre PE, Jarvis DA. Age is the best predictor of postoperative morphine requirements. *Pain* 1996; 64: 357–364.

26. Davies G, Kingswood C, Street M. Pharmacokinetics of opioids in renal dysfunction. *Clin Pharmacokinet* 1996; 31: 410–422.

27. Mercadante S, Arcuri E. Opioids and renal function. *J Pain* 2004; 5: 2–19.

28. AMH. *Australian Medicines Handbook*. Adelaide: Australian Medicines Handbook Pty Ltd, 2004.

29. Babul N, Darke AC, Hagen N. Hydromorphone metabolite accumulation in renal failure. *J Pain Sympt Manage* 1995; 3: 184–186.

30. Angst MS, Bührer M, Lötsch J. Insidious intoxication after morphine treatment in renal failure: delayed onset of morphine-6-glucuronide action. *Anesthesiology* 2000; 92: 1473–1476.

31. Stone PA, Macintyre PE, Jarvis DA. Norpethidine toxicity and patient controlled analgesia. *Br J Anaesth* 1993; 71: 738–740.

32. Simopoulos TT, Smith HS, Peeters-Asdourian C *et al.* Use of meperidine in patient-controlled analgesia and the development of a normeperidine toxic reaction. *Arch Surg* 2002; 137: 84–88.

33. MIMS. *MIMS Annual*. MediMedia Australia Pty Ltd, 2004.

34. Gammaitoni AR, Fine P, Alvarez N *et al.* Clinical application of opioid equianalgesic data. *Clin J Pain* 2003; 19: 286–297.

35. Klepstad P, Dale O, Kaasa S *et al.* Influences on serum concentrations of morphine, M6G and M3G during routine clinical drug monitoring: a prospective survey in 300 adult cancer patients. *Acta Anaesthesiol Scand* 2003; 47: 725–731.

36. Kaiko RF, Wallenstein SL, Rogers AG *et al.* Analgesic and mood effects of heroin and morphine in cancer patients with postoperative pain. *N Engl J Med* 1981; 304: 1501–1505.

37. Zhao SZ, Chung F, Hanna DB *et al.* Dose-response relationship between opioid use and adverse

effects after ambulatory surgery. *J Pain Symptom Manage* 2004; 28: 35–46.

38. Chaney MA. Side effects of intrathecal and epidural opioids. *Can J Anaesthesiol* 1995; 42: 891–903.

39. Hocking G, Cousins MJ. Ketamine in chronic pain management: an evidence-based review. *Anesth Analg* 2003; 97: 1730–1739.

40. Weinbroum AA. A single small dose of postoperative ketamine provides rapid and sustained improvement in morphine analgesia in the presence of morphine-resistance pain. *Anesth Analg* 2003; 96: 789–795.

41. Collins SL, Moore RA, McQuay HJ *et al.* Antidepressants and anticonvulsants for diabetic neuropathy and postherpetic neuralgia: a quantitative systematic review. *J Pain Symptom Manage* 2000; 20: 449–58.

42. McQuay HJ. Neuropathic pain: evidence matters. *Eur J Pain* 2002; 6(A): 11–18.

43. Sindrup SH, Bjerre U, Dejgaard A *et al.* The selective serotonin reuptake inhibitor citalopram relieves the symptoms of diabetic neuropathy. *Clin Pharmacol Ther* 1992; 52: 547–552.

44. Cymbalta summary of product characteristics. Eli Lilly and Company Ltd, 2006.

45. Theesen KA, Marsh WR. Relief of diabetic neuropathy with fluoxetine. *DICP* 1989; 23: 572–574.

46. Brannon GE, Stone KD: The use of mirtazapine in a patient with chronic pain. *J Pain Symptom Manage* 1999; 18: 382–385.

47. Sindrup SH, Grodum E, Gram LF, Beck-Nielsen H. Concentration-response relationship in paroxetine treatment of diabetic neuropathy symptoms: a patient-blinded dose-escalation study. *Ther Drug Monit* 1991; 13: 408–414.

48. Kiayias JA, Vlachou ED, Lakka-Papadodima E. Venlafaxine HCl in the treatment of painful peripheral diabetic neuropathy. *Diabetes Care* 2000; 23: 699.

49. Davis JL, Smith RL. Painful peripheral diabetic neuropathy treated with venlafaxine HCl extended release capsule. *Diabetes Care* 1999; 22: 1909.

50. Troy SM, Schultz RW, Parker BD *et al.* The effect of renal disease on the disposition of venlafaxine. *Clin Pharmacol Ther* 1994; 56: 14–21.

51. Backonja MM. Use of anticonvulsants for treatment of neuropathic pain. *Neurology* 2002; 59: S14–S17.

52. Jupert P, Almirall J, Casonovas A, Garcia M. Carbamazepine-induced acute renal failure. *Neurology* 1993; 43: 446–447.

53. Bone M, Critchley P, Buggy DJ. Gabapentin in postamputation phantom limb pain: a randomized, double-blind, placebo-controlled, cross-over study. *Reg Anesth Pain Med* 2002; 27: 481–486.

54. Neurontin summary of product characteristics. Pfizer Ltd, 2005.

55. Lamictal summary of product characteristics. GlaxoSmithKline, 2005.

56. Lyrica summary of product characteristics. Pfizer Ltd, 2006.

57. Moore A, Edwards J, Barden J *et al. Bandolier's Little Book of Pain.* Oxford: Oxford University Press, 2003: 14–18.

58. Epilim summary of product characteristics, Sanofi-Aventis, 2005.

59. Kalso E, Tramèr MR, McQuay HJ *et al.* Systemic local-anaesthetic-type drugs in chronic pain: a systematic review. *Eur J Pain* 1998; 2: 3–14.

60. Murphy EJ. Acute pain management pharmacology for the patient with concurrent renal or hepatic disease. *Anaesth Intens Care* 2005; 33: 311–322.

Further reading

Australian and New Zealand College of Anaesthetists and Faculty of Pain Medicine. *Acute Pain Management: Scientific Evidence.* Australian and New Zealand College of Anaesthetists, 2005.

Murphy EJ. Acute pain management pharmacology for the patient with concurrent renal or hepatic disease. *Anaesth Intensive Care* 2005; 33: 311–322.

16

Diabetes management in kidney disease

Mrudula Patel

Diabetes mellitus is a group of metabolic disorders characterised by chronic hyperglycaemia and is associated with disturbances of carbohydrate, fat and protein metabolism resulting in defects in insulin secretion, action or both. In type 1 diabetes mellitus, or insulin-dependent diabetes mellitus (IDDM), there is usually gross destruction of pancreatic beta cells (which produce insulin) while in type 2 diabetes mellitus, or non-insulin-dependent diabetes mellitus (NIDDM), insufficient insulin is produced to meet the metabolic needs. Type 2 diabetes mellitus usually occurs later in life than type 1.

Poorly controlled diabetes mellitus (hyperglycaemia, hypertension and dyslipidaemia are the key risks) can lead to serious and life-threatening long-term complications referred to as microvascular and macrovsacular complications. Microvascular complications arise from a cumulative damage to small blood vessels and include retinopathy, nephropathy and neuropathy. Macrovascular complications are the cardiovascular consequences of the metabolic abnormalities associated with diabetes mellitus which include coronary heart disease, cerebrovascular and peripheral vascular disease .

In the UK, the National Service Frameworks for both diabetes (2001) and renal services (2005) have highlighted the importance of ensuring tight blood glucose and blood pressure control to prevent patients with diabetes mellitus developing microvascular and macrovascular complications and then subsequently the detection and management of these long-term complications.[1,2]

Diabetic renal disease, often referred to as diabetic nephropathy, is the leading cause of chronic kidney disease (CKD) in Western Europe and develops in 40% of type 1 diabetes mellitus and 5–40% of type 2 diabetes mellitus.[3] This chapter discusses the issues around diabetic renal disease by reviewing the following areas:

- The definitions of the various stages of diabetic renal disease
- The actual structural changes that occur in the diabetic kidney
- The diagnosis of diabetic renal disease
- The prevention of diabetic renal disease
- The screening and referral process for diabetic renal disease
- The management of diabetes in renal disease.

Definitions of diabetic renal disease

Diabetic renal disease is a clinical condition of altered renal function accompanied by structural changes in the kidney. It progresses through a continuum of hyperfiltration and renal hypertrophy, increased protein excretion to declining renal function leading to end stage renal failure (ESRF).

Microalbuminuria

Microalbuminuria is defined as a persistent urinary albumin excretion between 30 and 300 mg/day. A good estimate is provided by the urinary albumin:creatinine ratio (ACR), with values ≥2.5 mg/mmol in men and ≥3.5 mg/mmol in women indicating microalbuminuria. An equivalent threshold on a timed urine collection is approximately 20 µg/min.

205

Clinical/overt diabetic nephropathy

Clinical/overt diabetic nephropathy is defined by a persistent urinary albumin excretion ≥300 mg/24 hours and corresponds to clinical proteinuria as reliably detected by albumin dipstick. An equivalent ACR on a random urine sample is about 25 mg/mmol.[4]

The actual structural changes that occur in the diabetic kidney

The structural changes that occur in the kidney are a continuum, as summarised in Table 16.1.

There is an initial basement membrane thickening of the glomerulus leading to altered pressures and function within the glomerular capillaries thus causing a leakage of proteins, particularly albumin. In the early stages many of the abnormalities are reversible, but eventually this increasing glomerular damage will lead to scarring, permanent loss of function and dramatically increasing proteinuria. Alongside

Table 16.1 The progressive changes with diabetic renal disease

Progressive changes	Status
Normal	GFR normal (e.g 100 mL/min) BP normal Well Albuminuria <20 mg/day
Hyperfiltration	Increased GFR (e.g 120 mL/min)
Microalbuminuria	Albumin excretion 30–300 mg/day Slight increase in BP
Persistent proteinuria	Progressive increase in proteinuria, albumin >300 mg/day Pronounced increase in BP Decrease in GFR Raised serum creatinine but within normal range

Adapted from ref. 4.

this renal damage there are hormonal changes occurring within the kidney that lead to raised blood pressure (BP) and this appears to amplify the damage process and the amount of proteinuria. At the microalbuminuria stage, sometimes referred to as incipient nephropathy, the renal function is normal but it should trigger a warning that the pathological process has started.[4]

The diagnosis of diabetic renal disease

A renal biopsy together with the classical clinical features should confirm the diagnosis of diabetic renal disease. The classical clinical features of established diabetic renal disease are:

• At least 5–10 years of diabetes mellitus, this includes the undiagnosed period
• Continuous significant proteinuria
• Mild–moderate increase in BP
• Rarely any other findings in the urine (haematuria, cells and casts are all uncommon)
• Normal or large size kidneys on ultrasound
• Usually significant retinopathy, but not always in type 2 diabetes.

Other causes of renal disease can be present in diabetic patients and sometimes co-exist:

• Renal disease long preceding diabetes
• Essential hypertension
• Renal stone disease
• Gout
• Congenital abnormalities
• Glomerulonephritis
• Pyelonephritis.

These should be excluded by basic investigations and then treated. Patients with a single kidney appear to be more vulnerable to diabetic renal disease.

The prevention of diabetic renal disease

Three landmark studies, one in type 1 diabetes, DCCT (Diabetes Control and Complication

Trial), and two in type 2 diabetes, UKPDS (UK Prospective Diabetes Study) and the Kumamoto study have all proven the substantial benefits of tight blood glucose control by showing a reduction in the risk of developing micro-albuminuria, proteinuria and rising serum creatinine.[5-7] Epidemiological analysis of the UKPDS cohort suggested that with every 1% reduction in glycated haemoglobin (HbA1c), the chance of developing nephropathy and retinopathy was reduced by 35%. The UKPDS also showed that by reducing blood pressure (154/87 to 144/82 mmHg), there was an associated decreased risk for developing microalbuminuria. The epidemiological analysis suggested a risk reduction of about 12% for each 10 mmHg decrease in mean systolic BP, with no lower threshold.

All patients who have microalbuminuria or proteinuria should be started on either an angiotensin-converting enzyme (ACE) inhibitor or an angiotensin II receptor antagonists, and this has shown to reduce the rate of progression to both diabetic nephropathy and non-diabetic nephropathy even when the BP is not obviously raised.[8] Serum creatinine and potassium should be checked before and after initiating treatment or after a dose increase. A small rise in serum creatinine is usually expected in the short term and should not be an indication to withdraw therapy, although renal artery stenosis should be considered if a marked creatinine rise is seen.

The major causes of death in type 2 diabetes are the cardiovascular-related illnesses and because of this high risk of macrovascular disease and premature mortality with worsening renal disease, all patients with microalbuminuria and clinical diabetic nephropathy should start treatment with a low-dose aspirin and a lipid-lowering agent for vascular protection.[9]

The screening and referral process for diabetic renal disease

Patients with diabetic renal disease are frequently referred too late to initiate treatment to reduce renal disease progression. These patients have the highest risk of mortality and morbidity of any subgroup in diabetes mellitus.

In patients with type 1 and type 2 diabetes, measure the urinary ACR or albumin concentration annually. If microalbuminuria or proteinuria is present then repeat the ACR or albumin concentration twice more within one month where possible. Serum creatinine is measured annually. A referral to a nephrologist is made for an opinion when the results are abnormal, together with a serum creatinine greater than 150 µmol/L. Controversy still remains around the standardisation of creatinine measurements to determine renal function. Serum creatinine is significantly lower in diabetes than non-diabetes patients because the muscle mass is lower. The result will show a better renal function but this may be incorrect as the severity of renal disease in diabetes is underestimated. The American Diabetes Association has now recommended that physicians use the Levey modification of the Cockcroft and Gault equation, also known as MDRD (see Chapter 2), to calculate an estimated glomerular filtration rate (eGFR) from serum creatinine, or of course the original Cockcroft and Gault equation, to stage the patient's renal disease. See Chapter 2 for equations. A referral should be made to the nephrologist when the eGFR has fallen to <60 mL/min/1.73 m^2 (stage 3 CKD). This highlights the fact that patients with stage 3 CKD often show a 'normal' serum creatinine and 42% will have a serum creatinine <120 µmol/L. In other words, just looking at the serum creatinine alone, without calculating the patient's GFR, the CKD would remain undiagnosed. See Chapter 2 for stages of CKD.

Once a referral is made to a nephrologist, long-term management plans can be made to optimise treatment both in the primary and secondary care setting, thus preventing any further life-threatening complications.

The management of diabetes in kidney disease

The management of diabetes in kidney disease should follow the same pathway as the management of diabetes mellitus, however considerations, and possibly adjustments, should be made to account for any renal impairment.

The aim of treatment in diabetes mellitus is to maintain effective glycaemic and BP control. The treatment plan for type 2 diabetes should be:

• Diet and exercise
• Oral monotherapy
• Oral combination therapy
• Insulin ± oral agents.

In type 1 diabetes, insulin therapy should be optimised to keep HbA1c as low as possible, ideally between 6.5% and 7% (the normal level for healthy individuals is <6%).

The major limitation of using intensive treatments in both type 1 and type 2 diabetes is the concern of hypoglycaemia, and this risk increases as HbA1c is driven down. The frequency of hypoglycaemia at any given HbA1c is much greater in type 1 compared with type 2 diabetes, although hypoglycaemia does not occur when metformin or the thiazolidinediones (or sometimes referred to as the glitazones) are used alone, and the risk is lower with the modern insulin regimens, human insulin analogues. Despite this concern of hypoglycaemia with tight blood glucose control, the target for HbA1c should still be as low as possible, as long as hypoglycaemia is not a major problem. Table 16.2 is a guide for the HbA1c targets.

Weight gain is also a common adverse outcome of intensive insulin treatment in type 1 diabetes, and apart from diet or metformin alone, in all other treatment options for type 2 diabetes.

For each individual, the potential benefits of intensive glycaemic control should be balanced against the actual or expected risks.

Lifestyle interventions for type 2 diabetes

In type 2 diabetes, lifestyle interventions are key in the prevention and treatment of the condition. The aims are to encourage weight loss, improve glycaemic control and improve the cardiac risk factors and potential outcomes by encouraging patients to increase the proportion of vegetables, fruit, nuts and oily fish in their diet, although patients with ESRF need to be cautious and avoid all foods that may increase potassium and phosphate, for example bananas and dairy products.

Dietary interventions should always be the first-line therapy in type 2 diabetes so patients do not receive the message that the major treatment is tablets. In the UKPDS study, dietary therapy was the sole intervention for the first three months and achieved a mean 2% decrease in HbA1c, more than that achieved by any single oral hypoglycaemic agent. When the initial blood glucose level is high, and the patient is not highly symptomatic, it is usually better to start with diet and exercise alone, except if there are important personal indications (exams, foreign travel for example), as the sole removal of large quantities of sugary drinks and simple sugars often leads to a rapid fall in blood glucose and control of the symptoms. In those patients with a persistent high blood glucose at diagnosis, then an oral hypoglycaemic agent together with diet should be started. Other lifestyle interventions would include exercise (need to counsel patients on hypoglycaemia with exercise and the undertaking of blood glucose monitoring during exercise), stopping smoking and reducing alcohol consumption.

Oral hypoglycaemic agents for type 2 diabetes

As discussed earlier, if the blood glucose level is still inadequately controlled, despite the life-

Table 16.2 Suggested HbA1c targets

Patient group	Approximate target	Action if
Diet alone, metformin or glitazones	<6.5%	>6.8–7%
Sulfonylurea or meglitinides	<7%	>7.5%
Insulin alone or in combination	<7.5%	≥8%

Adapted from ref. 4.

Sites of action for oral therapies for type 2 diabetes

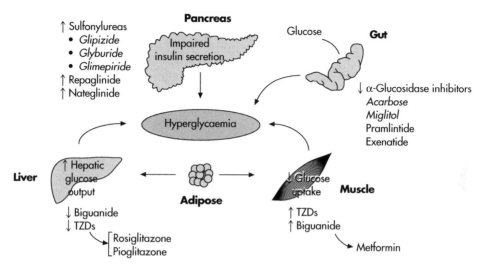

Figure 16.1   Sites of action for oral therapies for type 2 diabetes mellitus. From ref. 10.

style interventions, then an oral hypoglycaemic agent (OHA) should be commenced.[10] Figure 16.1 highlights the sites of action for the various OHAs.

Metformin (biguanide)

About 85–95% of newly diagnosed patients with type 2 diabetes in Western countries are overweight or obese and so the first-line oral agent is metformin (biguanide) unless it is contraindicated and this will be discussed later. Metformin targets the main problem of insulin resistance, and in the UKPDS, the obese group treated with metformin showed a much greater drop in vascular events than the sulfonylurea/insulin groups. Metformin is not associated with weight gain whereas all the other OHAs are (the exception are the thiazolidinediones). The mechanism of action of metformin is not fully understood, but it does decrease hepatic gluconeogenesis and enhances peripheral glucose utilisation and thus reduces appetite. It is only effective if there are some residual functioning pancreatic beta cells. The main drawback of metformin is the high incidence of gastrointestinal side-effects, nausea and diarrhoea,

together with flatulence, abdominal pain and a metallic taste. These effects are usually dose related and so always start the patient with a low dose, 500 mg twice a day, then increase over weeks. Always counsel the patients to take metformin with meals and never on an empty stomach and warn patients about the gastrointestinal side-effects. If the side-effects persist, halve the dose and then gradually increase but more slowly. An emphasis should be made to patients that it will take some days to weeks to become effective. The target for most patients is 1000 mg twice a day.

The contraindications for metformin are controversial,[11] and the main anxiety is lactic acidosis. Lactic acidosis associated with metformin is a rare condition but it should be withdrawn:

- If serum creatinine is higher than 150 µmol/L (this is a chosen cut-off point for renal failure so additional considerations for patients' muscle mass and protein turnover should be made)
- During periods of suspected tissue hypoxia (sepsis, myocardial infarction. etc.)
- Three days after contrast medium containing iodine has been given, and restart metformin only when renal function has been checked

- Two days before general anaesthesia and restart only when renal function is stable.

In diabetic kidney disease, metformin is still the first-line agent unless the eGFR falls below 60 mL/min/1.73 m^2 as discussed above. In an acute episode of renal failure, metformin should be stopped but can be safely restarted if the eGFR returns to above 60 mL/min/1.73 m^2 and the renal function routinely measured thereafter, if not an alternate OHA, usually a sulfonylurea, should be commenced. Other contraindications include pregnancy or breastfeeding.

Sulfonylureas

Sulfonylureas increase pancreatic insulin secretion, therefore are only effective when there is some residual pancreatic beta cell activity. The most commonly prescribed sulfonylureas are gliclazide, glipizide, glimepiride and glibenclamide; less commonly seen are chlorpropamide and tolbutamide. Hypoglycaemia is the main issue with sulfonylureas, especially in renal impairment, and sulfonylurea-induced hypoglycaemia may persist for many hours, often requiring hospitalisation. The long-acting sulfonylureas chlorpropamide and glibenclamide are associated with a higher risk of hypoglycaemia.

Chlorpropamide is contraindicated in severe renal impairment, eGFR <20 mL/min/1.73 m^2, but can be used with caution if the eGFR is between 20 and 50 mL/min, and as well as the increased risk of hypoglycaemia, there is a severe risk of metabolic acidosis. Glibenclamide in renal impairment, again should be used with caution and initially at low doses, 1.25–2.5 mg once a day with monitoring. The short-acting sulfonylurea gliclazide is the usual drug of choice in renal impairment, and doses start between 20 mg and 40 mg once a day (refer to the *Renal Drug Handbook* for further drug dosing information[12]). Again, as with renal impairment, sulfonylureas should be used with caution in elderly or frail patients or those living alone, as severe protracted hypoglycaemia can occur.

Other side-effects include weight gain, which is common especially in the first 3–6 months.

Otherwise they are well tolerated with occasional effects of rashes, nausea, vomiting, diarrhoea and constipation. They may rarely cause hepatic problems including cholestatic jaundice and eventual liver failure so are contraindicated in severe hepatic disease. Blood dyscrasias and severe skin rashes have also been seen rarely. They are contraindicated whilst breastfeeding and in patients with porphyria.

Patients should always be taught how to recognise hypoglycaemia and told weight gain is expected. There is no benefit at all in exceeding the maximum dose or using more than one sulfonylurea, so another group of OHAs should be added, usually metformin, unless it is contraindicated, in which case a glitazone is a good choice.

Thiazolidinediones (glitazones)

The thiazolidinediones, often referred to as the glitazones, are selective agonists at the peroxisomal proliferator-activated receptor gamma (PPARγ) nuclear receptor and reduce glycaemia by reducing insulin resistance at adipose tissue, skeletal muscle and liver. The glitazones have a synergistic action with other OHAs, so the National Institute for Health and Clinical Excellence (NICE) in the UK have sanctioned their use as second-line therapy with either metformin or a sulfonylurea, where the glitazone should replace whichever drug in the combination is poorly tolerated or contraindicated.

At present there are only two glitazones available for the management of type 2 diabetes, pioglitazone and rosiglitazone, both of which were licensed in the UK in 2000. The two landmark studies for patients with type 2 diabetes, UKPDS (1998) and Kumamato (1995), occurred well before the glitazones were manufactured, thus publication data on outcome results for their use have been fairly limited. In general the glitazones produce similar glycaemic improvements (1–1.5% HbA1c) to other OHAs either as monotherapy or as combined therapy, although as mentioned earlier, NICE guidelines restrict their use for dual therapy only. From the limited evidence available, they have been shown to maintain effect in the long term and preserve beta cell function, have beneficial effects on lipids and many other cardiovascular risk factors.

Originally there were concerns about hepatic toxicity, oedema and heart failure. The hepatic toxicity anxiety is probably unfounded and dates back to the first glitazone, troglitazone, that was licensed in the United States. Now there is increasing evidence that the glitazones may benefit fatty liver, although the manufacturers still recommend liver function tests (LFTs) should be carried out before therapy and every two months for the first year and periodically thereafter. The remaining side-effects are weight gain and oedema. There is concern about precipitation of heart failure, especially in patients on insulin, so the glitazones at present should not be used in patients with heart failure or at a very high risk for it. They are also contraindicated for co-administration with insulin, during pregnancy and while breastfeeding.

The glitazones are extensively metabolised in the liver, some of the metabolites are active, and are excreted mainly via the urine and 25% via faecal elimination. When using the glitazones in diabetic kidney disease, therefore, no dose adjustment is required if patients have mild to moderate renal impairment. The data for their use in ESRF are limited and the manufacturers recommend that the glitazones should be used with caution. In practice, the glitazones can be used at normal doses in ESRF, but blood glucose should be monitored especially during any acute episodes (refer to the *Renal Drug Handbook* for further drug dosing information[12]).

The glitazones take several months to show their full effect (up to six months), so doses should not be rapidly adjusted and patients should be encouraged to continue treatment. Some consultant diabetologists are trialling triple therapy (metformin + sulfonylurea + glitazone) for a 2–3 month period to account for this delayed effect from the glitazones and then stopping whichever initial drug (metformin or sulfonylurea) was ineffective. Around 25% of patients will show no blood glucose response to the glitazones; such patients tend to be more obese and have a long-standing insulin resistance with depleted pancreatic insulin reserves. In those non-responders there should not be a delay to move over to insulin.

The meglitinides

The meglitinides stimulate insulin secretion and are the newest group of antidiabetics licensed in the UK (2001). There are two drugs available, repaglinide and nateglinide. Both drugs have different mechanisms of action but predominately enhance first-phase insulin release, and therefore reduce immediate post-prandial hyperglycaemia. New patients should always be initiated on a small dose and then titrated according to blood glucose.

Repaglinide has been licensed as monotherapy or in combination with metformin, while nateglinide has a licence for combination with metformin only. Both drugs have a rapid onset of action, so patients should be advised to take the tablet up to 30 minutes prior to meals. The duration of activity is short, so omit the dose if a meal is missed.

Had the meglitinides been invented before the sulfonylureas and were less expensive, they would probably be preferred as they cause less hypoglycaemia and minimal weight gain, but they are more expensive, and this has limited their use.

The meglitinides in diabetic kidney disease require no dose adjustments in patients with renal impairment and as nateglinide is licensed only in combination with metformin, it would not be considered for patients with ESRF. Side-effects include gastrointestinal upsets and rashes and rarely hypoglycaemia. They are also contraindicated in severe hepatic impairment, during pregnancy and while breastfeeding.

Acarbose

Acarbose is an inhibitor of alpha-glucosidase, and therefore limits and delays the absorption of starches. It has a mild hypoglycaemic effect with a mean HbA1c reduction of around 0.5% but its gastrointestinal side-effects, mainly flatulence, makes it an unpopular choice. However, it may have a small role in patients unable to tolerate metformin and in combination therapy.

Combination therapy for type 2 diabetes

If monotherapy with a single OHA fails to control blood glucose, then a second OHA should be added. The most common combination for type 2 diabetes is metformin with a sulfonylurea, but if this combination is contraindicated, then the alternate options could be:

- Metformin with a glitazone
- Sulfonylurea with a glitazone
- Metformin with a sulfonylurea and a glitazone (triple therapy, not ideal for the long term and insulin would be a better alternative)
- Metformin with a meglitinide
- Metformin with acarbose.

However, most people with type 2 diabetes will eventually progress to needing insulin due to pancreatic beta cell exhaustion, and it is important to identify these patients promptly, thus preventing microvascular and macrovascular complications.

Insulin

Insulin therapy in type 2 diabetes
Insulin therapy, as mentioned earlier, should be initiated as promptly as possible if OHAs cannot achieve HbA1c <8%. If there is still some residual insulin secretion, then patients with type 2 diabetes will usually administer insulin at night (immediate or prolonged action) and continue with a daytime OHA (usually metformin or a sulfonylurea). This use of a nocturnal insulin will suppress hepatic glucose production overnight, therefore controlling the fasting blood glucose levels, whilst continuing a daytime OHA will minimise the weight gain. The new prolonged action basal insulin analogues glargine and detemir are increasingly being used to cover the overnight insulin as clinical trials have proven a reduction in nocturnal hypoglycaemia and weight gain compared with the older intermediate insulin.

For those patients with type 2 diabetes where there is complete pancreatic beta cell exhaustion insulin alone will be the only option. These patients will need to be carefully monitored and the dose adjusted in order to balance and prevent weight gain and hypoglycaemia from the insulin regimen.

Insulin therapy in type 1 diabetes
Most patients with type 1 diabetes continue to produce their own insulin for a year or so after diagnosis, which becomes apparent soon after starting insulin as the removal of glucose toxicity allows the pancreatic beta cells to recover, resulting in a reduction in the total amount of insulin required, sometimes referred to as the 'honeymoon period', lasting 6–12 months.

Insulin therapy in type 1 and type 2 diabetes
The aim of insulin treatment in both type 1 and type 2 diabetes is to maintain effective glycaemic and BP control.

Ideally, insulin regimens should mimic as closely as possible the insulin profile of healthy individuals, a prandial bolus insulin with a basal insulin, often referred to as a basal–bolus regimen (i.e. rapid/short-acting insulin to control postprandial spikes with a long-acting insulin to give a low-level background cover). The recent advances in insulin technology has led to the introduction of new human insulin analogues, thus revolutionising insulin treatment for diabetes and allowing specific tailoring for each individual.[13]

The insulin groups now available are:

- Rapid-acting analogues
- Short-acting
- Intermediate-acting
- Long-acting
- Prolonged-action analogue.

Insulin therapy in diabetic kidney disease
Insulin in a healthy individual circulates free as a monomer with a half-life of 4–5 minutes. It is metabolised by the liver and kidney. In the kidney, insulin is filtered by the glomeruli and reabsorbed by the tubules which also degrade it. In renal and hepatic disease, there is a decrease in the rate of insulin clearance, resulting in increased amounts of circulating insulin, thus increasing the risk of hypoglycaemia, so insulin doses should be reduced. In diabetic kidney disease this reduction in insulin requirement will vary depending on the degree of renal impairment. In ESRF, the insulin dosing may need a

further reduction as there is a complete failure of the kidney to remove insulin, together with the anorexia and weight loss associated with uraemia, which can lead to virtual starvation. Some patients in ESRF even manage to come off treatment completely.[14]

For those patients in ESRF the type of renal replacement therapy, haemodialysis or peritoneal dialysis, will also decide the type and dose of insulin required. Haemodialysis usually takes place three times a week for around 4 hours each session so this will interrupt the daily eating habit as well as the daily activity for these patients. Also, because insulin is a big molecule, it will not be removed by haemodialysis, thus increasing the incidence of hypoglycaemia. The options for the patient on haemodialysis are to reduce the dose of insulin on haemodialysis days or to use a once-a-day prolonged-acting basal insulin for a low-level 24-hour background cover.

Peritoneal dialysis occurs on a daily basis, at set times and is less aggressive. It will therefore have a minimal effect on the overall glycaemic control, although the peritoneal dialysis dialysate will contain glucose and its absorption can increase the blood glucose levels in patients on PD. Hence these patients generally require higher doses of insulin than haemodialysis patients.[15]

New agents

Inhaled insulin (Exubera)

The inhaled insulin Exubera has recently received a licence in the UK for certain patients with type 1 and type 2 diabetes. It is fast acting and when inhaled will reach the lungs within 10 minutes before starting a meal. NICE are in the process of formalising a technology guidance on the use of inhaled insulin, but the current evidence has shown that it is as effective as injectable insulin in blood glucose control in type 1 diabetes but the dosing regimen is complicated and wasteful and the equipment is not convenient.

At present there are no published data for its use in renal impairment.[16]

Rapid-acting insulin analogue, glulisine (Apidra)

The rapid-acting insulin analogue glulisine (Apidra) has been introduced and licensed for use in both type 1 and type 2 diabetes. Evidence to date has shown its advantage as an alternative for obese or overweight patients.[10]

Glucagon-like peptide 1 analogue (Exenatide)

The glucagon-like peptide 1 (GLP-1) analogue Exenatide has been available in the USA since 2005 but is awaiting a European regulatory review. Exenatide is an injection and a member of a new class of drugs which mimic the glucose-lowering action of human hormones called incretins. In the USA, it has been approved as adjunctive therapy for patients with type 2 diabetes with metformin or a sulfonylurea, or both. There are no published data for its use in renal impairment.[17]

Islet cell transplantation

Islet cell transplantation is currently available in some hospitals around the UK as a potential cure and or change to the natural history of the disease diabetes.

Pancreas transplantation

Pancreas transplantation is a solid organ transplant and a potential cure/change for diabetes. Again, as with islet cell transplantation, it is an option available in some hospitals around the UK.

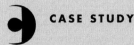

CASE STUDY

DP is a 76-year-old woman, weighing 99.1 kg, who presents with acute renal failure, shortness of breath, tachycardia and diarrhoea. She has a past medical history of hypertension, type 2 diabetes mellitus, chronic renal failure (diabetic nephropathy) and has recently been treated for cellulitis with flucloxacillin then cefalexin by her GP.

Drug history:

- Metformin 850 mg twice daily (stopped on admission)
- Gliclazide 160 mg every morning 80 mg every night (withheld)
- Rosiglitazone 4 mg every morning (withheld on admission)
- Atenolol 100 mg every morning (stopped on admission)
- Valsartan 40 mg every morning (stopped on admission)
- Atorvastatin 40 mg every night (stopped on admission)
- Aspirin 75 mg every morning (stopped on admission).

Family history:
Nil relevant.

Social history:
Lives alone and independent.

Biochemistry:

Day	1	2	3	4	10	11	12
Creatinine (μmol/L)	716	641	454	319	248	204	192
Urea (mmol/L)	49.2	34.3	35.2	30.2	25	23	23
Sodium (mmol/L)	136	139	137	138	137	137	134
Potassium (mmol/L)	7.1	5.7	4.8	4.5	3.0	3.2	3.2
Bicarbonate (mmol/L)	17	18	22	22	24	25	24
Calcium (mmol/L)	1.98	2.14	2.34	2.45	2.35	2.24	2.24
Phosphate (mmol/L)	2.39	2.54	1.64	1.38	1.07	0.89	0.90
Alb (g/L)	38	38	43	43	39	38	38
BP (mmHg)	70/40	85/31	110/50	115/50	130/75	120/80	120/75
Blood glucose (7 am) (mmol/L)	4.5	6.2	7.7	7.6	10.1	12	5.3
Blood glucose (noon) (mmol/L)	8.5	12.9	11	14.7	10.1	23.5	12
Blood glucose (10 pm) (mmol/L)	8.7	8.2	7.4	16	12.2	13.2	14
HbA1c (%)	9.0						
Hb g/dL	7.6	10.9	11.0	12.3	12.3	12	11
WCC (×10⁹/L)	12	9	9	9	9	9	9
Weight (kg)	99.1	94.4	92.5	91.1	90	90	90

→

◖ CASE STUDY (continued)

The main issues are the acute renal failure (anuric, hyperkalaemic, acidotic), shortness of breath and fluid overloaded, hypotension, tachycardia, diarrhoea and poor blood glucose control.

On day 1, patient DP is haemofiltered. Metformin, valsartan and atenolol are stopped and all other medicines are withheld. Ranitidine is commenced temporarily for uraemia. A chest X-ray shows pulmonary oedema but no signs of chest infection. Cultures are taken to rule out sepsis. Patient has signs of peripheral oedema. She is fluid restricted and furosemide 120 mg every morning is started. Tropium level is taken to rule out any cardiac event; the result is <0.2 µgram/L.

On day 2, DP is haemofiltered again although she has started to pass some urine and the peripheral oedema is improving. The diarrhoea has stopped.

On day 3, the patient has passed >2 L of urine and her biochemistry is improving. Blood cultures return as no growth; patient is apyrexial, C-reactive protein is returning towards normal. Blood glucose is reviewed, but as the patient is not eating much, she remains solely on gliclazide 80 mg every morning to control blood glucose. Her weight is down to 92.5 kg. Renal USS shows no new abnormalities.

On day 4, the patient continues to improve, passing good urine and eating well. Atorvastatin and aspirin are restarted.

On day 10, the patient is reviewed by the diabetologist for blood glucose control, and insulin, Novomix 30 twice daily, is recommended and oral antidiabetics are stopped.

On day 11, valsartan 40 mg every morning is restarted as results show no renovascular disease.

On day 12, the patient is responding well to insulin and discharge plans are made.

Q1. What might her causes of diabetes be?

Q2. What might her causes of chronic renal failure be?

Q3. Could it have been prevented?

Q4. What might her causes of acute renal failure be?

Q5. Explain her drug history and any possible reasons for stopping some of her medication on admission.

Q6. Why would this patient take atorvastatin and aspirin?

Q7. Why change this patient's diabetic regimen to insulin?

Q8. Would the regimen differ if the patient had ESRF?

Q9. Comment on BP control in diabetes.

Q10. What discharge plans should be made for this patient?

References

1. Department of Health. *National Service Framework for Renal Services, Part Two: Chronic Kidney Disease, Acute renal Failure and End of Life Care.* London: Department of Health, 2005.
2. Department of Health. *National Service Framework for Diabetes: Standards.* London: Department of Health. 2002.
3. Hasslacher C. *Diabetic Nephropathy.* London: Wiley, 2001: 22–27.
4. Drury P, Gatling W. *Your Questions Answered. Diabetes.* London: Churchill Livingstone, 2005.
5. The Diabetes Control and Complications Trial Research Group. The effect of intensive treatment of diabetes on the development and progression of long-term complications in insulin-dependent diabetes mellitus. *N Engl J Med* 1993; 329: 977–986.
6. Alder AI, Stevens RJ, Manley SE *et al.* Development and progression of nephropathy in type 2 diabetes: The United Kingdom Prospective Diabetes Study (UKPDS 64). *Kidney Int* 2003; 63: 225–232.
7. Ohkubo Y, Kishikawa H, Araki E *et al.* Intensive insulin therapy prevents the progression of diabetic microvascular complications in Japanese patients with non-insulin-dependent diabetes

mellitus: a randomised prospective 6-year study. (Kumamoto Study). *Diabetes Res Clin Pract* 1995; 28: 103–117.
8. Mogensen CE, Cooper ME. Diabetic renal disease: from recent studies to improved clinical practice. *Diabet Med* 2004; 21: 4–17.
9. National Prescribing Centre NHS. Drug management of type 2 diabetes: summary. *MeRec Bull* 2004; 15.
10. Medscape. Diabetes and insulin: Indications, initiation and innovations. http//medcape.com/viewprogram/5500_pnt (accessed 13 June 2006).
11. Alexander WD, Jones GC, Macklin JP. Contra-indications to the use of metformin. *BMJ* 2003; 326: 4–5.
12. Ashley C, Currie A. *The Renal Drug Handbook*, 2nd edn. Oxford: Radcliffe Medical Press, 2004.
13. Gummerson I. An update on insulin analogues. *Pharm J* 2006; 277: 169–172.
14. Bilous RW. End-stage renal failure and management of diabetes. *Diabet Med* 2004; 21: 12–14.
15. Atherton G. Specialism within a specialty: diabetes and dialysis. *Br J Renal Med* 2003/2004; 8: 10–11.
16. Barnett EJ, Morton-Eggleston E. Inhaled insulin. *BMJ* 2006; 332: 1043–1044.
17. Dungan K. Treating diabetes by modifying GLP-1 activity: Current options and new developments. *Diabet Microvasc Complic* 2006; 3: 43–46.

17

Myeloma and kidney disease

Elizabeth Lamerton

Myeloma is a cancer affecting plasma cells or white blood cells in the bone marrow. The cancerous plasma cells proliferate and fill more than 10% of the bone marrow, preventing the formation of normal blood cells. Patients with myeloma may present with a range of non-specific symptoms including kidney disease, anaemia and infections.

Myeloma cells produce an abnormal antibody protein known as paraprotein. The proliferation of plasma cells produces an excess of the abnormal proteins. In addition, incomplete immunoglobulins are produced, for example monoclonal immunoglobulin.

Kidney disease is a common complication of multiple myeloma with approximately 50% of patients having kidney disease at diagnosis. There are a number of possible mechanisms of kidney damage and often more than one mechanism will be involved.

The incidence of multiple myeloma in the UK and Scandinavian countries is approximately 50 cases per million.[1] The incidence rises with progressing age, with a mean of 70 years (Table 17.1).

An exact incidence of kidney disease associated with multiple myeloma is difficult to quantify. The definitions of kidney disease have varied in the UK and internationally and as a result comparison of data is somewhat unreliable. As an approximate guide, 43% of 998 patients in one study had a creatinine greater than 133 µmol/L and 22% of 423 patients had a creatinine greater than 177 µmol/L.[2,3] Advanced acute renal failure (ARF) requiring urgent dialysis therapy occurs in 3–12% of all cases.[4]

Myeloma and kidney disease are undoubtedly closely linked, with up to 30% of all myeloma patients having some degree of kidney damage at presentation and over 50% developing kidney damage during their illness.[2]

In myeloma the paraprotein light chains are filtered in the kidney across the glomerulus, where some will be reabsorbed by the tubular cells. Light chains that are incompletely reabsorbed by tubular cells are found in the urine as Bence-Jones protein. Urinary Bence-Jones proteins can be detected and quantified in the laboratory. Simultaneously, myeloma cast nephropathy may occur, where immunoglobulin light chains are deposited in the kidney as casts. In cast nephropathy, the filtered immunoglobulin light chains bind to a common site on Tamm-Horsfall protein. Aggregation of the protein complexes produces casts that can cause a physical obstruction in the tubular cells. This can result in kidney disease.

The presence of paraproteins and the deposition of fibrils causes related conditions such as amyloid disease, and crystals of abnormal protein light chains cause light chain deposition disease and Fanconi's syndrome.[1,2]

Myeloma kidney is associated with a high initial mortality of approximately 20% within one month of referral to a specialist centre. The poor survival rates reflect the large tumour burden often already present at diagnosis and is

Table 17.1	Incidence of myeloma by age	
Age <40 years	<2%
Age 40–60 years	15%
Age 60–65 years	15%
General population	50 cases per million

due to both underlying haematological malignancy and to ARF.[5]

Clinical presentation of multiple myeloma

Patients with multiple myeloma may present in a number of ways. Patients with symptoms of disease or organ damage require urgent referral, assessment and treatment. Some may present to hospital with an acute medical emergency, such as spinal cord compression, hypercalcaemia or acute kidney disease, especially ARF.

Other patients may present with non-specific clinical signs such as:

- Bone disease, in particular unexplained chronic back pain without an obvious precipitating cause
- Normochromic, normocytic anaemia with no clear cause
- Recurrent infection
- Hyperviscosity syndrome
- Features of amyloidosis such as nephritic syndrome and cardiac failure
- Raised erythrocyte sedimentation rate (ESR) or plasma viscosity
- Chronic kidney disease.

Investigation and diagnosis of myeloma

When myeloma is suspected, patients require at least the following tests and investigations:

- Full blood count
- Erythrocyte sedimentation rate
- Serum and plasma electrolytes
- Electrophoresis of serum and concentrated urine
- Quantification of immunoglobulin in urine and serum
- Skeletal survey – X-ray, CT or MRI
- Bone marrow aspirates or trephine biopsy and histological review under the microscope
- Immunofixation of serum and urine

- Quantification of monoclonal protein in serum and urine.

The presence of any monoclonal protein – m-protein or paraprotein – indicates a plasma cell abnormality and warrants detailed investigation and referral to a haemato-oncologist.[1]

Myeloma kidney

Myeloma kidney is a general term that is applied to both ARF and to chronic kidney disease associated with multiple myeloma.

Acute renal failure associated with myeloma

There are a number of factors responsible for ARF associated with myeloma. In up to 80% of cases, light chain-induced cast nephropathy is responsible and this is worsened by the presence of sepsis, hypovolaemia and hypercalcaemia. For further discussion on contributing factors to ARF see Chapter 3.[2]

Chronic renal disease associated with myeloma

The three most common kidney diseases associated with multiple myeloma are:

- Cast nephropathy
- Primary amyloidosis
- Light chain deposition disease.

They are all associated with overproduction of monoclonal immunoglobulin light chains.

Light chains

Light chains are not detected on routine urine dipstick. A 24-hour urine collection is usually sent to the biochemistry and immunology laboratories for detailed analysis using techniques such as immunoelectrophoresis and immunofixation. Light chains have a molecular weight of 22 000 Da and are therefore filtered freely across the glomerulus before re-absorption in the proximal tubular cells. In myeloma the light chain excretion rate is markedly increased from less than 30 mg/day to 100 mg–20 g in 24 hours.

The biochemical characteristics of the individual light chains determine the type of renal disease observed. Generally patients will exhibit only one type of light chain-associated kidney disease at any given time.

Renal tubular dysfunction

The glomerular filtration rate (GFR) may be relatively unaffected in some patients where the direct toxicity from the filtered light chains affects only the renal tubular cells. The clinical consequences of tubular disease in myeloma may include proximal renal tubular acidosis and phosphate losses, both of which are signs of Fanconi's syndrome.

Amyloidosis and light chain deposition disease

The proliferation of plasma cells in myeloma leads to an excess of monoclonal light chains and rarely heavy chains. The monoclonal chains can fragment and deposit immunoglobulin around the body. This process causes primary amyloidosis, light chain deposition disease and heavy chain deposition disease.

Hypercalcaemia

Increased bone resorption contributes to the presence of hypercalcaemia in 15% of patients with multiple myeloma. Hypercalcaemia alone may worsen ARF and must be treated urgently if it is one of the presenting features (see Chapter 3).

Hypercalcaemia may be treated with aggressive rehydration and intravenous bisphosphonates.

Bone pain

Pain is a common complaint in patients with myeloma due to the common skeletal manifestations of disease. Systemic analgesia require-

Table 17.2 Dose of pamidronate

Serum calcium (mmol/L)	Dose (mg)
Up to 3.0	15–30
3.0–3.5	30–60
3.5–4.0	60–90
>4.0	90

ments are high and may be given in combination with localised therapy such as radiotherapy or surgical intervention. Pain symptoms often improve following chemotherapy and associated disease regression. For detailed discussion on pain control in patients with kidney disease see Chapter 15.

In myeloma patients, bone pain may also be effectively treated with bisphosphonate therapy, and clodronate, pamidronate and zoledronic acid have all been used in both clinical trials and routine clinical settings.[1] See Table 17.2 for dose of pamidronate.

Patients with kidney disease may require modification of both the volume of bisphosphonate infusion and a reduction in the rate of administration. Intravenous bisphosphonates such as zoledronic acid should be used with caution in patients with any stage of kidney disease.

Treatment options

Treatment of myeloma is not usually curative but aims to control the disease by putting the patient in remission or slowing progression and to effectively control symptoms.

Regular monitoring of kidney function is essential to ensure speedy identification of developing kidney damage. Advise high fluid intake to promote good urine output, and allow correction of dehydration. Any abnormal electrolytes should be treated appropriately, including hypercalcaemia. It is important to avoid any potentially nephrotoxic agents where possible.

Therapy of myeloma may be considered in three stages: induction, maintenance and relapse.[1]

Induction therapy

Management of symptoms

At presentation, pain control is a common feature and requires immediate attention. Good pain control is usually achieved using a combination of factors:

- Analgesia
- Radiotherapy
- Orthopaedic intervention
- Chemotherapy to control the underlying pathological process.

Analgesia

Systemic analgesic options may be complicated by associated kidney disease (see Chapter 15). Alternative analgesic approaches include local radiotherapy for skeletal disease. Myeloma skeletal metastases have been found to be radio responsive and therefore this may be used for palliation.

Radiotherapy

High doses of radiation may be targeted at diseased bone marrow to treat severe localised problems. Radiotherapy is often used for symptom management, for example, as targeted therapy for bone pain caused by myeloma cells in the bone marrow.

Chemotherapy

Chemotherapy will be considered for patients with myeloma symptoms and for patients with myeloma-related organ damage, such as myeloma kidney, in the absence of other myeloma symptoms.

In patients for whom high-dose chemotherapy is planned, initial chemotherapy is given to reduce the cancer load, while maintaining a future possibility of stem cell mobilisation and transplantation. The commonly used regimens include, vincristine, doxorubicin and dexamethasone (VAD) given as a continuous infusion for 4 days or a combination of cyclophosphamide, doxorubicin, vincristine, methotrexate and prednisolone. These combinations have been shown to offer a higher response rate and cure rate of 10–25%.[1] There have been no large trials, however, comparing the different regimens with each other.[1,6,7] Doses may have to be adjusted according to renal function.

The infusional regimens have the significant disadvantage of requiring central venous access, usually through a permanent central venous catheter. This is associated with significant infection risks and may be particularly difficult in patients with end stage kidney disease who also require central access for haemodialysis.

Conventional chemotherapy is given to patients where a response is required but toxicity should be avoided. This treatment is generally expected to be less aggressive and oral treatment is often chosen rather than invasive parenteral therapy. One of the most common protocols used in this setting is melphalan and prednisolone, based upon the conclusions of the Myeloma Trialist's Collaborative Group in 1998. Patients must be monitored for signs of toxicity, and particular attention must be paid to the nadir cell counts and duration. Doses require modification for both toxicity and in patients with decreased renal function.[8]

Chemotherapy for patients presenting with organ damage to the kidneys aims to reduce the quantity of paraprotein and light chains and thereby minimise organ damage.

Melphalan

Melphalan is predominantly excreted by the kidney and therefore as for conventional therapy, requires careful monitoring and adjustment for bone marrow suppression. Retrospective analysis of the Nordic Myeloma Study Group (NMSG) trials[9] prompted the authors to propose a 25% initial dose reduction of melphalan and individualisation of doses thereafter according to bone marrow suppression.[1]

Cyclophosphamide

Cylophosphamide is a pre-drug whose metabolites are cleared by the kidney. Manufacturers recommend dose reductions of 25% in stage 4 chronic kidney disease (CKD) and 50% in stage 5 CKD (see Chapter 2 for classification of CKD). It is recommended that doses should be monitored and adjusted according to effect and toxicity.

Dexamethasone

Dexamethasone is often given as single-agent initial therapy for patients with myeloma while future chemotherapy regimens are decided. No dose reduction is necessary and pulsed high-dose oral doses are given for 4 days.[7]

Combination regimens – infusional chemotherapy

Infusional chemotherapy regimens discussed above, such as VAD chemotherapy, may also be administered to patients with kidney disease without dose modification.[6]

Thalidomide

The exact mechanism of action for thalidomide is uncertain. There are a number of actions:

- Direct suppression of the growth and survival of myeloma cells
- Direct kill of myeloma cells
- Alteration of the molecules that allow myeloma cells to attach themselves and grow within the bone marrow
- Alteration of the production and activity of chemicals involved in the growth and survival of myeloma cells
- Inhibition of angiogenesis – growth of new blood vessels
- Stimulation of lymphocytes to attack myeloma cells.

Thalidomide undergoes non-enzymatic hydrolysis to multiple degradation products and is not dependent on renal clearance. It is therefore not necessary to adjust doses for kidney disease.[1]

Lenalidomide

Lenalidomide has both immunomodulatory and anti-angiogenic properties, with multiple mechanisms for this action. It is rapidly absorbed orally and approximately 65% of the parent drug is excreted unchanged in the urine. Patients with kidney disease may require a dose modification to avoid accumulation and should be carefully monitored for adverse effects and toxicity.

Bortezomib

Bortezomib is a new agent being used in the therapy of myeloma. It is a proteasome inhibitor. There are on-going clinical trials to establish the optimum combination and most efficacious stage at which this therapy should be given.[1]

Maintenance phase

Chemotherapy may be required for a prolonged period of time – often at least 12 months until the patient's disease is in the plateau phase, with stable M-proteins in serum and urine and no clinical or laboratory evidence of progression. The plateau phase describes a period of disease stability of at least 4–6 months following chemotherapy. Maintenance chemotherapy is usually not recommended in the plateau phase although some patients will continue to receive drugs such as thalidomide long term.

During the maintenance phase of therapy patients will be monitored for disease relapse and progression.

Relapse of disease

When patients relapse and symptoms return, rapid reduction of paraprotein excretion is the first aim of therapy. Initial therapy is given immediately using high dose steroids such as pulsed dexamethasone 40mg daily for 4 days for a rapid response.

In the presence of ARF, patients will usually receive pulsed steroid therapy in addition to plasmapheresis or plasma exchange to filter excessive amounts of paraprotein from the blood. Haemodialysis or haemofiltration may be required as a life saving intervention in ARF.

Treatment of hypercalcaemia

During active myeloma disease, hypercalcaemia may be found in up to 30% of patients. Hypercalcaemia is directly nephrotoxic and exacerbates light chain-mediated nephrotoxicity. Management strategies include adequate hydration and intravenous bisphosphonate therapy.

Fluid replacement may be complicated in patients with fluid restriction due to kidney disease.

Parenteral bisphosphonates must be used with caution as they have been associated with nephrotoxicity. Consequently bisphosphonates require reduction in both dose and rate of administration in the presence of kidney disease. Individual assessment of the risks and benefits must be made on each occasion.

Treatment of kidney disease in multiple myeloma

The MERIT trial is a multicentre study to evaluate the effectiveness of plasma exchange in patients with newly diagnosed myeloma and ARF.[10] Plasma exchange has been used to reduce serum light chain levels and minimise long-term kidney damage. Plasma exchange is a similar process to dialysis, but is significantly more at removing plasma proteins.

Long-term kidney damage may be reduced by prompt intervention and correction of early signs of kidney disease. Urine output over 3 L in 24 hours should be maintained where possible, guided by the patient's fluid status. Central venous pressure monitoring may be required and is a useful guide to fluid replacement. Hypercalcaemia should be corrected as described above with fluids and bisphosphonate therapy.

Infection must be aggressively managed as sepsis is the commonest cause of mortality in all stages of myeloma kidney disease.[1,4]

Treatment of anaemia

Sixty per cent of patients with myeloma will have normochromic, normocytic anaemia at presentation. The incidence of anaemia increases in patients with recurrent or aggressive progressive disease who have received previous chemotherapy.[1]

Previously, anaemia was managed with regular and repeated red blood cell transfusions. This method of management was associated with significant transfusion risks, hospital admission time and the additional risk of accentuating hyperviscosity in patients with high paraprotein levels. It is therefore preferable to avoid admission to hospital for blood transfusions and outpatient alternative therapy has been sought.

The growth in the use of erythropoiesis-stimulating agents (ESA) in the therapy of renal anaemia over the past 10 years has led to further investigation and evaluation in the oncology and haematology settings. There is strong evidence for the use of recombinant human erythropoietin in the treatment of chemotherapy-related anaemia in myeloma.

The use of ESAs in patients with myeloma is recommended by the American Society of Clinical Oncology (ASCO) and the American Society of Hematology (ASH) and the British Society of Haematologists.[1]

Dose of erythropoietin-stimulating agents

In contrast to patients with anaemia of chronic kidney disease, the starting doses of ESA for patients with myeloma is notably higher: epoetin beta 30 000 units per week or darbepoetin 150 µg each week. This dose should be doubled if no improvement in haemoglobin is observed after 4–6 weeks.

Treatment of infections

The combined effects of haematological disease, kidney disease and chemotherapy result in immunosuppression and leave patients at a very high risk of infections. Infections carry an associated high morbidity and mortality in this patient group and must be treated aggressively with appropriate antibiotics.[1]

Summary

The management of multiple myeloma poses a challenge for the healthcare professions and for patients. The role of the pharmacist is essential both in the treatment of myeloma with chemotherapy and in the prevention and treatment of associated kidney disease. Perhaps the most important role is ensuring kidney disease is not exacerbated by myeloma therapies and in ensuring patients are not unnecessarily exposed to increased adverse effects from medicines.

 CASE STUDY

Mr CB is a 64-year-old man transferred to the renal ward for further investigation of kidney disease. He was admitted to another hospital via his GP with sepsis. He has no relevant past medical history.

His blood results on admission to hospital were:

- Serum creatinine 450 µmol/L
- Urea 25 mmol/L
- Potassium 5.6 mmol/L
- Sodium 140 mmol/L
- Corrected calcium 2.8 mmol/L
- Haemoglobin 10.1 g/L
- WCC 15×10^9/L.

Q1. He has been transferred to your ward. As the ward pharmacist, what further information would you like to know?

Q2. At the previous hospital he was given gentamicin, vancomycin and pamidronate? Could any of these contribute to his renal failure?

Q3. What would be your pharmaceutical care plan at this stage?

The 24-hour urine collection shows the presence of Bence-Jones proteins and the medical team plan to biopsy a kidney. The biopsy shows myeloma cast cell nephropathy. The medical team refer the patient to the haemato-oncology team for treatment options.

The patient is commenced on haemodialysis and plasma exchange on alternate days. The haemato-onocologist recommends C-Thal-Dex therapy.

Q4. Would your pharmaceutical care plan change at this stage? Outline a new pharmaceutical care plan.

Q5. After 10 days Mr CB remains haemodialysis-dependent as his renal function has not improved. The renal team would like to treat Mr CB's anaemia and commence an erythropoesis-stimulating agent. What dose would you recommend? Are there any other factors to consider?

References

1. Smith A, Wisloff F, Samson D. Guidelines on the diagnosis and management of multiple myeloma 2005. *Br J Haematol* 2005; 132: 410–451.
2. Winearls CG. Acute myeloma kidney. *Kidney Int* 1995; 48: 1347.
3. Blade J, Fernandes-Llama P, Bosch F *et al.* Renal failure in multiple myeloma. Presenting features and predictors of outcome in 94 patients from a single institution. *Arch Intern Med* 1998; 158: 1889.
4. Clark AD, Shetty A, Soutar R. Renal failure and multiple myeloma: pathogenesis and treatment of renal failure and management of underlying myeloma. *Blood Rev* 1999; 13: 79–90.
5. Pozzi C, Pasquali S, Donini U *et al.* Prognostic factors and effectiveness of treatment in acute renal failure due to multiple myeloma: a review of 50 cases. *Clin Nephrol* 1987; 28: 1–9.
6. Aitchison RG, Reilly IAG, Morgan AG, Russell NH. Vincristine, adriamycin and high dose steroids in myeloma complicated by renal failure. *Br J Cancer* 1990; 61: 765–766.
7. Alexanian R, Dimopoulos MA, Delasalle K, Barlogie B. Primary dexamethasone treatment of multiple myeloma. *Blood* 1992; 80: 887–890.
8. Myeloma Trialists' Collaborative Group. Combination chemotherapy versus melphalan plus prednisone as treatment for multiple myeloma: an overview of 6633 patients from 7 randomised trials. *J Clin Oncol* 1998; 16: 3832–3842.
9. The Nordic Myeloma Study Group. Interferon-alpha 2b added to melphalan-prednisone for initial and maintenance therapy in multiple myeloma. A randomized, controlled trial. *Ann Intern Med* 1996; 124: 212–222.
10. MERIT (Myeloma Renal Impairment Trial). A randomized controlled trial of adjunctive plasma exchange in patients with newly diagnosed multiple myeloma and acute renal failure. Renal Association and the UK Myeloma Forum, Protocol 1.6, September 2005.

18

Palliative care

Fliss Murtagh, Emma Murphy and Hayley Wells

Technological and medical advances bring new possibilities for prolonging life. In the UK in 1951 there were 300 people aged 100 and over; by the year 2031, it is estimated that this figure will reach 36 000.[1] The World Health Organization warns that the health impact could be enormous, predicting a big rise in the prevalence of chronic diseases, including renal disease. The percentage of the population on dialysis is increasing by around 10% per annum and this increase contains disproportionate numbers of older patients with poor functional status and extensive co-morbidity.[2]

There is a greater recognition within renal teams that dialysing these patients may not greatly improve survival but can negatively impact on quality of life[3,4] and growing numbers of patients are therefore being managed conservatively (choosing, in conjunction with their renal team, not to have dialysis). The National Service Framework (NSF) for Renal Services requires that people with renal failure should receive information about the choices available, including conservative management, and that, if appropriate, they should have a palliative care plan built around their needs.[5] The NSF also states that people who choose a non-dialysis pathway should continue to receive all other medical care and that a '"no-dialysis" option is not a "no-treatment" option;[5] maximal conservative management including active symptom management can relieve many symptoms and substantially improve quality of life.'

Patients choosing this management option may survive for months or even years, but when end of life does approach, healthcare professionals have a duty to ensure that each patient's death is as gentle and symptom-free as possible. During the last stages of a patient's life, medical responsibility shifts from sustaining life to enabling a person to die comfortably. Removal of active treatment is not abandonment of the patient, but rather ensures that the patient is as comfortable as possible and has a dignified death, with appropriate family support.

There is also a group of dialysis patients, again particularly older people and those with co-morbidity, who decide to withdraw from dialysis therapy. The mean survival time from the last dialysis session has been stated to be about 9 days, although the range extends from 1 to 42 days.[6] Advance planning, good symptom management and high-quality end of life care is also critical for this group of patients.

In the literature, patients with renal failure who follow a conservative management pathway have underreported symptoms, but work at Guy's and King's College Hospitals has demonstrated a high burden of symptoms with over half of the patients reporting poor mobility, weakness, pain and itching and over one-third reporting poor appetite, difficulty sleeping, drowsiness, dyspnoea and constipation (personal communication). This study also indicated that these symptoms became more prevalent as renal function worsened.

Established palliative care services are increasingly accepting referrals of patients with renal failure but compared to malignant conditions the numbers of patients are small. However, the help of the local specialist palliative care team should always be sought if symptom control is difficult.

Prescribing for symptom control in patients with stage 5 chronic kidney disease managed without dialysis

The main principles of symptom management in patients with stage 5 chronic kidney disease (eGFR <15 mL/min/1.73 m^2) being managed without dialysis are common to other palliative care areas, but there are specific issues that arise, including the very altered pharmacokinetics and pharmacodynamics when eGFR is less than 15 mL/min/1.73 m^2. These patients have increased sensitivity to drugs, with reduced renal excretion, accumulation of metabolites, decreased protein binding and increased permeability of the blood–brain barrier, all increasing risk of toxicity. In the latter stages of treatment the renal function is often unknown as blood samples may not be taken, so drugs need to be initiated at low doses, often with increased dosing intervals, and then titrated slowly to effect with the knowledge that the drug may accumulate very rapidly.

The symptoms most likely to occur are anorexia, constipation, dyspnoea, fatigue, nausea and vomiting, pain, pruritus and restless legs syndrome. It is important to identify the cause of any symptoms as far as possible and treat the underlying cause if feasible before considering purely symptomatic management.

Anorexia

Anorexia is an inevitable consequence of advanced renal failure and uraemia, and a distressing symptom for patients and family.

Management

There may be contributing reversible factors to loss of appetite (e.g. constipation, diarrhoea, oesphagitis, nausea and vomiting, gastroparesis, dry mouth, oral candidiasis, dysphagia and anxiety), which should be actively treated before considering direct pharmacological measures. Dry mouth should be treated by ensuring the patient is not dehydrated, if possible stopping drugs that exacerbate dry mouth, using ice to moisten the mouth in fluid-restricted patients, using artificial saliva, and, if persistent, pilocarpine 5 mg three times daily can be considered. Relaxation of dietary restrictions may be appropriate with referral to a renal dietician for advice. Addition of zinc 220 mg four times daily may be effective to treat taste disturbances.

If these options fail, direct pharmacological measures can be used to treat anorexia. These include:

• Dexamethasone 2–4 mg daily for up to four weeks. Prolonged use is not recommended as the effects are relatively short lived. If an improvement is noted the dose can be weaned down gradually over several weeks; if no benefit is noted it can be reduced and stopped over a much shorter period of time.
• Medroxyprogesterone 100–200 mg daily improves appetite but has an unknown mode of action, with more prolonged benefit than cortico steroids. It is therefore more suitable for those with a lengthier prognosis. A 1–2 week trial is recommended but it is contra-indicated in those patients with a thrombo-embolic risk.
• Thalidomide and omega-3 fatty acids have also been suggested, but there is currently insufficient supporting evidence.

Constipation

Constipation is common in this group of patients with multifactorial causes: drugs, poor dietary intake, reduced mobility, dehydration, depression and reduced muscle tone through immobility.

Management

A thorough assessment is required to treat reversible causes of constipation where possible, with acute management to treat current constipation and active management to prevent further recurrence. Mobility, adequate dietary intake including sufficient fibre and fluid should be encouraged before laxatives are prescribed.

If these measures fail, laxatives are required. The most commonly prescribed laxatives are

Table 18.1 Commonly prescribed laxatives used to treat constipation in palliative care patients with renal failure

Drug	Dose	Mode of action	Comments
Lactulose	10–20 mL BD/TDS	Osmotic – softens by retaining fluid in bowel	Should be used with a stimulant laxative when prescribed with opioids
Senna	2–4 tablets BD	Stimulant	
Bisacodyl	5–10 mg OD/BD	Stimulant	
Co-danthramer	5–20 mL BD	Stimulant and softener	Avoid in urinary or faecal incontinence as can cause danthron burns
Docusate sodium	100–200 mg BD	Stimulant and softener	
Movicol	1–3 sachets daily	Osmotic	Fluid restrictions and/or poor oral intake may constrain use

BD, twice daily; OD, once daily; TDS, three times daily.

listed in Table 18.1. If the patient is on opioid medication, it is usual to require both a 'softener' and a stimulant in moderate to high doses.

Dyspnoea

The most common causes of dyspnoea in patients with renal impairment are anaemia or fluid overload (related to renal disease), pulmonary oedema (usually related to co-existing cardiovascular disease) or co-existing respiratory disease. Active management of the underlying cause of the dyspnoea is the most important strategy, although as the patient reaches the end of life and dyspnoea is likely to become more problematic, active treatment of any underlying cause may no longer be feasible, and purely symptomatic management becomes important.

Management

Significant symptoms of dyspnoea can be caused by anaemia and although any anaemia is likely to be due to renal failure, other causes should be considered and excluded. If patients have months to live, anaemia should be actively managed (see Chapter 5). Planning with the patient how they would like to be treated in the future is essential if they become acutely symptomatic, as not all patients will choose to be admitted to hospital for aggressive intravenous

diuretics. Table 18.2 lists some of the more commonly used diuretics.

Bronchodilators and other therapy may be useful for symptomatic treatment if there is co-existing respiratory disease and bronchospasm.

There are some simple non-drug measures that can also be used to reduce dyspnoea:

- Position – sitting upright rather than lying increases the vital capacity of the lungs
- Cool air from a fan or an open window
- Oxygen therapy if hypoxia is confirmed or suspected (usually when there is co-existing cardiac or respiratory disease)
- Reassurance and active anxiety management, including work with families.

Dyspnoea is very commonly associated with anxiety, often in an escalating cycle (anxiety causing worsening dyspnoea, which triggers worsening anxiety, and so on). It is important to inform, educate and support the patient and family and to identify psychological and physical triggers to episodes. Regular use of relaxation techniques (e.g. aromatherapy, massage) and cognitive behavioral therapy can help to reduce anxiety and may be effective in reducing dyspnoea.

When treatment of the underlying cause and other measures can offer no more relief, then pharmacological interventions to control the symptoms are indicated. Untreated moderate or severe dyspnoea at the end of life is particularly distressing; no patient should be allowed to

Table 18.2 Commonly prescribed diuretics used to treat fluid overload in palliative care patients with renal failure

Diuretic	Dose	Mode of action	Comments
Furosemide	Oral 80 mg–2 g daily (2 g rarely used) IV 40 mg–1 g daily (Note: 500 mg orally = 250 mg IV)	Loop diuretic	Furosemide acts within 1 hour of oral administration and diuresis is usually complete within 6 hours. Doses at the higher end of the range are often used in this group of patients
Bumetanide	Oral 1–5 mg in severe cases IV 1–2 mg repeated after 20 min	Loop diuretic	1 mg of bumetanide = 40 mg furosemide at low doses (avoid direct substitution at high doses)
Metolazone	5–10 mg increased to 20 mg daily	Acts synergistically with loop diuretics – not used alone	Introduce cautiously – may result in profound diuresis. Monitor fluid balance carefully and review patient soon after commencement. Monitor for hypokalaemia, dehydration and rising urea

remain dyspnoeic and distressed in their last days of life. The mainstay of pharmacological symptomatic management is benzodiazepines. Uraemic patients are more sensitive to the cerebral effects of these drugs, and often very small doses are sufficient. If the patient is still able to take oral medication, then a shorter acting benzodiazepine such as sublingual lorazepam 0.5 mg is often effective. If the patient is too ill for oral medication and in the last few days of life, then midazolam 2.5 mg subcutaneously is usually effective. The dose should be repeated as required, but is rarely needed more than every 4–6 hours, and sometimes much less frequently.

Opioid medications are used for breathlessness in patients with cardiac and respiratory dyspnoea – in much lower doses than for pain, but with supporting evidence.[7] There is no supporting evidence for the use of opioids for dyspnoea in renal patients, and there are many constraints on the use of opioids in patients with eGFR less than 15 mL/min who are not dialysed (see Chapter 15), but nevertheless, for a dyspnoeic renal patient near the end of life and who perhaps has co-morbid cardiac or respiratory disease, they may be very useful. Starting doses are usually half those for pain.

Nausea and vomiting

Nausea and vomiting is common in patients with end stage renal failure, resulting in the inability to take diet or drugs orally, and patients can quickly become dehydrated. Nausea and vomiting may frequently be multifactorial and specific causes need to be identified. Drugs (e.g. opioids) or toxins such as high serum urea or calcium may cause nausea, which is usually persistent and not relieved by vomiting. In this situation retching may feature more prominently than actual vomiting. Gastric motility problems (especially common in diabetic patients) usually cause post-prandial vomiting of undigested food, which often relieves the nausea and may be accompanied by bloating, epigastric fullness, flatulence, hiccough or heartburn. Nausea and vomiting associated with gastritis is often associated with heartburn or epigastric pain, which is sometimes worse after eating. Emesis can also be associated with movement or constipation.

If nausea is established and vomiting frequent or severe, then oral drugs will not be absorbed and a continuous subcutaneous infusion is indicated. Once symptoms have settled (but not before) subcutaneous antiemetics can then be replaced by oral antiemetics.

Management

The aim of treatment is to identify and treat the suspected cause as shown in Table 18.3.

Pain

Pain is underrecognised and undertreated in this group of patients.[8,9] It is hard to manage due to the constraints reduced renal function puts on the use of medicines. The little evidence that is available on pain in this group of patients suggests the pain is often due to co-morbidities rather the impaired renal function.[8] Examples include neuropathic pain in, for example, diabetic neuropathy, and bone pain from osteoporosis, but these pains still need active management. Anxiety or depression should be treated actively as pain may sometimes not improve until this is addressed.

The principles of the World Health Organization analgesic ladder should be followed for primary analgesia as in other palliative care patients, and constant or frequent pain should be treated with regular, not 'as required' analgesia.[10] Initially step 1 analgesia (e.g. paracetamol) should be started, unless pain is severe. The next step (step 2 opioids for moderate pain) should be proceeded to if the analgesic from the current step has not controlled the pain adequately. Step 3 opioids for severe pain should be used if step 2 medication is not enough. At each step, another drug within the same step should not be tried if pain is inadequately controlled at that step. Using opioids when eGFR is less than 15 mL/min/1.73 m^2 is challenging, and can be complex, but it is important not to leave pain untreated

Table 18.3 Commonly prescribed antiemetics used to treat nausea and vomiting in palliative care patients with renal failure

Suspected cause	Drug of choice	Dose	Comments
Drug-induced or uraemia (First step is to stop causative drugs if possible. Opioid-induced nausea usually settles spontaneously after about 7–14 days of treatment)	Haloperidol	0.5–2 mg daily	Sedating, accumulation and increased cerebral sensitivity in renal failure
Gastric motility problems	Metoclopramide	5–10 mg TDS	Do not use in bowel obstruction with colic. Do not use with cyclizine
	Domperidone	10–20 mg TDS	Rectal route available
Gastritis	Lansoprazole	30 mg OD	
	Omeprazole	20 mg OD	
	Ranitidine	150 mg BD	
Second line (if severe or unknown or multifactorial causes)	(Consider asking advice of specialist palliative care team at this stage)		
	Levomepromazine may be appropriate but needs cautious use in low doses because of increased cerebral sensitivity	Starting dose: ^{a}3 mg–6.25 mg OD orally or 2.5 mg subcutaneously	Very sedating at higher doses

BD, twice daily; OD, once daily; TDS, three times daily. ^{a} 6 mg tablets available on named-patient basis.

because of this. The analgesics discussed are outlined in Table 18.4.

Adjuvant medicines, such as non-steroidal anti-inflammatory drugs (NSAIDs) (for musculoskeletal or soft tissue pain), antidepressant or anticonvulsant medication (for nerve pain), are important considerations. NSAIDs can be used if the benefits of analgesia outweigh the risk of potential further reduction in renal function. If NSAIDs are used, a gastro-protective agent (e.g. omeprazole) should be co-prescribed.

Step 1 analgesia

Paracetamol (maximum dose 1 g three times daily if eGFR less than 15 mL/min/1.73 m^2).

Step 2 analgesia

Codeine and dihydrocodeine

Codeine and dihydrocodeine are hepatically metabolised with the majority of the metabolites pharmacologically active and renally excreted. In end stage renal failure this renal clearance is reduced and there have been reports of serious side-effects, including severe hypotension and respiratory arrest.[11–13] If possible, both these analgesics should be avoided in patients with an eGFR less than 15 mL/min/1.73 m^2 who are not dialysed, but this may not always be practical. If used, the dose should be reduced to 25–50% of normal with careful monitoring of blood pressure and respiratory rate. Constipation should be anticipated and therefore laxatives co-prescribed.

Tramadol

Tramadol acts peripherally and centrally on mu-opioid receptors and by inhibiting monoamine (noradrenaline (norepinephrine) and serotonin) reuptake. Ninety per cent of the drug is excreted renally and there is a twofold increase in the elimination half-life in end stage renal failure.[14] In this group of patients both the dose should be reduced and the dosing interval increased, to a maximum of 50 mg every 12 hours.[15] Tramadol may also lower fit threshold in this group of patients with a high urea so use in those at risk of convulsions for other reasons should be avoided. Clinically, tramadol may

have a high incidence of drowsiness and lethargy but it can be a very useful step 2 analgesic in this group of patients.

Step 3 analgesia

The choice of step 3 analgesic will depend on the severity and acuteness of the pain, whether the patient is in primary or secondary care, appropriate route of administration, and availability of drugs and preparations.

If the patient has severe pain and is in hospital, then the subcutaneous route is preferable to gain rapid control of the pain. Once severe pain is controlled by the subcutaneous route, analgesia can either be switched to the trans-dermal routes or oral routes, or (if the patient is unable to take oral drugs) continued in a continuous subcutaneous infusion via syringe driver.

Buprenorphine

Buprenorphine acts as a potent partial mu-opioid receptor antagonist, kappa-opioid receptor antagonist and a weak delta-opioid receptor agonist. The parent drug is excreted via the biliary system, but the metabolites buprenorphine-3-glucuronide and norbuprenorphine, are excreted renally.[18] There has been little published pharmacokinetic data in patients with renal impairment so it cannot be wholly recommended. The effects and possible toxicity of the metabolites is unclear. However, the partial biliary excretion may make it more appropriate for use in renal impairment; if used, it should be prescribed cautiously, with dose reduction, increased dosing interval, and careful monitoring, pending further evidence.

Fentanyl and alfentanil

Fentanyl is a potent synthetic opioid that is hepatically metabolised to norfentanyl and other inactive metabolites with less than 10% of the parent drug excreted renally.[14,16] When single bolus doses are given to patients with renal impairment no dose modifications appear to be required.[19] However, there are few data on the pharmacokinetics when the drug is given repeatedly or by infusion. Studies have shown that fentanyl may accumulate with extended administration and that there is considerable

Table 18.4 Analgesics used to treat pain in palliative care patients with eGFR <15 mL/min and without dialysis

Drug	Dose	Route	Frequency	Comments
Step 1				
Paracetamol	1 g	PO	TDS	
Step 2				
Codeine				Not recommended
Dihydrocodeine				Not recommended
Tramadol	50 mg	Orally	Every 12 hours	Use with caution
Step 3				
Buprenorphine	200–400 µg	Sublingual	Every 8 hours	Safer than morphine or diamorphine
	'5' patch upwards	Transdermal	every 7 days	but limited evidence so use with
	'35' patch upwards	Transdermal	every 72–96 hours	caution. Greater incidence of nausea than other step 3 opioids, so consider avoiding if patient already nauseous. Theoretically, 'ceiling' effect, and both agonist and antagonist properties, so perhaps avoid if pain is escalating, or alternative step 3 opioid likely to be used later
Fentanyl	Starting dose 25µg as required	Subcutaneous	3–6 hourly according to need	No appropriate oral preparation available for chronic pain. (Oral transmucosal fentanyl is only suitable for breakthrough or incident pain.)
	'25' patch upwards	Transdermal	every 72 hours	The patch is effective once pain is stable on other opioid, but is not advisable if the patient is opioid naïve
Alfentanil				Use in continuous SC infusion, when volume makes larger doses of fentanyl impractical
Hydromorphone:				Limited evidence of safety, but like
As Palladone	1.3 mg upwards	Oral	Every 6–8 hours	oxycodone, may be used by some practitioners despite limited evidence
As Palladone SR	2 mg upwards	Oral	Every 12 hours	of safety. Monitor for accumulation with long term use
Methadone	Reduce dose by 50–75%			Safe when eGFR <15 but needs specialist palliative care or pain team advice on prescribing, as wide inter-individual variations and risk of (late) accumulation
Morphine	Starting dose 2.5 mg	Subcutaneous	4–12 hourly as required	Not recommended (but see text re. short-term use)
Diamorphine	Starting dose 1.25 mg	Subcutaneous	4–12 hourly as required	Not recommended (but see text re. short-term use)
Oxycodone:				Used but limited evidence of safety.
as OxyNorm	2.5 mg upwards	Oral	Every 8–12 hours	No upper dose limit, provided it is titrated slowly, is effective for the pain,
as OxyContin	5 mg upwards	Oral	Every 12 hours	and there are no adverse effects. Start with OxyNorm, to gain rapid control of the pain, and consider switch to OxyContin later for ease of administration (but beware accumulation with longer term use)

inter-patient variability.[16] Alfentanil has a much shorter half-life than fentanyl, but similarly has inactive metabolites, and, with fentanyl, perhaps the best evidence for safety in severe renal impairment.[14,16]

For the management of moderate or severe chronic pain in advanced renal impairment, fentanyl or alfentanil are therefore probably the optimal step 3 opioids. In order to prevent accumulation, the dose should be reduced (e.g. 75% of usual dose when eGFR is between 15 and 50 mL/min/1.73 m^2 and 50% dose when eGFR is less than 15 mL/min/1.73 m^2), with careful and frequent monitoring for adverse effects. Alfentanil, however, has the disadvantage of a short half-life (1–2 hours). This makes it inappropriate for prn (as required) use – pain will recur quickly and additional doses may need to be given frequently. For this reason, fentanyl is a better choice. At the end of life, however, if large doses of fentanyl are required in a continuous subcutaneous infusion (after careful titration of analgesic requirements against the pain), then it is sometimes necessary to switch to alfentanil, because it is available in more concentrated preparations.

Hydromorphone

Hydromorphone is a morphine analogue with a short duration of action and is hepatically metabolised to its main metabolite hydromorphone-3-glucuronide (H3G). This is cleared renally and accumulates in renal failure.[20,21] There is evidence that H3G is neuroexcitatory in both animals[22] and humans.[23] There are concerns about the use of hydromorphone in this group of patients as a single-dose study indicated accumulation of the drug and its metabolite in renal failure.[20] Other reports in mild renal failure suggested that the drug was better tolerated.[24] However, the evidence for hydromorphone in renal failure is limited, and dose reduction, titration and monitoring is essential. It may be preferable to morphine or diamorphine, but (like oxycodone) cannot be recommended in the absence of evidence of safety.

Methadone

Methadone is hepatically metabolised and the metabolites are predominantly faecally excreted, although renal excretion of the unchanged drug is also an important route of elimination. There is a large inter-patient pharmacodynamic and pharmacokinetic variation with methadone treatment, and it accumulates on repeated administration due to its high volume of distribution. There is evidence in two patients with chronic renal failure that plasma concentrations were no higher than in those with normal renal function, suggesting that faecal excretion may compensate for impaired renal excretion.[25] For this reason, methadone may be a good choice of opioid in severe renal impairment, but because of the problems with inter-patient variability and accumulation, it is advisable that it is only prescribed by specialists familiar with its use and monitoring. Dose reduction of 50–75% and close monitoring is advised.[15]

Morphine and diamorphine

Morphine is metabolised hepatically to renally excreted metabolites, morphine-3-glucuronide (M3G) and morphine-6-glucuronide (M6G), which accumulate in significant renal impairment.[14,16] The metabolite M6G may be more potent than morphine and depresses the central nervous system. M6G also crosses the blood–brain barrier slowly and once there its action is prolonged. M3G appears to have little analgesic activity but may antagonise the effect of M6G. Diamorphine is rapidly deacetylated to morphine and M6G and acts similarly to morphine.

Because alternative strong opioids (such as fentanyl) are now available, morphine and diamorphine are no longer first-choice opioids when eGFR is less than 15 mL/min and patients are not dialysed. In the last few days of life, morphine and diamorphine use can increase the risk of terminal agitation due to accumulation of metabolites.[17] They should therefore only be used where there is moderate or severe pain and alternative opioids are unavailable (e.g. in the community setting), and in the short term (e.g. for one or two doses). Efforts should be made to try and anticipate the requirements for a step 3 opioid before it occurs, and to provide the most appropriate drug (e.g. fentanyl) in case of need. This requires anticipation and planning, ensuring that patients nearing death at home have prn medication provided before need, so that district nurses and GPs can then administer when required. If morphine or diamorphine is used, the initial dose should be small (e.g. 2.5 mg SC morphine) and titrated to response. If a continuous SC infusion is required, morphine or diamorphine are not the opioids of choice as they will be excreted slowly, if at all; any CNS effects will be prolonged.

Oxycodone

Oxycodone is metabolised hepatically to the active metabolites noroxycodone and oxymorphone, with less than 10% of the parent drug excreted in the urine. A study of 10 uraemic patients demonstrated a reduced elimination in renal failure patients with a large inter-patient variation.[26] There is currently insufficient evidence to confirm the safety of oxycodone in renal failure patients and if used it should be monitored carefully with reduced doses of 75% of normal dose when eGFR is 10–50 mL/min/1.73 m^2, and 50% of normal dose when eGFR is less than 10 mL/min/1.73 m^2.[15] Like hydromorphone, it is a better choice than morphine or diamorphine.

Pruritus

Pruritus is a difficult symptom to manage, and advice should be sought early from a specialist palliative care team if the first options are not successful. Although uraemia is the most likely cause, other common causes of pruritus need to be considered if the symptoms are not resolving (e.g. other skin disorders, scabies, liver impairment).

Management

Management of renal failure should be optimised and for certain patients, high serum phosphate levels may contribute to pruritus, so a referral to a renal dietician for dietary advice, and prescription of phosphate binders to reduce phosphate levels should be considered. Hyperparathyroidism may also be a contributory factor so parathyroid hormone should be monitored and treated with alfacalcidol as appropriate, while monitoring for hypercalcaemia.

Dry skin both causes and contributes to pruritus, and should be treated very actively using liberal emollients (e.g. aqueous cream). Nails should also be kept short and patients advised to keep cool with light clothing, tepid baths or showers. There is limited evidence for drug therapy with no one preparation recommended.[27] However, individual patients do report significant benefit, with some of treatments outlined in Table 18.5. Time should be taken to discuss with the patient the need to persist with any one drug, and to explaining how to minimise side-effects where possible.

Restless legs syndrome

There are limited studies on uraemic restless legs syndrome, so much evidence is extrapolated from management of idiopathic restless legs. In uraemia, restless legs are thought to be associated with anaemia, iron deficiency and hyperphosphataemia.[28,29] Psychological factors may also play a role.

Management

Treatment should involve the reduction of potential exacerbating drugs (tricyclic antidepressants, selective serotonin uptake inhibitors, lithium and dopamine antagonists) and correction of anaemia, iron deficiency and hyperphosphataemia. Drugs used to treat restless leg syndrome are outlined in Table 18.6.

Prescribing in the last few days of life

When managing a patient in the last few days of life, care is modified to focus on making the patient as comfortable as possible with stopping of all unnecessary blood tests, monitoring and non-essential medicines. At the end of life, not only do the symptoms discussed previously continue to require management but other symptoms also require treatment, such as restlessness/agitation, or retained respiratory secretions. Midazolam subcutaneously is effective for restlessness and agitation but patients with severe renal impairment are much more sensitive to the cerebral effects of all benzodiazepines – doses should be reduced and monitored

Table 18.5 Commonly prescribed drugs used to treat pruritus in palliative care patients with renal failure

Drug	Dose	Comments
Emollients	Topical, ad lib	Long standing use, but limited evidence of benefit. May be important for those with dry skin
Antihistamines		
Chlorphenamine	4 mg QDS (TDS if eGFR <15 mL/min)	Some patients benefit from a sedative effect for nocturnal pruritus – if this is the case, use a sedating antihistamine such as chlorphenamine
Cetirizine	10 mg OD (5 mg if eGFR <15 mL/min)	
Immune modulators		
Thalidomide	100 mg at night	There is evidence that thalidomide may give notable benefit, especially in more severe pruritus. The drug is unlicensed and caution is required to ensure no pregnant or potentially pregnant woman are exposed to the drug (even the handling of it). There is also risk of (reversible) neuropathy
Ondansetron	2–8 mg BD	A few very small trials have been undertaken with conflicting results. If used, it is also helpful for nausea, but note it is very constipating (laxative should be co-prescribed).
Capsaicin	0.025% cream applied four times daily	Impractical unless pruritus is localised. If used, local burning may occur, and deter continuation
Gabapentin	After dialysis	Not advisable for use in the non-dialysed patient with eGFR <15 mL/min due to near 100% renal clearance and rapid accumulation

OD = once daily, BD = twice daily, TDS = three times daily, QDS = four times daily.

Table 18.6 Commonly prescribed drugs used to treat restless legs syndrome in palliative care patients with renal failure

Drug	Starting dose	Comments
Co-careldopa	12.5/50 at night	Restless legs syndrome may become, with time, worse in about 80% of cases. This correlates with greater accumulated dose of levodopa, so the lowest dose for shortest duration should be used. Pulsed dosing can be considered
Pergolide	25 μg OD	Nausea is a common side-effect
Clonazepam	250–500 μg	Very limited evidence of benefit. Can cause day-time drowsiness and cognitive impairment
Opioids		Extremely limited evidence of benefit, but may be appropriate to consider if there is concurrent pain. Follow the guidelines in the pain section as to opioid selection and dosing

OD = once daily.

carefully. Often 2.5 mg 6–8 hourly is sufficient. For retained respiratory secretions it is advisable to avoid hyoscine hydrobromide (because of possible cerebral effects), and use either hyoscine butylbromide 20 mg as required or glycopyrronium 0.2 mg as required.

Every patient should have an analgesic, antiemetic, sedative and medication for retained secretions available for prn use in the last few days of life, whether or not they have required these medications before. This is important, especially if patients are discharged from hospital to die at home, and hospital pharmacists will need to facilitate this anticipatory prescribing of additional medications to take home.

Conclusions

For patients following a conservative pathway or withdrawing from dialysis, symptom management and prescribing can be challenging.

Specialist palliative care services see very few of these patients and this is a newly recognised area for renal teams. Pharmacists, as part of this team can have a great influence on improving management of patient symptoms and ensuring a patient's end of life is as comfortable as possible.

Acknowledgements

We would like to thank Mee-Onn Chai, renal pharmacist at King's College Hospital, for her help with this chapter.

 CASE STUDY

Mr RP is a 63-year-old man with a history of end stage renal failure secondary to diabetic nephropathy. Complications of IDDM include nephropathy, retinopathy and neuropathy. He was diagnosed with metastatic prostate carcinoma in late 2005. His PSA was over 900 on diagnosis, then dropped but has been rising again despite goserelin (Zoladex). Further hormone manipulation did not improve disease control. Subsequent investigations with CT and bone scan showed him to have bone metastases. He has been informed by the urology team that he has a poor prognosis and a likely life expectancy of 1 year. He has opted for conservative management of his renal failure. He has no follow-up outpatient appointment with oncology. He was keen to attend the renal palliative clinic to discuss symptoms and the future. Biochemistry review reveals serum creatinine 430 μmol/L, urea 25 mmol/L and eGFR 13 mL/min/1.73 m^2.

His current medications are:

- Lansoprazole 30 mg once daily
- Gliclazide 40 mg once daily
- Alfacalcidol 0.5 μg once daily
- NeoRecormon 5000 units weekly
- Simvastatin 10 mg every night
- Ramipril 2.5 mg once daily
- Adcal 1 three times daily
- Lactulose 10 mL twice daily
- Senna 2 tabs at night
- Docusate sodium 2 tablets twice daily
- Co-danthramer 10 mL twice daily
- Zoladex every 3 months
- Co-codamol 2 tablets four times daily.

(continued overleaf)

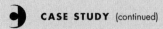

CASE STUDY (continued)

When seen in clinic his main complaint is of pain. He has severe pain related to his left lower limb. He complains of aching over his anterolateral thigh and lateral leg. This pain is graded 8 out of 10 at its worst. It is exacerbated by sitting for long periods of time, walking and by trying to extend his hip or knee. He also complains of severe pain related to his right shoulder, which is aching in nature and radiates all the way down his right arm to his wrist. He grades this pain 7 out of 10 and it is exacerbated by lying down. At present he is taking co-codamol maximum dose particularly at night for pain. He finds this has very little impact on the pain and reduces it by approximately 20% at the most. He tolerates it fine.

Q1.   What are the possible causes of his pain?
In addition to his pain he complains of nausea and vomiting. This is not related to his constipation and there is no associated colic. He becomes increasingly nauseous after eating and can only manage a few mouthfuls before feeling full. His vomiting is occasional, consists of undigested food, and relieves his nausea. This pattern of nausea and vomiting is suggestive of gastric stasis which may be related to his diabetes. He also complains of constipation. He can go 7–10 days without opening his bowels and then alternates to diarrhoea due to an increase in his laxatives.

Q2.   How would you manage his nausea and vomiting?
He sleeps poorly largely due to his pain. His sleep is particularly interrupted by a stabbing pain in his left forefoot which occurs at night but is not helped by sitting out and lowering his leg. He is known to have calcified vessels on recent Doppler scans.

Q3.   What might be causing his pain? What other treatment would you consider to relieve his pain?
He lives with his wife at home. He manages reasonably well and his wife is clearly very involved in his care. Due to his visual impairment his wife organises his dosette box on a weekly basis. He can manage to go up and down the stairs at home but this wears him out. He does not have a bathroom downstairs at home, which can present some difficulties. His wife works full time. They have two children who do not live at home.

He is reviewed one month later in the renal palliative clinic and his main concern is his low mood. He feels quite hopeless and negative and gains no pleasure from anything. He acutely feels the loss of his physical fitness and his former role. He also suffers somatic symptoms in the shape of early waking and poor appetite and lethargy. He acknowledges he is depressed. He does not have a past history of treatment for this. On further questioning he describes suicidal ideation and intent. He requests that this is not discussed with his GP.

When reviewed in clinic two months later he has clearly deteriorated. He finds the transport issues particularly difficult due to his poor mobility and finds this has significant impact on his quality of life. His general level of functioning is now very poor. He is essentially wheelchair- or bed-bound. He has had several falls and recent fracture of his right humerus. He feels much more vulnerable and unsafe at home. His wife is out at work during the day and so he spends long periods of time on his own. He is keen to know if he has any rehabilitation potential with his legs and mobility.

Q4.   What would you discuss at this stage? What medications could you ensure were prescribed for the last few days of life?

References

1. Government Actuary's Office. *National Population Projections*. Series PP2 No 20. London: Office for National Statistics, 1996.
2. Ansell D, Feest T, Rao R *et al. UK Renal Registry Report 2005*. Bristol: UK Renal Registry, 2006.
3. Munshi SK, Vijayakumar N, Taub NA *et al.* Outcome of renal replacement therapy in the very elderly. *Nephrol Dial Transplant* 2001; 16: 128–133.
4. Smith C, Silva-Gane M, Chandna S *et al.* Choosing not to dialyse: evaluation of planned non-dialytic management in a cohort of patients with end-stage renal failure. *Nephron Clin Pract* 2003; 95: c40–c46.
5. Department of Health. *National Service Framework for Renal Services – Part 2 Chronic Kidney Disease, Acute Renal Failure, and End of Life Care*. London: Department of Health, February 2005.
6. Cohen LM, McCue JD, Germain M, Kjellstrand CM. Dialysis discontinuation. A 'good' death? *Arch Intern Med* 1995; 155: 42–47.
7. Jennings AL, Davies AN, Higgins JP *et al.* A systematic review of the use of opioids in the management of dyspnoea. *Thorax* 2002; 57: 939–944.
8. Davison SN. Pain in hemodialysis patients: prevalence, cause, severity, and management. *Am J Kidney Dis* 2003; 42: 1239–1247.
9. Andreucci VE, Fissell RB, Bragg-Gresham JL *et al.* Dialysis Outcomes and Practice Patterns Study (DOPPS) – data on medications in hemodialysis patients. *Am J Kidney Dis* 2004; 44 (Suppl 2): S61–S67.
10. Launay-Vacher V, Karie S, Fau JB *et al.* Treatment of pain in patients with renal insufficiency: The World Health Organization three-step ladder adapted. *J Pain* 2005; 6: 137–148.
11. Parke TJ, Nandi PR, Bird KJ, Jewkes DA. Profound hypotension following intravenous codeine phosphate. Three case reports and some recommendations. *Anaesthesia* 1992; 47: 852–854.
12. Talbott GA, Lynn AM, Levy FH, Zelikovic I. Respiratory arrest precipitated by codeine in a child with chronic renal failure. *Clin Pediatr (Phila)* 1997; 36: 171–173.
13. Matzke GR, Chan GL, Abraham PA. Codeine dosage in renal failure. *Clin Pharm* 1986; 5: 15–16.
14. Mercadante S, Arcuri E. Opioids and renal function. *J Pain* 2004; 5: 2–19.
15. Broadbent A, Khor K, Heaney A. Palliation and chronic renal failure: Opioid and other palliative medications – dosage guidelines. *Prog Palliative Care* 2003; 11: 183–190.
16. Davies G, Kingswood C, Street M. Pharmacokinetics of opioids in renal dysfunction. *Clin Pharmacokinet* 1996; 31: 410–422.
17. Kirkham SR, Pugh R. Opioid analgesia in uraemic patients. *Lancet* 1995; 345: 1185.
18. Hand CW, Sear JW, Uppington J *et al.* Buprenorphine disposition in patients with renal impairment: single and continuous dosing, with special reference to metabolites. *Br J Anaesth* 1990; 64: 276–282.
19. Coral IM, Moore AR, Strunin L. Plasma concentrations of fentanyl in normal surgical patients with severe renal failure. *Br J Anaesth* 1980; 52: 101P.
20. Durnin C, Hind ID, Wickens MM *et al.* Pharmacokinetics of oral immediate-release hydromorphone in subjects with renal impairment. *Proc West Pharmacol Soc* 2001; 44: 81–82.
21. Babul N, Darke AC, Hagen N. Hydromorphone metabolite accumulation in renal failure. *J Pain Symptom Manage* 1995; 10: 184–186.
22. Wright AW, Mather LE, Smith MT. Hydromorphone-3-glucuronide: a more potent neuro-excitant than its structural analogue, morphine-3-glucuronide. *Life Sci* 2001; 69: 409–420.
23. Fainsinger R, Schoeller T, Boiskin M, Bruera E. Palliative care round: cognitive failure and coma after renal failure in a patient receiving captopril and hydromorphone. *J Palliat Care* 1993; 9: 53–55.
24. Lee MA, Leng ME, Tiernan EJ. Retrospective study of the use of hydromorphone in palliative care patients with normal and abnormal urea and creatinine. *Palliat Med* 2001; 15: 26–34.
25. Kreek MJ, Schecter AJ, Gutjahr CL, Hecht M. Methadone use in patients with chronic renal disease. *Drug Alcohol Depend* 1980; 5: 197–205.
26. Kirvela M, Lindgren L, Seppala T, Olkkola KT. The pharmacokinetics of oxycodone in uremic patients undergoing renal transplantation. *J Clin Anesth* 1996; 8: 13–18.
27. Lugon JR. Uremic pruritus: a review. *Hemodial Int* 2005; 9: 180–188.
28. Dinwiddie LC. Restless legs syndrome: not just a problem for dialysis patients. *ANNA J* 1997; 24: 655–662.
29. Wetter TC. Restless legs syndrome: a review for the renal care professionals. *EDTNA-ERCA J* 2001; 27: 42–46.

19

Dietary management of kidney disease

Diane Green

Dietary treatment is one of the cornerstones of treatment for patients with end stage renal disease. In the 1960s many patients were treated with diet alone, using very low-protein diets. The renal diet was adapted to dialysis and transplantation when renal replacement therapy became available in the 1970s and 1980s. Today, protein–energy malnutrition, hyperphosphataemia, chronic fluid overload and obesity are the most common challenges, leading to long-term complications and adversely affecting the outcome of treatment.

This chapter covers the important issues of dietary management and the role diet plays in the treatment of patients with end stage renal failure (ESRF).

Historic pre-dialysis dietary intervention

Historically, the dietary treatment for patients with ESRF was a very low-protein diet (VLPD). The best known was the Giovanetti diet which contained 20 g of high biological protein to cover the essential amino acid requirements. It was also necessary to ensure the diet provided 50 kcal/kg to prevent loss of lean body mass and to maintain nitrogen balance.[1] This was commonly prescribed to patients with ESRF and was the only treatment available to patients until regular haemodialysis became available.

In the 1980s there was a renewed interest in low-protein, high-energy diets as partially nephrectomised rats showed that protein restriction delayed the progression of renal disease. In 1985 the National Institutes of Health

(NIH) in the USA initiated a large multicentre study – the Modification of Diet in Renal Disease (MDRD) study – to investigate the effect of protein restriction on the progression of kidney failure. It used four different levels of protein diets ranging from VLPD supplement with keto acids and phosphorus restrictions to normal intakes. The results were published in 1994.[2] The results of the study initially showed a slower rate in decline of kidney function in the absence of severe proteinuria and hypertension, but there appeared to be no further advantage to using VLPD.[2]

As a result of these findings, treatments became focused on the prevention of complications due to uraemia, improving blood pressure control, prevention of malnutrition and dietary phosphorus restriction to prevent renal bone disease. In the absence of malnutrition, healthy eating principles are also discussed to help reduce the incidence of cardiovascular disease. Research continues into the effects of protein restriction on reducing symptoms of uraemia and the progression of kidney failure.

Protein restrictions combined with a very high calorie diet are again becoming a treatment option for patients opting not to have dialysis but to follow a conservative medical management route.

Pre-dialysis dietary management

The nutritional content of a diet for a patient with chronic kidney diseases should be specifically adapted to their individual needs and personal circumstances. Dietary management of kidney disease is very patient-specific. The diet prescribed will depend upon:

- Stage of chronic kidney disease
- Biochemistry
- Medical history – diabetes, hypercholesterolemia
- Medical treatment plan
- Nutritional status
- The patient's normal dietary intake.

The diet needs to provide sufficient flexibility to enable the patient to continue to lead a normal life and to aid compliance of the dietary restrictions. The main dietary components of the renal diet are: protein, energy (fat and carbohydrate), phosphorus, potassium, sodium, fluid and other minerals, such as calcium and iron. Patients may be advised to follow none, some or all of the aspects of the diet.

Protein

Protein is an important nutrient in growth and the repair and maintenance of tissue.

In the pre-dialysis diet the level of restriction should maintain nitrogen balance and nutritional status. The amount of protein prescribed is dependent on the patient's ideal body weight (IBW) and taking the patient's residual kidney function into consideration (Table 19.1). The average daily consumption of protein in the UK is 88 g for men and 64 g for women,[3] which means that most patients are advised to reduce their intake of protein foods in their diet. To ensure that essential amino acids are available in the diet about 60% of protein needs to

obtained from high biological value proteins, such as meat, fish, eggs and milk. Once the protein in the diet is reduced, the serum urea and creatinine levels often decrease. Some patients notice an improvement in well-being; others notice a change in taste acuity.

A daily protein intake of 0.8–1.0 g/kg IBW is recommended,[4] with at least 60% from high biological value protein sources.

Energy

The energy values of the different food types are as follows:

- Fat 1 g = 9 kcal
- Carbohydrate 1 g = 4 kcal
- Protein 1 g = 3.8 kcal.

The amount of energy required in the diet is as important as the amount of protein. Inadequate energy will lead to protein catabolism, weight loss and protein–energy malnutrition. Energy requirements will depend on activity levels and body size, but a daily intake of 35 kcal/kg will be adequate for most patients' needs.[5]

To achieve a satisfactory energy intake with patients on a protein restriction diet, high intakes of fat and/or sugar are often recommended. This often includes fried food, addition of cream, high-fat snacks, such as cakes and biscuits, and sugary fizzy drinks to be included in a patient's diet.

Obesity should be treated in the early stages of renal failure with a low-calorie diet as this can help control a patient's blood pressure, but

Table 19.1   Protein and energy requirements for pre-dialysis patients

GFR (mL/min)	Protein (g/kg IBW)	Energy (kcal/kg IBW)
>30	Normal	30–35
20–30	0.6–1.0 (EDTNA/ERCA)	30–35
<19 (not on dialysis)	0.6–1.0 (EDTNA/ERCA)	30–35

GFR, glomerular filtration rate; IBW, ideal body weight; EDTNA/ERCA, European Dialysis and Transplant Nurses Association/European Renal Care Association.
From ref. 9.

this needs to be carefully monitored as obesity can often mask malnutrition.

Phosphorus (1 mmol = 31 mg P)

Phosphate is a major constituent of plants and animals and so is present in most foods. Inorganic phosphorus is added to processed foods, particularly baked goods and carbonated drinks, and these provide about 10% of total phosphorus intake. The main sources of phosphorus in the UK diet[3] are:

- Milk and milk products (24%)
- Cereal products (23%)
- Meat and meat products (21%)
- Vegetables and potatoes (10%).

Approximately 60% dietary phosphorus is absorbed.

Hyperphosphataemia contributes to the development of renal bone disease through the stimulation of parathyroid production.[6] Dietary phosphorus restriction is an essential part of controlling serum phosphate levels. However, the need to provide both adequate dietary protein and a palatable diet limits the degree to which dietary phosphate can be restricted.[7] The appropriate prescription of phosphate binders is equally important in controlling phosphate.

All foods with high protein content also contain a fair amount of phosphorus. However, some of these foods are an essential part of the diet and cannot be eliminated. Table 19.2 lists examples of foods that can be excluded from the diet without altering the nutritional quality of the diet.

Potassium (1 mmol = 39 mg K)

Potassium is predominantly an intracellular cation and plays a fundamental role in acid–base regulation, fluid balance, muscle contraction and nerve conduction. Ninety-five per cent of the body's potassium in found within the cells.

In the average UK diet,[3] potassium is derived from:

- Vegetables and potatoes (28%)
- Beverages, particularly coffee (15%)

- Milk and milk products (13%)
- Cereal products (13%)
- Meat and meat products (15%)
- Fruit (5%).

Progressive renal failure is often complicated by hyperkalaemia and may occur when renal function has declined to a glomerular filtration rate (GFR) of 5 mL/min with normal urine output.

A dietary intake of no more than 60–70 mmol/day (1 mmol/kg IBW) is sufficient to prevent or treat hyperkalaemia. However an anuric non-dialysed patient on a diet containing 50 mmol K could raise serum potassium by 1 mmol/day despite gastrointestinal adaptation to eliminate dietary potassium in chronic renal failure (CRF).[8]

A low potassium diet should only be initiated either to prevent or treat hyperkalaemia as well as correcting other possible causes which may have contributed to the rising serum potassium levels. Some examples of non-dietary causes for hyperkalaemia are:

- Drugs such as angiotensin-converting enzyme (ACE) inhibitors, potassium-sparing diuretics, non-steroidal anti-inflammatory drugs (NSAIDs)
- Constipation (avoid drugs that contribute to constipation, i.e. phosphate binders)
- Metabolic acidosis
- Increased catabolism
- Endocrine abnormalities
- Excessive exercise, heat stroke and rhabdomyolysis, causing hyperkalaemia due to tissue cell destruction.[8]

Most foods contain potassium, but the majority is found in vegetables and fruit. Some varieties contain more than others: basic fruits such apples or pears contain 4 mmol of potassium per portion, whereas a banana contains 8 mmol potassium. Staple foods such as potatoes, sweet potatoes and yam, plantain and green bananas are also high in potassium but should be included in a potassium-reduced diet. Cutting up vegetables and potatoes into small pieces and boiling in large volumes of water will significantly reduce the potassium content of those foods (Table 19.3).

Table 19.2 Low phosphorus diet sheet

Foods with a high phosphorus content	Foods with a low phosphorus content
Cereals	
Bran, All-Bran, Bran Flakes, cereals containing nuts, rye bread, oatcakes, scones	All other breakfast cereals, porridge, puri, chapatti, nan, pitta bread, pasta, rice, noodles
Dairy products	
Milk, yoghurt, evaporated and condensed milk, milk powder, Horlicks, hard cheese, cheese spread, eggs	Cream, crème fraiche, fromage frais, quark, cottage cheese and curd cheese, full fat or reduced fat cream cheese such as Philadelphia, roule, Boursin, mascarpone, ricotta, egg white, meringue
Meat and meat products	
Liver, kidney, liver pate and liver sausage, black pudding	Beef, veal, lamb, pork, chicken, turkey, sausages
Fish and fish products	
Fish with edible bones such as anchovies, herring, kippers, sprats, whitebait, fish roe, fish paste	Fresh or smoked fish such as cod, haddock, salmon
Vegetables	
Pulses such as dried peas, dried beans, lentils, baked beans, chick peas	All other vegetables
Cakes and biscuits	
Any cake or biscuit containing chocolate, nuts or marzipan	All other types of cakes, biscuits, pastries, doughnuts, cream cakes
Puddings	
Milk pudding, custard, bread pudding, Christmas pudding, chocolate mousse, ice-cream	Fruit jelly, sorbet, cheesecake
Savoury snacks	
Nuts, Bombay mix, chevra, chana, ganthia, poppadoms	Popcorn, corn snacks
Sweets	
Chocolate, cocoa powder, halva, burfi with nuts, Bounty, Snicker	Mints, barley sugars, wine gums, Turkish delight, jelly babies, chewing gum, lollipops
Beverages	
Milk and milk drinks, Build-up, Complan, drinking chocolate	Tea, coffee, fruit squash, lemon barley, Lucozade, soft drinks
Miscellaneous	
Meat and yeast extracts such as Marmite and Bovril, marzipan, seeds such as sesame, tahini	Jam, honey, tomato ketchup, lemon juice, vinegar, mustard, salad cream, herbs and spices

Sodium (1 mmol = 23 mg Na) and fluid

It is helpful to consider sodium and fluid together since they are closely associated in the body and the mechanisms for regulating their balance are integrated. The body's sodium and fluid status is a main determinant of blood pressure and therefore is of clinical significance. People with renal failure lose their ability to adapt to changes in dietary sodium intake; high levels may promote salt and fluid accumulation, while low intakes may lead to depletion and dehydration.

Dietary restriction should be implemented if patients are hypertensive, oedematous or require a fluid restriction for other reasons to an intake of <100 mmol sodium per day.

The major sources of sodium in the UK diet are:[3]

Table 19.3   Low potassium diet sheet

Foods with a high potassium content	Foods with a low potassium content
Cereals All-Bran, Bran Flakes, fruit and fibre, Raisin Splitz, Sultana Bran	Rice, noodles, pasta, bread, pitta bread, croissants, puri, chapatti, Cornflakes, Rice Krispies, Flour, barley, sago, semolina, tapioca
Meat substitutes Fresh soya bean products, vegetarian meat substitutes, bean milk	
Vegetables Ackee, artichokes, beetroot, mushrooms, spinach, celeriac, squash, tomatoes, parsnips, brussel sprouts, okra, plantain and green bananas, dried pulses such as dried beans, red kidney beans, broad beans, butter beans, black-eyed beans, chick peas, lentils	Runner beans, cauliflower, carrots, cabbage, peas, spring greens, asparagus, leeks, mangetout, courgette, sweetcorn
Fruit Avocado pear, banana, fresh blackcurrants or redcurrants, dried fruit such as dried apricots, dried banana chips, currants, figs, prunes, raisins, sultanas	Apple, clementine, pear, satsuma, tangerine, passion fruit, peach
Cakes and pastries Fruit cake, mince pies, Christmas cake, ginger nuts, oat cakes, rye crispbread, all biscuits and cakes containing dried fruit, nut and chocolate	Plain cake and biscuits, cream crackers
Puddings Bread pudding and Christmas pudding, desserts containing chocolate	Fruit jelly, sorbet, cheesecake
Savoury snacks Bombay mix, curu snacks, peanuts and raisins, potato crisps, Twiglets, vegetable samosas, nuts	Popcorn, corn snacks
Sweets Chocolate, all sweets containing chocolate or cocoa, liquorice, toffees, fudge and other sweets containing nuts, chocolate and dried fruit	Mints, barley sugars, wine gums, Turkish delight, jelly babies, chewing gum, lollipops, fruit pastilles, sherbets, marshmallows
Beverages Coffee, milk powder and drinks containing milk powder such as Ovaltine, Horlicks, Complan, Build-up, drinking chocolate, milk shakes, cocoa powder, fruit juices unless exchanged for fruit, tomato juice, carrot juice, mango juice, strong ale (e.g. Guinness)	Tea (black or with a little milk), soft drinks such as tonic, lemonade, soda water, ginger beer, sparkling orange, fruit squash, lemon barley. Whisky, gin, vodka, brandy, rum
Miscellaneous Tomato ketchup, tomato chutney, tomato puree, tomato sauce, meat and yeast extract, salt substitutes containing potassium chloride (i.e. low-salt products)	Jam, honey, vinegar, Worcester sauce, mustard, horseradish, sweet pickles, fresh herbs, spices

- Bread and other cereals (35%)
- Meat and meat products (26%)
- Milk and milk products (8%)
- Pickles and sauces (7%).

The remaining 22% is derived from a wide range of other foods.

Concentrated sources of sodium are fairly obvious because of their associated salty taste and include: ham, bacon, smoked fish, products canned in brine, cheese, salted butter, salted foods (e.g. nuts, salted biscuits), yeast extract spreads, stock cubes and bottled sauces.

Less obvious but significant sources of sodium include many meat and fish products, canned and packaged soups, 'instant' foods and ready meals. The majority of manufactured foods now provide nutritional labelling information which includes information on the sodium content. 1.25 g salt (0.5 g sodium) or more per 100 g is a lot of salt; 0.25 g salt (0.1 g sodium) or less per 100 g is a little salt.

Dietary management of renal replacement therapy

Haemodialysis

Protein

During haemodialysis there must be adequate dietary protein to prevent malnutrition. An intake of 1.0 g protein/kg IBW has been recommended[4] and appears adequate for stable patients. However others advocate 1.2 g/kg day as a safer level, as this helps cover the needs of individuals with increased requirements. Patients are provided with individual advice on the amount and type of protein they need to include within their diet.

Energy

Energy requirements are not altered by haemodialysis and an intake of 35 kcal/kg IBW is recommended.[9] When assessing a patient's calorie intake a dialysis day and non-dialysis day must be taken into consideration as there can be significant differences in terms of a patient's dietary intake.

Potassium

The aim of dietary restrictions is to maintain pre-dialysis blood levels within the range of 3.5–6.5 mmol/L.[4] To avoid hyperkalaemia, dietary potassium should be restricted. For a patient with some remaining residual renal function, a more liberal potassium intake may be allowed. Serum biochemistry and frequent dietary assessments are necessary to prevent hyper- or hypokalaemia.

Phosphorus

Hyperphosphataemia is a problem encountered in the majority of patients. Low-phosphorus diets together with phosphate binders will be needed to maintain pre-dialysis target range of <1.8 mmol/L.[4]

Sodium and fluid

Soon after starting haemodialysis, urine output in the majority of patients will cease or reduce to very low volumes. Fluid and salt intakes need to be restricted if hypertension and oedema are to be avoided. Patients often need reminding that foods such as soup, milk puddings, ice-cream have to be included within their fluid restriction. Many find that restricting their fluid allowance is the hardest part of their diet.

Useful tips for patients on a fluid restriction diet include:

- Use a little salt in cooking and avoid adding salt to food at the table.
- Avoid or minimise the use of processed food.
- Use herbs and spices to flavour food.
- Measure the fluid allowance into a jug and use throughout the day.
- Use a small cup or glass instead of a mug.
- Drink half a cup each time.
- Rinse the mouth with water, gargle, but do not swallow.
- Stimulate saliva production by sucking a slice of lemon, sherbets or chewing gum.

Peritoneal dialysis

Continuous ambulatory peritoneal dialysis (CAPD) is the most popular form of peritoneal dialysis, so most work on nutritional status and requirements has been undertaken in patients on CAPD.

Protein

Large amounts of protein are lost during the dialysis process with an average daily loss of 15 g across the peritoneum.[10] The amount of protein lost can vary greatly between patients but during episodes of peritonitis protein losses increase significantly. To compensate for the high protein losses, a dietary protein intake of >1.2 g/kg IBW is recommended. The consequence of this is that a patient's diet is often higher in calories and phosphate.

Energy

Glucose absorption from the dialysate across the peritoneum will provide approximately 300 kcal daily. The energy gain may be of benefit to some patients who are undernourished. A combined (oral and dialysate) energy intake of >35 kcal/kg IBW is recommended.

Potassium

The aim is to maintain serum levels with the range of 3.5–5.5 mmol/L.[4] Hyperkalaemia is less of a problem in CAPD than in intermittent forms of dialysis and a more liberal potassium intake is allowed. However, high levels are monitored and a potassium restriction is initiated if required.

Phosphorus

Foods with high protein content commonly also have high phosphorus content. Consequently, the high protein diet recommended with CAPD will also contain more phosphorus. To achieve the target range of <1.8 mmol/L[4] a dietary restriction will usually be required and phosphate binders prescribed.

Fluid and sodium

Dietary intakes of both fluid and sodium will need to be limited to prevent excessive fluid retention. The restrictions depend on the amount of fluid dialysis is able to remove (Table 19.4).

Transplantation

A well-functioning graft enables the restrictive dietary regimens imposed in the pre-dialysis and dialysis period to be relaxed. Nutrition though still remains an important aspect of their care both in the peri-operative phase and over the long term.

Both under- and overnutrition in the peri-operative phase can adversely affect outcome in the kidney transplant recipient. Death rates are significantly increased in patients with a body mass index (BMI) <18 kg/m^2 and the risk of graft failure rises with increasing BMI.[11] Obese recipients also suffer from significantly higher rates of delayed graft function, new-onset diabetes and higher mortality rates.[12] Some kidneys work immediately post transplant, but most take a few days to function. As the kidney function improves, a patient's appetite and well-being will improve and previous restrictions can be relaxed once serum biochemistry has normalised.

Longer term weight gain following transplantation is well documemented. Average weight increases of 14% in the first year post transplant have been reported.[13] Dietary intervention at an early stage has been shown to limit weight gain successfully in this patient group.[14]

Hyperlipidaemia occurs in 25% of transplant patients, therefore a cardioprotective diet based on healthy eating principles is appropriate.[15,16]

Acute renal failure

The aims of dietary treatment for patients in acute renal failure (ARF) are the same as for all patients with kidney failure, that is to maintain nutritional status and limit the complications of renal failure. Malnutrition can develop rapidly in this patient cohort and changes in fluid, electrolyte and acid–base balance are more

Table 19.4 Nutritional requirements for patients with chronic renal failure or on renal replacement therapy

	Protein (g/kg IBW)	Energy (kcal/kg IBW)	Fat	CHO	Phosphate (mg/day)	Potassium (mmol/kg IBW)	Sodium (mmol/day)	Fluid
CRF	0.6–1.0	30–35	40% of energy Reduced SFA Increased PUFA and MUFA	50% of energy Increase fibre	600–1000 (19–31 mmol/L) use binder if required	Approx. 1.0 with hyperkalaemia	80–110 (1800–2500 mg)	If required, to a volume as medically indicated
Haemodialysis	1.0–1.2	30–35	Reduced SFA Increased PUFA and MUFA	30–35	1000–1400 (31–45 mmol/L) use binder if required	1.0	80–110	500 mL + PDUO
Peritoneal dialysis	1.2–1.5	30–35	Reduced SFA Increased PUFA and MUFA	30–35	1000–1400 (31–45 mmol/L) use binder if required	1.0	80–110	800 mL + PDUO + UF capacity
Transplant	EAR	EAR	EAR – decreased SFA	EAR	Free	Free	80–110	Free

IBW, ideal body weight; HBV, high biological value protein; SFA, saturated fatty acid; PUFA, polyunsaturated fatty acid; MUFA, mono-unsaturated fatty acid; PDUO, previous day's urine output; EAR, estimated average requirements (national agreement).
Based on ref. 9.

pronounced. Patients' nutritional requirements can be broadly categorised according to the disorder causing the kidney failure. ARF from a catabolic cause such as sepsis or trauma is accompanied by increased protein turnover and dietary needs. Macronutrients requirements in ARF caused by an obstruction or non-catabolic event are not elevated.

Patients with catabolic ARF are often extremely ill. Mortality rates are high (40–80%) but appropriate feeding is associated with improved survival.[17,18] Each patient therefore requires an individual dietary assessment and treatment plan based on the degree of catabolism, organs affected, biochemistry and renal replacement therapy used. Artificial nutrition is frequently required, with daily assessment of fluid status and biochemistry.

Vitamins and minerals

Magnesium (1 mmol = 24 mg Mg)

Magnesium functions in many enzyme systems, such as those involved in decarboxylation or phosphate group transfer and energy release. It plays a vital role in skeletal development, protein synthesis, muscle contraction and neurotransmission. Metabolically, it is closely linked with calcium. Homeostatasis is largely controlled by the kidneys.

Iron (1 mmol = 56 mg Fe)

The major role of iron is as an oxygen carrier in haemoglobin in the blood and myoglobin in muscle. It is also required for many metabolic processes, including the citric acid cycle and amino acid metabolism.

The human body contains 3–5 g iron, about two-thirds of which is in haemoglobin.

The UK recommended nutrient intake (RNIs) for iron for adults are are follows:

- Men >19 years: 8.7 mg/day
- Women 11–50: 14.8 mg/day
- Women >50: 8.7 mg/day.

Dietary iron exists in two forms: haem and non-haem. Haem iron, which is contained in the haemoglobin and myoglobin of foods derived from animals, is relatively available and its absorption is relatively unaffected by other food items. The absorbability of non-haem iron present in plant-derived foods depends on other dietary components such as tannins, phytates and fibre, making it less readily solubilised and available than haem iron. Tea and eggs are notable inhibitors of non-haem iron, whereas vitamin C can enhance the absorption.

Good sources of haem iron are:

- Red meat
- Liver and offal meats.

Good sources of non-haem iron are:

- Bread and cereal foods made from UK fortified white flour
- Fortified breakfast cereals
- Green leafy vegetables
- Pulses
- Dried fruit
- Nuts and seeds.

Vitamins

Vitamins regulate the metabolic pathways of protein, carbohydrate and fat, and end stage renal failure alters the serum levels, body stores and function of many of these vitamins. Deficiencies also occur due to the dietary restrictions imposed on patients.

The B vitamins – B_6, folic acid and B_{12} – are more likely to be affected by drug interactions. These vitamins may improve poor erythropoietic responses in patients on dialysis.

An average of 125 mg vitamin C is lost during each dialysis session and supplementation is often required, especially in malnourished patients. However a supplement of 200 mg vitamin C may increase oxalate levels. Oxalate deposits as crystals in soft tissues such as muscle and vital organs and may increase the risk of myocardial infarction, muscle weakness and bone disease.

Vitamins A, D, E and K are the fat-soluble vitamins and vitamin supplements containing these are contraindicated in patients with renal failure. Vitamin A metabolites are excreted poorly and can accumulate over time.

High-dose vitamin E supplementation may be a potential risk factor affecting the clotting mechanism. Vitamin K is contraindicated unless a patient is on chronic antibiotic treatment.[19]

Malnutrition

There have been many papers published since the early 1980s on the consequence of malnutrition, including:

- Increased morbidity
- Delayed wound healing
- Increase risk of infection
- Electrolyte imbalance
- Prolonged hospitalisation
- Increased mortality.

In the renal population various factors lead to a risk of protein–energy malnutrition, including existing malnutrition, uraemia, depression, co-existing gastrointestinal disease such as gastroparesis, cancer, heart failure, anorexia, financial constraints, increases in nutritional losses due to proteinuria, and losses during dialysis. Routine nutritional assessment and individual advice is essential to identify patients at risk of developing malnutrition.[20]

Assessment of nutritional status

Assessment of nutritional status means determining the extent to which an individual's nutritional needs have been or are being met.

There is no single or standard way of assessing nutritional status. Nutritional status is a dynamic entity reflecting physiological requirements, nutritional intake, body composition and function and all these have to be considered and the findings interpreted in conjunction with one another.

Dietary considerations

These focus on the extent to which dietary intake is likely to meet nutritional needs. Factors to be assessed include:

- Current food and fluid intake
- Duration and severity of any changes in appetite and oral intake
- Presence of factors that may be affecting food and fluid intake.

Methods of dietary assessment include asking a patient to recall in as much detail as possible everything consumed in the last 24 hours or asking patients to keep food diaries, usually for 5–7 days, which are then assessed.

Anthropometric consideration

Anthropometric methods are used to assess body composition in living people. Anthropometric parameters reflect both health and nutritional status and can predict performance, health and survival. For practical purposes, body composition can be considered to be comprised of lean body mass, fat stores and body water. Ways in which these can be measured are summarised in Table 19.5.

Table 19.5 Anthropometric measurements of body composition

Protein status	Fat stores	Body water
Mid-arm muscle circumference	Triceps skin fold thickness	Bioelectrical impedance
Grip strength	Body mass index	Biochemistry
Nitrogen balance		Fluid balance charts
Plasma proteins		Rapid weight changes
Plasma urea		Girth (asites)
		Pitting oedema

Body mass index

Height and weight measurements are easy to perform and BMI can be calculated using the following formula:

$$BMI = weight\ (kg)/height\ (m)^2$$

The BMI reflects body fat stores and has important predictive values in terms of morbidity and mortality in those classified as underweight or obese:[21]

- Severely underweight <16
- Underweight <18.9
- Normal range 19–24.9
- Overweight 25–29.9
- Obese class I 30–34.9
- Obese class II 35–39.9
- Obese class III 40–60.

Subjective global assessment

Subjective global assessment is an assessment of nutritional status. It is based on the patient's history and physical examination. The medical history involves asking the patient questions about: weight changes, dietary intake, gastrointestinal symptoms and functional impairment. The physical evidence includes signs of: loss of subcutaneous fat, muscle wasting, oedema and ascites. These are observed at several locations on the body, including the face, clavicle, back, hands, arms, legs and ankles. The overall rating depends on the scores given, from normal to mild malnutrition to severely malnourished.[22]

Nutritional support

Nutritional support does not just mean the use of supplements or enteral/parenteral nutrition. The first step in the process of providing nutritional support is simple dietary advice focused on improving the quality and quantity of food which may be sufficient to correct or avert the problem. Food enrichment (with fat, sugar and/or protein) may help improve nutrient density. Some people may need further support in the form of sip-feed and other supplements. Only a few will require artificial nutritional support in the form of enteral or parenteral nutrition.

Nutritional supplementation

Many sip-feed supplements are available on an ACBS (Advisory Committee on Borderline Substances) prescription for severe undernutrition as detailed in the *British National Formulary* (*BNF*). Some are designed to meet higher energy or protein needs or with particular clinical indications such as renal disease. One potential problem with nutritional supplements is that few of the products are suitable for vegans (or people who strictly follow Vegetarian Society guidelines) or for Kosher diets. Oral supplements should be tried initially, although their efficacy has been shown to be greatest in those with a BMI <20 (Table 19.6).[23]

Enteral feeds

Feeding enterally is superior to the parenteral route in terms of physiology, immunology and cost, and has numerous clinical advantages such as helping to maintain normal intestinal function and structure.[24] Mechanical obstruction, prolonged ileus and cardiovascular instability are the only absolute contraindications to enteral nutrition.[24] Guidelines on the management of enteral nutrition in the adult patient have been produced by the British Society of Gastroenterology.[25] Specialist renal feeds with reduced electrolyte content are available. These are useful where the control of serum phosphate, potassium or fluid balance proves difficult.

Complications of enteral tube feeding include:[26]

- Aspiration – This may occur with no obvious vomiting or coughing, and pneumonia can develop silently.
- Gastrointestinal symptoms. Nausea occurs in 10–20% of patients and abdominal bloating and cramps from delayed gastric emptying are also common. Diarrhoea occurs in up to 30% of enterally fed patients; this can create serious problems from nutrient, fluid and electrolyte losses, and from infected pressure sores and general patient distress.

Table 19.6 Nutritional content of oral dietary supplements

Nutritional supplement	Ensure Plus	Fortisip	Fresubin Energy	Enlive Plus	Provide Extra	Complan	Renilon 7.5	Maxijule	Calogen	Formance	Nepro
Quantity	220 mL	200 mL	200 mL	220 mL	200 mL	230 mL	125 mL	100 g	100 mL	113 g	100 mL
Energy (kcal)	330	300	300	330	250	244	250	400	466	167	200
Protein (g)	13.8	12.0	11.3	10.6	7.5	9.4	9.4	0	0	3.96	7.0
Fat (g)	10.8	11.6	11.6	0	0	9.0	12.5	0	50	4.97	9.6
CHO (g)	44.4	36.8	37.6	71.9	55	31.3	25.0	0	4	27.1	22.2
Sodium (mmol)	11.5	105 mg	7.0	1.05	2.4	5.7	3.2	0	<0.4	4.67	3.67
Potassium (mmol)	11.3	210 mg	7.0	0.92	2.4	11.8	0.4	0	0	3.91	2.72
Phosphate (mg)	202	108	100	24.2	80	270	7.5	0	0	99.4	69.0

CHO = carbohydrate.

- Blocked feeding tubes. Tubes can block easily, especially if they are not flushed with fresh tap, cooled boiled or sterile water before and after every feed or medication. Any drugs administered through a tube should ideally be suspensions rather than syrups. Hyper-osmolar drugs, crushed tablets, potassium and iron supplements are particularly likely to cause problems. A tube can often be unblocked by flushing with warm water.

Parenteral nutrition

Parenteral nutrition is a method of providing nutritional support to an individual whose gastrointestinal tract is not functioning or is inaccessible. Nutrients are delivered directly into the circulatory system via a dedicated venous catheter. Although parenteral nutrition is essential and a potentially life-saving therapy, it is expensive and carries life-threatening complications (sepsis and metabolic disorders), so must be monitored and administered correctly. The main complications of parenteral nutrition are:

- Metabolic – fluid overload, hyperglycaemia and electrolyte abnormalities.

- Physiological – rise in serum bilirubin, secondary to reduced bilirubin binding capacity and increased free circulating bilirubin due to free fatty acids from the lipid emulsion of the parenteral nutrition. Excessive glucose can lead to a fatty liver.
- Infections – either secondary to the catheter or non-catheter concurrent infections.

Intradialytic parenteral nutrition

Intradialytic parenteral nutrition (IDPN) is given whilst a patient is undergoing haemodialysis using the same vascular access. This may improve nutritional status and protein kinetics.[27] Parenteral formulas containing approximately 65–70 g protein and 1000 kcal (mainly glucose) can be safely delivered during haemodialysis treatment. Glucose monitoring during treatment is essential to prevent hyperglycaemia. The fluid balance can be adjusted accordingly. IDPN still remains a controversial mode of nutritional support, but an evidence-based evaluation by Foulks[28] showed it to be of benefit. The cost of IDPN is 10 times that of enteral nutrition or oral supplementation.

CASE STUDY

Mr Smith is a 63-year-old man referred to the dietetic outpatient service with stage 4 chronic kidney disease for a renal diet. His biochemistry is within expectable ranges, with no reported weight loss but he is hypertensive.

Q1. What advice would you give him?
At his next review his serum phosphate has increased (PO_4 2.10 mmol/L) and the consultant has started him on phosphate binders.

Q2. What advice would you give him now?
Twelve months later his eGFR has dropped to 14. His serum potassium has increased (K 6.4 mmol/L).

Q3. What further dietary measures would be needed?
As Mr Smith approaches dialysis his weight begins to decrease and the doctor has requested some nutritional supplements for a renal patient.

Q4. Which supplements would you suggest?

References

1. Berlyne GM. *A Course in Renal Disease*, 2nd edn. Oxford: Blackwell Scientific Publications, 1968.
2. Klahr S, Levey AS, Beck GJ *et al.* The effects of dietary protein restriction and blood-pressure control on the progression of chronic renal disease. *N Engl J Med* 1994; 330: 878–884.
3. National Diet and Nutrition Survey (NDNS). Adults aged 19–64 years. Medical Research Office/Office for National Statistics, 2003/2004.
4. Renal Association. *Treatment of Adult Patients with Renal Failure. Recommended Standards and Audit Measures*, 3rd edn. London: The Royal College of Physicians, 2002.
5. Kopple JD, Monteon FJ, Shaib JK. Effect of energy intake on nitrogen metabolism in nondialyzed patients with chronic renal failure. *Kidney Int* 1986; 29: 734–742.
6. Slatapolsky E, Delmez JA. Pathogenesis of secondary hyperparathyroidism. *Nephrol Dial Transplant* 1996; 3 (Suppl 11): 130–135.
7. Rufino M, Bonis ED, Martin M *et al.* Is it possible to control hyperphosphataemia with diet, without inducing protein malnutrition? *Nephrol Dial Transplant* 1998; 13 (Suppl 3): 65–67.
8. Bansal VK. Potassium metabolism in renal failure: nondietary rationale for hyperkalaemia. *J Ren Nutr* 1992; 2: 8–12.
9. European Dialysis and Transplant Nurses Association/European Renal Care Association (EDTNA/ERCA). *Nutritional Guidelines 2001*. www.edtna-erca.org (accessed 7 November 2001).
10. Blumenkrantz MJ, Gahl GM, Kopple JD *et al.* Protein losses during peritoneal dialysis. *Kidney Int* 1981; 19: 593–602.
11. Chertow GM, Lazarus JM, Milford EL. Quetelet's index predicts outcome in cadaveric kidney transplantation. *J Ren Nutr* 1996; 6: 134–140.
12. Holley JL, Shapiro R, Lopatin WB *et al.* Obesity as a risk factor following cadaveric renal transplant. *Transplantation* 1990; 49: 387–389.
13. Przygrodzka F, Rayner HC, Morgan AG, Burden RP. Change in nutritional status after successful renal transplantation. *J Ren Nutr* 1992; 2: 18–20.
14. Patel MG. The effect of dietary intervention on weight gains after renal transplantation. *J Ren Nutr* 1998; 8: 137–141.
15. Lawrence IR, Thompson A, Hartley GH *et al.* The effect of dietary intervention on the management of hyperlipidemia in British renal transplant patients. *J Ren Nutr* 1995; 5: 73–77.
16. Nelson J, Beauregard M, Gelinas M *et al.* Rapid improvement of hyperlipidemia in kidney transplant patients with a multifactorial hypolipidemic diet. *Transplant Proc* 1988; 20: 1264–1270.
17. Rainford DJ. Nutritional management of acute renal failure. *Acta Chirurg Scand* 1981; 507 (Suppl): 327–329.
18. Bartlett RH, Mault JR, Dechert RE *et al.* Continuous arteriovenous hemofiltration: improved survival in surgical acute renal failure? *Surgery* 1986; 100: 400–408.
19. Rocco MV, Makoff R. Appropriate vitamin therapy for dialysis patients. *Semin Dial* 1997; 10: 272–277.
20. Malnutrition Advisory Group of the British Association for Parenteral and Enteral Nutrition (BAPEN). *Guidelines for the Detection and Management of Malnutrition*. Maidenhead: BAPEN, 2000.
21. de Onis M, Habicht JP. Anthropometric reference data for international use: recommendations from a World Health Organization Expert Committee. *Am J Clin Nutr* 1996; 64: 650–658.
22. Detsky AS, McLaughlin JR, Baker JP *et al.* What is subjective global assessment of nutritional status? *J Parenter Enteral Nutr* 1987; 11: 8–13.
23. Stratton RJ, Elia M. A critical systemic analysis of the use of oral nutritional supplements in the community. *Clin Nutr* 1998; 18 (Suppl 2): 29–84.
24. McClave SA, Snider HL, Spain DA. Preoperative issues in clinical nutrition. *Chest* 1999; 115: 64S–70S.
25. Kirby DF, Teran JC. Enteral feeding in critical care, gastrointestinal diseases and cancer. *Gastrointest Endosc Clin N Am* 1998; 8: 623–643.
26. Stroud M, Duncan H, Nightingale J. Guidelines for enteral feeding in adult hospital patients. *Gut* 2003; 52 (Suppl 7): vii1–vii12.
27. McCann L, Feldman C, Hornberger J et al. Effects of intradialytic parenteral nutrition on delivered Kt/V. *Am J Kidney Dis* 1999; 33: 1131–1135.
28. Foulks CJ. An evidence-based evaluation of intradialytic parenteral nutrition. *Am J Kidney Dis* 1999; 33: 186–192.

20

Travelling and vaccines

Zoe Thain

This chapter discusses issues in relation to travel for the patient with renal disease based in the UK. It begins with general considerations to be taken when booking holidays for different groups of renal patients, and goes on to examine both general travel health advice and specific advice relating to travelling abroad with medication. It also addresses the requirements for malaria prophylaxis and travel vaccinations. Patients have various reasons for travel. They may wish to visit relatives abroad, may be required to travel for business reasons, or may just want to go on holiday. The key message is that with appropriate planning and advice, kidney patients can travel and that destinations worldwide are possible.

Planning holidays

The first priority when a renal patient wants to go on holiday is to assess if they are fit to travel. All patients, even transplant patients, will require a letter from their renal unit confirming this in order to obtain suitable travel insurance. This also provides a first point of contact for the patient for advice on reducing illness and health risks whilst travelling, including advice on suitable malaria prophylaxis and vaccinations if required.

Most renal units now have a designated member of staff with the role of holiday co-ordinator who can assist with arranging the holiday, and suggest suitable destinations. Whilst last-minute bookings are certainly not an option for a holiday-dialysis patient, most destinations are possible with good planning. It can sometimes prove difficult, however, to accommodate a specific destination with specific travel dates, and patients may have to be quite flexible. Patients awaiting transplant who go abroad may be suspended from the transplant list for the duration of their holiday, depending on the destination.

Haemodialysis

Patients can usually choose their travel destination, although this will have to be close to a dialysis unit that can accommodate visitors. It is often easier to find dialysis space abroad than in the UK, as NHS hospital units tend to work at full capacity. Private units in the UK may provide a suitable option, usually at a similar cost to NHS units. All holiday dialysis sessions in the UK are paid for by the patient's purchasing authority.

There are various holiday directories on the Internet to help patients and co-ordinators locate suitable dialysis units. Eurodial is a helpful guide to dialysis units for patients travelling to Europe, and Holiday Dialysis International and Global Dialysis will locate units worldwide, including cruises. Recommendations for suitable units may also be provided by other patients, based on their own travel experiences.

There may be a charge per dialysis session depending on the destination. Most countries that accept the European Health Insurance Card (EHIC) within the European Union have a reciprocal arrangement with the UK; however a portion of the cost may still need to be paid, and some private clinics may not accept the EHIC. For countries not covered by the EHIC, charges may vary from between £150 and £200 for each dialysis session in Turkey, to £500 per session in the USA. Patients themselves have to pay for these dialysis costs.

Patients should be prepared for differences in the equipment and procedures used in units in other countries, and in some cases may have to take their own dialysers and medications for dialysis, such as heparin and erythropoietin. Transport between hotel and dialysis unit will not necessarily be provided, and patients will need to pay for and organise this themselves. It is essential, therefore, that patients are provided with full details of when their dialysis sessions will be before travel.

Recent blood results, including MRSA, HIV, hepatitis B and hepatitis C status will be required by the holiday-dialysis unit. These are usually requested to be taken within four weeks of travel. When planning trips to high-risk areas for blood-borne viruses, it must first be established that the base unit will be able to accommodate the traveller to dialyse in isolation on return to the UK. Each renal unit in the UK will have a policy for the isolation of patients returning from overseas dialysis.

Peritoneal dialysis

Patients who require peritoneal dialysis have a greater freedom to travel, the only restrictions being whether the dialysis fluids can be delivered to the destination of choice, and that they can be stored appropriately in the holiday accommodation selected. Delivery is arranged by the manufacturer of the particular fluid, and renal units will help to co-ordinate this for patients. It may take up to three months to make the necessary arrangements; the notice required for delivery of fluids is generally 2–4 weeks for the UK, 8 weeks for Europe and 12 weeks for worldwide destinations. Patients should call the destination a few days before travel to ensure supplies have arrived safely, and know who to contact if there are any problems with supplies during the holiday. Patients may be responsible for transporting their machines and ancillary products themselves, and will

require a letter from their renal unit to explain the need for excessive hand luggage and that it is required for medical treatment.

The need to carry out an exchange during the journey will depend on the itinerary, although it is always advisable to carry one dialysis bag in hand luggage in case of delays. The peritoneal dialysis nurse can advise on a suitable exchange plan whilst travelling, and give advice on where to carry out exchanges to reduce the risk of peritonitis. Renal units may provide patients with antibiotics to take with them in case of peritonitis, particularly if they are travelling to places that are not in close proximity to medical assistance, or are on a cruise ship. Appropriate equipment for administration and full instructions for treatment should also be provided.

Transplant patients

Transplant patients are advised not to travel to countries where the risk of catching an infection is high; otherwise they are not restricted in their choice of destination. Precautions should always be taken to reduce the risk of infection whilst on holiday, such as drinking only bottled or boiled water, and avoiding salads and ice-cubes. Transplant patients are at increased risk of skin cancer because of immunosuppressant drugs,[1] so sun exposure should be kept to a minimum. It is vital that sun protection measures, including the use of high-factor sun block, are taken.

General travel health advice

Any traveller should consider taking a basic first aid kit containing items such as plasters and dressings, antiseptic, sun block, insect repellent, and water-sterilisation tablets. Other medicines that can be bought over the counter (OTC), which may only be required occasionally, should also be considered by the traveller with kidney disease. These should be purchased before travel so that suitable OTC medicines can be recommended. It should be confirmed that there are no interactions with prescribed medicines, that doses and medicines are appropriate for the degree of renal impairment, and that they are not likely to worsen renal function. The exact content of the kit will be determined by the type of traveller, the destination and likely activities; factors which may affect whether a person will develop a travel-associated illness. Over-the-counter medicines suitable for renal patients are listed in Table 20.1.[2]

Apart from their usual medications it may be necessary to provide renal patients with medicines for self-treatment in emergency situations, particularly if travel is to remote areas or far from medical facilities. For example, renal units may supply continuous ambulatory peritoneal dialysis (CAPD) patients with antibiotics, based on their own protocol, for the initial treatment of peritonitis. These may be required if patients are travelling outside Europe, where appropriate antibiotics may not be readily available, or on cruise ships which do not carry supplies of such drugs on board. Full instructions should be given to the patient, so that they understand when and how to use these medications.

For travel to resource-poor areas where needles and other equipment may be in short supply or not always sterilised, patients may consider taking an emergency medical travel kit. These can be purchased from pharmacies and contain sterile needles, syringes, and dressing packs, which can be handed to a doctor or nurse for use in an emergency.

Traveller's diarrhoea

Traveller's diarrhoea is the most common illness contracted abroad by travellers generally, with incidence estimated to be between 30 and 50%. It is usually defined as the passage of three or more unformed stools in a 24-hour period, with at least one other symptom of enteric disease such as nausea, vomiting, abdominal pain, fever, faecal urgency, or blood or mucus in the stools.[3] Traveller's diarrhoea, along with hepatitis A and typhoid, is contracted through contaminated food and water. The risk of contracting diarrhoea can be reduced by taking the following simple precautions:[4]

- Wash your hands after using the lavatory and before handling and eating food.

Table 20.1 Over-the-counter medicines for renal patients

Ailment	Recommended	Avoid	Other information
Headache	Paracetamol Co-codamol	Aspirin Ibuprofen	Effervescent tablets contain sodium so avoid
Coughs and colds	Paracetamol Simple linctus	Decongestants	Steam inhalation, menthol or olbas oil may help congestion
Muscle aches	Ralgex Deep heat	Topical and oral NSAIDs	
Indigestion	Gaviscon	Aluminium- or magnesium-containing indigestion remedies	Gaviscon for short-term use only as contains sodium
Hayfever	Antihistamines		Nasal sprays and eye drops may also be effective
Constipation	Senna	Fybogel (if fluid restricted)	Seek medical advice if symptoms persist
Diarrhoea	Loperamide	Oral rehydration salts	Seek medical advice if symptoms are severe or persist

- Use bottled water or boiled or sterilised tap water for drinking, washing food or cleaning teeth in countries where sanitation may be poor.
- Avoid ice in drinks and ice used to keep food cool.
- Hot tea, coffee, wine, beer, carbonated water and soft drinks, and packaged juices are usually safe.
- Eat freshly cooked food which is piping hot.
- Avoid food which has been kept warm.
- Avoid salads or uncooked fruit or vegetables, unless you can peel or shell them yourself.
- Avoid unpasteurised milk, ice-cream and dairy products.
- Avoid food from unreliable sources such as street vendors.
- Avoid raw seafood and shellfish.
- Avoid food likely to have been exposed to flies.

Most cases of traveller's diarrhoea are mild, lasting a few days, and most travellers will recover with symptomatic treatment. Oral rehydration solutions contain both sodium and potassium, so should be avoided in people with kidney disease, although travellers should be advised to maintain their usual fluid intake. The antimotility agent loperamide is suitable for use by renal patients and will reduce symptoms of faecal frequency and stomach cramps. However, constipation can develop if loperamide is taken at maximum dose for more than a day or so. There is also a risk that infection may be prolonged by the use of antimotility agents due to retention of the organism, so loperamide should be avoided if there is fever or bloody diarrhoea. Quinolone antibiotics such as ciprofloxacin have been used for the treatment of traveller's diarrhoea.[3] They may be carried by those considered to be most at risk, such as immunosuppressed patients, for immediate self-treatment, although this is not a licensed indication. Doses of quinolone antibiotics need to be adjusted according to renal function.[5]

Medical advice should be sought if symptoms do not improve within a few days, if there is blood in the stools, or if a fever or confusion develops.

Insect bites

The risk of infection spread by insects, including malaria, can be reduced by good protection against insect bites.

Clothing

Travellers should be advised to wear long-sleeved clothing, long trousers, and socks out of doors between dusk and dawn.

Insect repellent

Of the products available on the market DEET (diethyltoluamide)-based products are the most effective, and should be used first line for travel to malarious areas. They are available in different concentrations for use on skin or clothing. There have been safety concerns as DEET can be absorbed after application to the skin, but as long as recommended concentrations of 20–50% are not exceeded and it is used as directed by the manufacturer, then clinical experience shows it is safe to use.[6] It should only be used on exposed areas of the skin and applied with care to the face, avoiding the mouth and eyes. It should not be used on broken or irritated skin. Hands should be washed after application and the repellent should be removed with soap and water when no longer required. Use of sunscreen which contains repellent should be avoided as repeated administration may result in excessive use of DEET.

Insecticides

Clothes and mosquito nets can be treated with an insecticide such as permethrin. Sprays, plug-in devices and coils can also be used to rid sleeping areas of insects. Mosquito nets should be used unless the room has screened windows and doors. Air-conditioned rooms are also advised.

Treatment of bites

Bites and stings are commonly experienced by travellers, although the response may vary from a mild allergic reaction to anaphylaxis. Most bites can be treated with application of a mild topical steroid cream to reduce swelling and oral antihistamines to relieve itching. Bites should be kept clean and not scratched, to reduce the risk of infection. Oral cortico steroids may be a consideration if severe reactions are likely, and epinephrine (adrenaline) should be carried by those who have previously experienced anaphylaxis with bites.[3]

Sun protection

Overexposure to the sun can cause sunburn and heatstroke. General measures such as covering up with suitable clothing and wearing a wide-brimmed hat and sunglasses that block UV radiation should be taken. Staying in the shade and avoiding direct sun between 11 am and 3 pm will also help reduce exposure. Patients should be advised to take extra care if they are also prescribed medications (e.g. doxycycline) that sensitise the skin to UV light. The correct use of appropriate suncream is vital, and travellers should use suncream with a sun protection factor (SPF) of at least 15.[3] The National Kidney Federation advises transplant patients to use SPF 25 or higher. The appropriate amount to apply is often underestimated; 100 mL will cover the body approximately three times. Suncream should be applied at least 30 minutes before sun exposure and reapplied frequently, at least every 2 hours.

Calamine lotion or cream can be used to soothe mild sunburn, and paracetamol taken if analgesia is required.

Travel sickness

Medications used to prevent motion sickness include cinnarizine, hyoscine and promethazine. All are suitable for use by renal patients at usual doses.[5] They differ in duration of action and side-effects which may help determine the most appropriate agent to use. For long journeys cinnarizine may be useful as it has a long duration of action, whereas hyoscine has a short duration. Cinnarizine causes least drowsiness, whereas promethazine, which induces a high degree of drowsiness, may be useful for night-time journeys.

Deep vein thrombosis

The risk of deep vein thrombosis (DVT) in relation to travel can be reduced by regular flexing of the ankles to encourage blood flow in the lower legs, avoiding alcohol and maintaining adequate fluid intake.

Additional measures may be considered for those at high risk of DVT such as those with a history of DVT, recent surgery or heart disease, pregnancy or hormonal medication, malignancy, haematological disorders, varicose veins, obesity, dehydration, or age over 40 years.[3]

Well-fitting compression stockings may reduce the risk of DVT in high-risk patients, as may the use of low-molecular-weight heparin. A suitable regimen should be discussed with medical staff as dose adjustment is required for renal impairment. British Medical Association guidelines[7] support the view that aspirin should not be used for the prevention of DVT in travellers due to insufficient evidence.

Travelling abroad with medication

Renal patients are often required to take a multitude of different medications. When planning a holiday, particularly abroad, it is essential that preparations are made well in advance of travel in order to arrange sufficient supplies.

Patients should see their GP to arrange a prescription to cover the holiday period, plus a few extra days in case of delays. British GPs can prescribe a maximum of three months' supply on an NHS prescription for overseas travel. After this time the individual ceases to be registered with the GP.[8]

It is advisable that patients obtain a letter from their GP detailing all medications (with generic names not just brand names), any equipment required (such as needles and syringes), and the medical conditions for which they are being used, to confirm the patient's need for the medication. Although not compulsory, it is likely to prove helpful when going through customs. As a minimum patients should at least take a copy of their prescription.

Many countries, particularly those outside Europe, such as India, Pakistan, Turkey and some Middle Eastern countries, have lists of medicines which they do not allow to be brought in. These might even include medicines available over the counter in the UK as the legal status of medicines varies between countries. The relevant Embassy in the UK should be contacted well before travel, to ensure the patient will have no problems taking the medicines they need. The UK Foreign and Commonwealth (FCO) website has contact details for Embassies and High Commissions in the UK.

Controlled drugs

For any medication classed as a controlled drug in the UK, a Home Office licence may be required to take it abroad. The HM Revenue and Customs leaflet, 'Taking medicines with you when you go abroad', available via www.hmrc.gov.uk, gives a list of permitted allowances for controlled drugs. If the patient needs to take more than the permitted allowance, they must apply in writing to the Home Office for a licence giving the following details:

- Patient's name, address, and date of birth
- Country/countries of destination
- Dates of departure from and return to UK
- A letter from the prescribing doctor confirming the drug details (name, form, strength and total quantity).

This should be done at least two weeks before travel to allow time for the licence to be issued.

Packing and storage

All medication should be stored in hand luggage, so that it is readily accessible, with each item in a correctly labelled container, as issued by the pharmacist. It may be tempting for the patient to carry loose tablets or pack medication down into smaller containers, but this could lead to problems at customs. It will also prove useful if the patient needs to consult a doctor overseas, that full instructions and information leaflets for their medications are available. For extra protection, travellers could consider storing items in a sealable plastic box or, if this is too bulky, then in resealable plastic bags to protect against moisture. Items such as erythropoietin or insulin which need to be kept cool can be carried in small cool bags or boxes, although care should be taken to avoid direct contact with ice packs. For long flights, airlines may provide cool storage. Documentation, such as a letter from the GP, will be required for patients to carry syringes and needles in their hand luggage (Box 20.1).

Consideration should also be given to how the medication will be stored at the holiday destination, particularly for long trips. For items

---

Box 20.1 Travel documentation which may be required by a renal patient

- Doctor's letter – detailing medications, medical equipment and medical conditions
- Copy of prescription
- Home Office licence – if required for controlled drugs
- European Health Insurance Card (EHIC) – replaced the E111 as from 1 January 2006. This entitles the traveller from the UK to reduced-cost, sometimes free, medical treatment that becomes necessary, because of illness or accident. It also covers treatment which may be needed for a chronic disease or pre-existing illness. Arrangements will need to be made in advance for dialysis
- Travel insurance – must cover for pre-existing medical conditions (the National Kidney Federation can recommend suitable insurance) and/or have specific health insurance
- Letter for airline if carrying excess hand luggage (CAPD patients)
- Copy of blood results and medical information – if requested by the holiday dialysis unit

that require refrigeration, patients should consider booking a room with a fridge, using a cool box, or if necessary, storing such items in the coolest, darkest area possible. The stability of medicines exposed to extremes of temperature has not been studied, so patients should consider discarding unused medicines after returning from a long trip to particularly warm or cold climates.[8]

Purchase of medicines overseas

Patients should be advised to take all their medications with them, including those prescribed and any OTC medicines which are likely to be required. This is particularly important if travel is to remote areas or developing countries where counterfeit or poor-quality medicines may be supplied.[8] Specific medicines to treat chronic conditions may not be marketed in other countries or availability could be unreliable. There is also the problem of communication, as travellers may be unable to adequately express their requirements, or may not be able to follow information about how to take medicines they have been supplied or prescribed whilst abroad.

If purchase of medicines is unavoidable, then reliable retailers recommended by an Embassy or Consulate should be used.

Malaria

Malaria is a significant health risk of travel abroad with approximately 2000 cases reported in the UK each year. Almost all malaria deaths, on average nine per year in the UK, are preventable.[9] Most cases of malaria occur in those who fail to comply with malaria prophylaxis, so it is essential that renal patients are counselled as to the importance of taking another drug in addition to their usual medications. The degree of renal failure and the drugs taken by renal patients should be taken into account when considering the most suitable prophylaxis for a particular patient.

Healthcare workers who advise travellers about malaria prophylaxis should refer to the guidelines formulated by the Health Protection Agency (HPA) Advisory Committee on Malaria Prevention (ACMP) for UK Travellers.[9] A full update of the current guidelines was carried out in 2006, but specific updates and notices are available on the ACMP web pages (http://www. hpa.org.uk/publications/2006/Malaria/Malaria_ guidelines.pdf). There are separate guidelines produced by the ACMP for advising long-term travellers (longer than six months) on malaria prophylaxis.[10]

Taking appropriate chemoprophylaxis is only one aspect of malarial prevention. The guidelines give four essential ABCD steps,[9] which are the same throughout the world, and relevant to any traveller regardless of their medical history.

Awareness of risk

The risk of malaria is determined by the destination, duration of the visit, and likely degree of exposure due to intended activities and style of travel. The risk in a particular country may also vary depending on the time of year, and between rural and urban destinations. Particularly at risk are ethnic groups in the UK (or long-term visitors to the UK) who visit friends and relatives in their country of origin. These travellers may assume they still possess some immunity, which actually fades quickly, and so do not take adequate, if any, preventative measures.

Bites by mosquitoes: prevent or avoid

Taking effective measures to reduce mosquito bites will significantly reduce the risk of contracting malaria, and will also protect against other insect-borne infections. Bite prevention measures should be taken by all travellers as no malaria prophylaxis regimen will provide complete protection.

Compliance with appropriate chemoprophylaxis

Patients should be counselled on the importance of taking the medication regularly and for the correct duration. Malaria is as likely to occur in those who take prophylaxis irregularly as in those who take no prophylaxis at all. Weekly regimens should be started at least one week (three weeks for mefloquine) before travel. Malarone (atovaquone/proguanil) can be started one to two days before travel into an endemic area. This will allow identification of any adverse effects before travel, and provide sufficient time to switch to an alternative medication. Travellers should be advised of possible side-effects and to seek advice if severe. Antimalarials should be taken while in a malarious area and for four weeks after leaving (one week for Malarone). This will protect against malaria contracted at the end of travel.

Daily doses should be taken at the same time each day, and weekly doses at the same time each week. Taking after meals will help reduce side-effects and provide a prompt to aid compliance. Travellers should obtain their full course of medication before travel, as the strength of antimalarials abroad may differ and could therefore provide inadequate protection.

Diagnose malaria swiftly and obtain treatment promptly

Early symptoms of malaria can be non-specific. Although symptoms usually occur within three months of being bitten by an infected mosquito, malaria can present at any time between one week and one year after exposure.[11] Travellers should be advised to seek medical attention immediately and mention their possible exposure to malaria if they develop any of the following symptoms:

- Fever
- Flu-like illness
- Backache
- Diarrhoea
- Joint pains
- Sore throat
- Headache.

Choice of chemoprophylaxis

There are currently six prophylactic regimens described in the ACMP guidelines for UK travellers.[9] These are given, along with usual adult doses, in Table 20.2. Doses of prophylactic antimalarials for children, based on weight, can also be found in the ACMP guidelines, and in the *BNF for children*.

The ACMP guidelines give the recommended prophylaxis regimen for specific areas and countries based on geographical resistance patterns. Also, where possible, there are alternative regimens suggested for those unwilling or unable to follow a recommended regimen. In some instances there are several regimens of equivalent efficacy. The choice between them then is determined by the particular circumstances of the traveller. The guidelines consider the importance of balancing the risk of malaria and the risk of adverse reaction to antimalarials, including observing the contraindications to the use of specific antimalarials. They also include recommendations for prophylaxis in

Table 20.2 Prophylactic regimens for malaria

Regimen	Dose for adults	Dose adjustment for renal function
Mefloquine	250 mg weekly	No
Doxycycline	100 mg daily	No
Atovaquone/proguanil	1 tablet daily	Do not use if GFR <30 mL/min
Proguanil plus chloroquine	200 mg daily plus 300 mg (base) weekly	Yes for proguanil
Chloroquine	300 mg (base) weekly	No
Proguanil	200 mg daily	Yes

people with other medical conditions, including renal failure.

Additional factors to consider for renal patients

Dose adjustment

Proguanil is excreted by the kidney and therefore requires dose adjustment according to renal function (Table 20.3).[5] Patients with renal failure receiving proguanil should also be prescribed folic acid 5 mg daily to reduce haematological side-effects.[5]

Malarone (atovaquone 250 mg/proguanil 100 mg) is not recommended at GFR <30 mL/min. The dose of proguanil would need to be reduced, but full dose of atovaquone would be required. This is clearly not possible with a combined product. No dose adjustments are required for any of the other agents when used at prophylactic doses.

Interactions

Renal patients often take multiple medications. It is important to check carefully for possible interactions when selecting the most appropriate antimalarial agent. Interactions could result in antimalarial effects being reduced or blood levels of immunosuppressants being altered. For example:[12]

- Ciclosporin, tacrolimus and sirolimus plasma concentration levels can be increased by both doxycycline and chloroquine.

Table 20.3 Dose of proguanil in renal impairment

GFR (mL/min)	Prophylactic dose of proguanil for adults
>60	200 mg daily
20–59	100 mg daily
10–19	50 mg alternate days
<10	50 mg once a week
CAPD/haemodialysis	50 mg once a week

- Ferrous sulfate may reduce the serum levels of doxycycline by up to 90%.
- Chloroquine absorption may be reduced by calcium carbonate.
- Calcium- and aluminium-based phosphate binders may reduce doxycycline levels by 50–100%.

Specialist advice

When taking into account all the above factors it may prove difficult to decide which, if any, is the most appropriate antimalarial for a particular patient. In such cases detailed advice is available from the Malaria Reference Laboratory (at the London School of Hygiene and Tropical Medicine) or the National Travel Health Network and Centre. All options should also be discussed with the renal clinician. It may be that the advice is not to travel to a particular area.

Travel vaccinations

The requirement for travel vaccinations will be determined by the disease risk to the traveller. All travellers should undergo a full risk assessment before travel. Travel-related hazards and risks may be determined not only by the country or countries to be visited, but also the area to be visited within that country (city or rural, altitude or jungle, etc.), type of accommodation, and proposed activities to be undertaken. Some risks may also be seasonal. It is vital, therefore, that guidance is given based on current recommendations. The National Travel Health Network and Centre (NaTHNaC) telephone advice line provides guidance for health professionals advising travellers who have a complex medical history or travel itinerary or both. Information about travel-related health issues, including clinical updates and disease outbreaks, can be found at the NaTHNaC website (www.nathnac.org). The on-line Travax database (www.travax.scot.nhs.uk – requires subscription) provides up-to-date country-by-country advice regarding travel vaccinations, malaria, disease outbreak news and other travel health-related issues. Fit for Travel (www.fitfortravel.scot.nhs. uk) is provided by NHS Scotland and is intended as a travel health resource for the general public. All the websites have links to other valuable travel health-related websites.

Renal patients have special immunisation requirements and contraindications, so it is important that the traveller provides full medical details as well as a detailed travel itinerary when accessing travel advice. The advising health professional should confirm that a traveller's primary courses and boosters have been received as recommended in the full British schedule. In addition, the Department of Health recommends that patients with chronic kidney disease receive influenza and pneumococcal immunisation. All patients being considered for, or who are on, dialysis should also be vaccinated against hepatitis B.

Immunosuppressed patients, including both transplant patients and those on dialysis, should not receive live vaccines. Inactivated vaccines can be administered, although the response may be reduced. Patients with end stage renal disease (ESRD) have a reduced response to vaccination because of the general suppression of the immune system associated with uraemia. The response of transplant patients to vaccination will depend on their degree of immunosuppression and underlying disease. See Table 20.4 for live/inactivated vaccines.

Hepatitis B

The hepatitis B status of a haemodialysis patient (in addition to other blood-borne viruses such as hepatitis C and HIV) may be requested by the holiday dialysis centre within a certain number of weeks before travel, and boosters may be required. Each haemodialysis unit in the UK will have a policy for the isolation of patients returning from dialysis in high-risk areas outside Europe and North America.

Yellow fever

Yellow fever vaccination is recommended for travel to some African and South American

Table 20.4 Vaccines given for travel when indicated (doses may differ for children and adults)

Inactivated vaccines	Live attenuated vaccines
Hepatitis A	Yellow fever
Hepatitis B	BCG
Typhoid	Typhoid (oral)
Oral cholera	MMR
Influenza	Varicella (rarely used in UK)
Pneumococcal	
Polio	
Diphtheria, polio and tetanus (combined)	
Japanese encephalitis	
Meningococcal meningitis – ACW135Y	
Rabies	
Tick-borne encephalitis	
Haemophilus influenzae type B	

countries where the disease is endemic.[13] Many countries, although not the UK, require an International Certificate of Vaccination or Prophylaxis from travellers arriving from, or who have passed through, an endemic area, before entry is allowed. However, countries for which the vaccine is recommended may not themselves request a vaccination certificate, so the absence of a requirement for a vaccination certificate does not imply that there is no risk in that country.

Yellow fever is a live vaccine, and as such, should not be given to immunosuppressed travellers. Renal patients who are immunosuppressed should avoid travel to yellow fever endemic areas as they cannot be protected against the disease by vaccination. A letter of medical exemption may be provided if an individual should not be vaccinated on medical grounds, and is visiting low-risk areas where a certificate requirement exists.

Yellow fever vaccine can only be administered at designated yellow fever centres. Designated centres in England and Wales are listed on the National Travel Health Network and Centre website (www.nathnac.org). Information on country requirements for yellow fever is published annually by the World Health Organization in International Travel and Health, Vaccination Requirements and Health Advice (www.who.int). International Certificates of Vaccination or Prophylaxis are valid for 10 years starting 10 days after the date of vaccination.

Vaccination summary

Although not always possible, travellers should plan vaccinations at least eight weeks ahead of travel, to ensure that the recommended time interval between doses and vaccines is followed. This will also allow immunity to develop before departure.

It may be necessary to discuss immunisation requirements for a renal patient with the supervising clinician in addition to a specialist centre such as NaTHNaC. The advice, based on vaccination requirements and contraindications, may be that the patient should not travel to a particular destination.

Conclusion

This chapter has given a brief overview of some of the considerations for which travellers from the UK with renal disease may seek advice. Although there are some restrictions, in the main, patients with renal disease are able to travel to many areas of the world, provided they make appropriate arrangements, take the required medications, and follow closely the travel health advice they are given.

Acknowledgements

With thanks to Hilary Simons, Claire Stringer, and Dr Lisa Ford for their comments and advice.

 CASE STUDIES

These cases are given as examples only. Always use up to date reference sources when advising actual patients. Seek expert medical opinion for complex patients and/or complicated travel plans.

Case 1
Ellen is a 43-year-old English woman who plans a 10-day cruise which will incorporate travel to the USA, Mexico, Panama Canal, Colombia (Cartegena only), and Barbados. She has chronic renal failure secondary to systemic lupus erythematosus, but does not yet require dialysis. Her current medication includes prednisolone.

Q1. What are the vaccinations required for travel to these areas?

Q2. What other considerations need to be taken into account when recommending appropriate vaccinations for Ellen?

Q3. What malaria prophylaxis is appropriate?

(continued overleaf)

CASE STUDIES (continued)

Case 2

Dorothy is a 56-year-old woman with renal failure secondary to diabetes, now requiring haemodialysis. She is planning a three-week trip through South Africa (Cape Town, Durban, Kruger Park) and onward overland to Zambia (Victoria Falls), returning to South Africa via the Chobe National Park, Botswana. Her current medications are: ramipril, amlodipine, calcium carbonate, alfacalcidol, doxazosin, furosemide and insulin.

Q1. What would be appropriate malaria prophylaxis for travel to these areas?

Q2. Which would be the most appropriate chemoprophylaxis for Dorothy?

Q3. What advice about malaria prophylaxis should be given to Dorothy?

Q4. Which vaccinations are required for travel to these areas?

Case 3

Mary plans a two-week all inclusive hotel holiday to Punta Cana in the Dominican Republic. She had a renal transplant in 1997 and is taking ciclosporin. Her GFR is now 55 mL/min. She is currently well, although she has been treated in the past for post-natal depression. On a previous trip 2 years ago, during which she took proguanil 200 mg daily, there was significant disturbance to her renal function.

Q1. What would be appropriate malarial prophylaxis for travel to Punta Cana?

Q2. Which agent would be most appropriate for Mary?

Q3. Would any other antimalarial be suitable?

Q4. What advice would you give to Mary?

References

1. Bordea C, Wojnarowska F. Educating renal transplant patients about skin cancer. *Br J Ren Med* 2003; 8: 23–26.
2. Paterson P, Hart S, Cahill S. What we tell our patients about OTC medicines. *Br J Ren Med* 1999; 4: 13–16.
3. Mason P. What advice can pharmacists offer travellers to reduce their health risks? *Pharm J* 2004; 273: 651–656.
4. NaTHNaC Travel Health Information Sheet, Prevention of Food and Water Borne Diseases April 2005. www.nathnac.org/pro/factsheets/food.htm (accessed 16 April 2006).
5. Ashley C, Currie A, eds. *The Renal Drug Handbook*, 2nd edn. Oxford: Radcliffe Medical Press, 2004.
6. NaTHNaC Travel Health Information Sheet, Insect Bite Avoidance April 2005. www.nathnac.org/pro/factsheets/iba.htm (accessed 16 April 2006).
7. British Medical Association Board of Science and Education. The impact of flying on passenger health: a guide for healthcare professionals. May 2004. www.bma.org.uk/ap.nsf/Content/Flying?OpenDocument&Highlight=2,impact,flying (accessed 16 April 2006).

8. Goodyear L. Medical kits for travellers. *Pharm J* 2001; 267: 154–158.

9. Chiodini P, Hill D, Lalloo D *et al.* Guidelines for malaria prevention in travellers from the United Kingdom. 2006. http://www.hpa.org.uk/publications/2006/Malaria/Malaria_guidelines.pdf

10. Hughes C, Tucker R, Bannister B, Bradley DJ. Malaria prophylaxis for long-term travellers. *Commun Dis Public Health* 2003; 6: 200–208.

11. Department of Health. *Health Information for Overseas Travel. The Yellow Book.* London: HMSO, 2001.

12. Baxter K, ed. *Stockley's Drug Interactions*, 7th edn. London: Pharmaceutical Press, 2006.

13. NaTHNaC Travel Health Information Sheet, Yellow Fever August 2005. www.nathnac.org/pro/factsheets/yellow.htm (accessed 16 April 2006).

Further information

Guidelines for the prevention of malaria in travellers from the United Kingdom. *Commun Dis Public Health* 2003; 6: 180–199. Available online at www.hpa.org.uk/infections/topics_az/malaria/menu.htm

World Health Organization: *International Travel and Health* – covers vaccination requirements and travel health advice. ISBN: 9241580275. Annual publication available online at: www.who.int/ith/index.html

Department of Health. *Immunisation against infectious disease. The Green Book.* London: HMSO 2006. Also available online at www.dh.gov.uk/PolicyAndGuidance/HealthAndSocialCareTopics/fs/en

Department of Health. *Health Information for Overseas Travel. The Yellow Book.* London: HMSO, 2001. Available at www.nathnac.org (Due for update soon)

Electronic information

British Foreign Office travel warnings: www.fco.gov.uk

NHS Scotland Fit for Travel website: www.fitfortravel.scot.nhs.uk

Health advice for travellers leaflet available free from Post Offices and online: www.dh.gov.uk/travellers

National Kidney Federation holiday pages: www.kidney.org.uk

National Travel Health Network and Centre (NaTHNaC): www.nathnac.org

Travax travel database (requires subscription): www.travax.scot.nhs.uk

World Health Organization: www.who.int

Case study answers

Chapter 3

Q1. What patient and pharmaceutical factors may have precipitated acute renal failure in this patient?

- The patient is elderly.
- He has previously been prescribed bendroflumethiazide on an escalating dose. This in turn precipitated an episode of gout. At this point the thiazide should have been stopped, since thiazide diuretics are contraindicated in gout. This did not happen.
- The colchicine prescribed to treat the gout caused the patient to vomit repeatedly, thus dehydrating him.
- The GP then added in indometacin, which further compromised renal perfusion. The combination therapy of an NSAID, an ACE inhibitor and a diuretic in an already dehydrated patient induced a state of acute renal failure.
- A previous medical history of non-insulin-dependent diabetes mellitus (NIDDM) and hypertension are added risk factors for developing acute renal failure, as they will predispose the patient to having a degree of chronically impaired renal function.
- Acute gout could cause urate uropathy, whereby uric acid crystals are deposited within the renal tubules, causing intrinsic renal damage.

Q2. What are the main pharmaceutical problems and how might they be managed?

- Main pharmaceutical problems are acute renal failure, hyperkalaemia, metabolic acidosis, hyperglycaemia and dehydration.
- There is no actual treatment per se for acute

renal failure. Just provide supportive measures, treat the symptoms and, if possible, the underlying cause, and wait to see if renal function is recovered.

- Stop all oral medications except the ranitidine – the patient is at risk of developing stress ulceration.
- Treat the hyperkalaemia – this is the most life-threatening symptom at present. Initially, the patient could be given salbutamol nebs, followed by insulin and glucose (± calcium gluconate IV), then, if necessary, Calcium Resonium and lactulose.
- Blood glucose levels should be very closely monitored, especially considering the treatment of the hyperkalaemia, and the switch from gliclazide to insulin.
- Although the patient is usually hypertensive, the fact that he is currently severely dehydrated would tend towards a state of hypotension. Therefore, all antihypertensive medications should be stopped temporarily until the patient is euvolaemic, and then reintroduced as necessary.
- Treat the metabolic acidosis with sodium bicarbonate, either IV or PO.
- The hyperglycaemia will respond to the insulin and glucose used to treat the hyperkalaemia. The patient could then be put on a sliding scale insulin infusion, until such time that he is considered stable enough to reintroduce the gliclazide.
- Since the patient is dehydrated, he should receive crystalloid by IV infusion until euvolaemic. Ideally, his CVP should be monitored in order to assess fluid balance. Once the patient is rehydrated, if he still fails to pass urine, stop giving large volumes of fluid replacement. To continue to administer large

volumes of fluid would put the patient at risk of developing severe hypertension and pulmonary oedema. Furosemide should only be given if the patient is euvolaemic or fluid overloaded, and if the drug fails to induce a diuresis, then it should be discontinued, as further use merely increases renal damage. There is no evidence that either mannitol or dopamine are of any benefit.

Q3. Comment on the appropriateness of the prescribed antibiotic therapy. What advice would you provide regarding this?

Mr VC has recovering renal function after an episode of acute renal failure, but at this stage any futher nephrotoxic insults should be avoided.

Ideally, Mr VC should have been prescribed prophylactic antibiotics to cover the insertion of the catheter. Suitable agents would include ciprofloxacin 500 mg PO, or if gentamicin was warranted, a single dose of 80 mg would have been sufficient.

Since Mr VC developed urinary sepsis, even without benefit of cultures and sensitivities, it would be reasonably safe to assume that the patient has a Gram-negative sepsis. As such, oral (500 mg twice daily) or IV (200 mg twice daily) ciprofloxacin would be a good choice. An aminoglycoside would not be first-choice therapy since the associated nephrotoxicity would damage the recovering kidneys, and the accumulated aminoglycoside also puts the patient at increased risk of ototoxicity. However, if it were deemed to be necessary, the dose should be adjusted according to the patient's renal function.

Some centres may wish to use an alternative, less nephrotoxic antibiotic, for example, a second- or third-generation cephalosporin IV, co-amoxiclav, ciprofloxacin, etc. Trimethoprim will probably not be potent enough to treat fullblown urinary sepsis. In addition, anaerobic cover may be required, for example, with metronidazole.

Since Mr VC has fairly rapidly changing renal function, the Cockcroft and Gault equation should be used with great caution. However, as a rough calculation of his current degree of renal impairment:

$$CrCl = \frac{1.23\ (140 - Age) \times Weight}{Serum\ creatinine}$$
$$= \frac{1.23\ (140 - 65) \times 68}{272}$$

i.e. CrCl = approx 23 mL/min.

At this level of renal function, a dose of gentamicin 3–4 mg/kg once every 24 hours could be used, and trough levels monitored, to ensure they are below 1.5–2.0 mg/L before the next dose is given.

Chapter 4

Q1. What are the metabolic abnormalities?

- Renal impairment – acute on chronic
- Hyperkalaemia – life threatening
- Low bicarbonate – from renal impairment causing metabolic acidosis
- Hyperphosphataemia
- Anaemia.

Q2. What has caused the abnormalities?

- Angiotensin II receptor blocker – most likely. The history of ischaemic heart disease and peripheral vascular disease with hypertension suggests renovascular disease.
- Could possibly have any other cause (i.e. volume depletion, obstruction, sepsis, etc.) but this is unlikely given the patient's history.

Learning points

- ACE/angiotensin II blockers are **not** contraindicated in renal impairment. They are the only antihypertensive agents to reduce the progression of renal disease significantly in proteinuric patients. All renal failure patients should be on them – especially those with diabetes, the commonest cause of ESRF. In addition, the majority of ESRF patients die of a cardiovascular event, and many on dialysis develop left ventricular hypertrophy, often secondary to chronic fluid overload. ACE inhibitors are the drug of choice to aid left ventricular remodelling and decrease left ventricular hypertrophy. Renal artery stenosis is the only renal contraindication to their use. Mild hyperkalaemia is relative and usually controllable.

- Angiotensin II blockers, like ACE inhibitors, are contraindicated in renovascular disease.
- Angiotensin II blockers do cause hyperkalaemia but perhaps to a lesser extent than ACE inhibitors.
- The combination of ACE inhibitors/ angiotensin II blockers gives synergistic reduction in blood pressure and proteinuria but also increases the risk of hyperkalaemia.
- Most patients will show some mild deterioration in function after starting ACE/ angiotensin II blocker but do not necessarily have renal artery stenosis

Q3. What is the life-threatening complication and how would you treat it?

Hyperkalaemia.

Learning points

- Calcium gluconate – to stabilise myocardium – competition between potassium and calcium for cardiac muscle binding sites. Calcium gluconate does **not** reduce potassium and is **very** venotoxic. Should be given into a large vein.
- Insulin and dextrose – shifts potassium into cells. Insulin receptor has a potassium channel associated with it. This is very effective at reducing plasma levels of potassium, but does not get rid of potassium. It is only a temporary measure which lasts a few hours before potassium levels will begin to rise again. Patients must receive close monitoring of blood glucose levels.
- Salbutamol (nebulised or IV) – effective, especially if patients are bradycardic with hyperkalaemia. There is a potassium channel associated with the beta receptor.
- Lactulose +++ – diarrhoea is a very effective way to reduce excess fluid and potassium in the body. Beware if already intravascular volume deplete as it will cause profound hypotension.
- Diuretics – high-dose furosemide is a good

way of clearing potassium (e.g. 500 mg to 1 g per day).
- Calcium Resonium – works well but compliance is a problem. Needs to be administered with lactulose to stop bowel congestion. Takes a few days to work
- Dialysis/haemofiltration – in uncontrollable potassium – is the only way to rapidly remove potassium. Has associated risks for patient on dialysis.

Q4. What is the rest of his medication for and how much does it cost per year?

- Calcium carbonate – primarily used as a phosphate binder to limit the amount of dietary phosphate absorbed from the gut. Any excess calcium can be absorbed to treat the hypocalcaemia associated with ESRF. Other phosphate binders commonly used are: calcium acetate, magnesium carbonate, aluminium hydroxide, sevelamer hydrochloride.
- Alfacalcidol – for control of PTH aim for 2–3 times upper limit of normal. Vitamin D is a steroid hormone, and there are vitamin D receptors on the parathyroid glands which help regulate the production of PTH, and hence control bone turnover. ESRF is associated with decreased active vitamin D levels, which coupled with hypocalcaemia and hyperphosphataemia, eventually leads to the development of secondary hyperparathyroidism and hence to renal bone disease.
- Amlodipine – high blood pressure affects almost all chronic renal failure patients. Ischaemic heart disease is much higher than in general population (50–500 times risk). Risk of a 35 year old on dialysis dying of ischaemic heart disease is the same as that of an 85 year old in the general population.
- Atorvastatin – see above. Lipid profiles are different in renal failure. Lower total cholesterol but adverse LDL:HDL ratios. Also higher triglycerides.
- Vitamin supplementation (Ketovite) – ESRF patients are notorious for having poor nutrition. Hyperkalaemia can be life-threatening, so fruit, vegetables and foods generally containing water-soluble vitamins

are on a restricted diet list, therefore patients may require supplements. There is a difference between the tablet and liquid forms. Tablets are water-soluble vitamins, whereas liquid contains fat-soluble vitamins – you cannot interchange them.

- Iron sulfate – due to increased red cell turnover, reduced absorption, increased need with erythropoietin (EPO) therapy. Assessment of iron status in CRF patients is notoriously difficult. There is evidence of altered gut pH in renal patients, which coupled with gut oedema from fluid overload makes renal patients very poor absorbers of oral iron.
- Furosemide – for control of fluid status and salt load. Doses of 500 mg to 1 g daily are not uncommon. Still works even if GFR <5 mL/min.
- Sodium bicarbonate – to reduce acidosis and therefore reduce protein breakdown and bone buffering of H^+ ion. It may lead to a huge salt load (8.4% sodium bicarbonate = 1 mmol/mL therefore 1 L will give a load of 1000 mmol Na^+. One 600 mg tablet contains approx. 7 mmol bicarbonate). May help with hyperkalaemia, but only in minor way.
- EPO – target haemoglobin is approximately 11 g/dL.
- Cost is approximately £4000–6000 per annum.

Chapter 5

Q1. The Senior House Officer (SHO) asks if Mrs AP could be started on ESA therapy. Give three reasons why you might advise against this at this point.

- Her blood pressure is currently uncontrolled – it would make sense to control this before initiating a drug that can elevate blood pressure further.
- No iron studies have been performed at this point. It could be that she is iron depleted and this is the cause of her anaemia. At this level of renal impairment, it may be that erythropoietin deficiency is more likely, but unless any iron deficiency is corrected then ESA therapy will not be effective in raising haemoglobin.

- It could be that she has had an acute bleed – she has CKD, is on an NSAID, and has no gastro-protection. Has the fall in haemoglobin been acute or chronic?

Q2. If ESA therapy is to be initiated, what are the choices in terms of initial dose and monitoring?

Since Mrs AP is not on haemodialysis, she needs her therapy administered by the subcutaneous route, and at the time of preparation this meant therapy with either NeoRecormon (epoetin beta) or Aranesp (darbepoetin). NeoRecormon could be started at 60 units/kg weekly – if Mrs AP were 60 kg this would be 3600 units weekly. Most centres would prescribe this at 2000 units twice a week, to reduce the number of injections that Mrs AP needs, though three times a week would be more efficient. Haemoglobin should rise at 1–2 g/dL monthly, and if this is not happening most prescribers would increase to 4000 units twice weekly, and eventually to 6000 units twice a week. Blood pressure, full blood count, iron stores and potassium need monitoring. If Aranesp is used, the initial dose of 0.45 µg/kg weekly suggests a prescribed dose of 30 µg weekly, monitored and adjusted in a similar manner.

Q3. What factors might contribute to reduced efficiency of ESA therapy in Mrs AP?

The above answer assumes that her iron stores are adequate to ensure erythropoiesis, and if not have been corrected with intravenous iron therapy. In a non-haemodialysis patient, oral iron supplementation with ferrous sulfate may maintain adequate transferrin saturation during erythropoiesis. Care should be taken to avoid interactions between phosphate binders and iron salts. In addition, Mrs AP has a degree of uraemia and hyperphosphataemia, both of which impair erythropoiesis, and factors such as her PTH, folate, B_{12} and so forth are unknown. If angiontensin-converting enzyme (ACE) inhibitors were initiated for her hypertension, these can affect erythropoiesis as well, and finally aluminium from her AluCap capsules may be having an adverse effect. Infections and inflammation can reduce response to ESAs dramatically.

Q4. What factors affect the choice of ESA for Mrs AP?

All the companies have evidence that their product offers certain advantages in different situations, but in general, both Aranesp and NeoRecormon achieve similar responses to therapy, have similar rates of adverse drug reactions and cost about the same (depending on local contracts). Aranesp offers reduced dosing frequency without loss of efficiency, which means fewer injections for non-haemodialysis patients. NeoRecormon has a longer track record, a range of different administration devices, and a very fine needle on the pre-filled syringe and pen device which patients report favourably upon. With the rise of the regional contract in the UK, the choice of product is increasingly being removed from individual prescribers.

Chapter 6

Q1. Why is this patient's hyperphosphataemia worsening?

The progression of CKD further impairs the urinary excretion of phosphate. Compensatory mechanisms to promote phosphate clearance can no longer cope as renal function declines and serum phosphate will continue to rise.

Q2. Are there any symptoms she may now experience secondary to her elevated phosphate?

Hyperphosphataemia contributes to uraemic itching and can also cause redness and soreness in the eyes.

Q3. What would you advise as first-line phosphate-binding agent for Mrs A? What dose would you recommend? How would you educate the patient on why phosphate binders are important, how they work, when to take them and what side-effects to expect?

Calcium-based phosphate binders are currently the first-line agents in many CKD patients, espe-cially in the case of Mrs A because she has co-existing hypocalcaemia. For example, calcium carbonate (Calcichew) at a dose of one or two tablets 5–10 minutes pre-meals may be pre-scribed. Patients need to have some knowledge of why a high phosphate is important (e.g. con-tributes to bone damage), how the drugs work by binding dietary phosphate in the gut (so are very different from their other medicines as they are taken at mealtimes only and dose may vary according to type of meal) and the most common binder side-effects (e.g. gastrointest-inal disturbances).

Q4. What do you think is a realistic target serum phosphate level for Mrs A?

It is generally accepted that achieving a normal phosphate level is unlikely for the majority of CKD patients. Realistic targets in current guide-lines are serum phosphate less than 1.7 or 1.8 mmol/L. Patients should be aware of what their target phosphate is.

Q5. Is vitamin D therapy indicated for Mrs A at this point? If yes, which vitamin D agent and what starting dose would you recommend? If no, why do you think it is appropriate to leave her on Calcichew alone at present?

Ideally, Mrs A would not be commenced on vitamin D at this stage. Her mild hypocalcaemia could be corrected by Calcichew alone, through gastrointestinal absorption of calcium and reduction in serum phosphate, which will increase the proportion of free serum calcium. In practice, some patients would be commenced on vitamin D at this stage – alfacalcidol 0.25 µg daily is a commonly prescribed regimen.

Q6. What other biochemical investigation(s) would you request at this stage in the management of Mrs A's renal bone disease? How would knowledge of the result(s) influence your decision to initiate or hold off vitamin D therapy?

A serum parathyroid hormone (PTH) is indi-cated for Mrs A. It is a vital part of the bio-chemical bone profile used to guide prescribing of phosphate binders and particularly vitamin

D. A high PTH would indicate a significant degree of secondary HPT is already present – requiring prescription of vitamin D for its direct and indirect effects to suppress PTH secretion. In CKD patients, vitamin D is used mainly for its actions to control secondary HPT, not simply correcting hypocalcaemia. A mildly raised PTH would mean less need for vitamin D at present – controlling phosphate alone will directly suppress PTH secretion.

Q7. What are the other two commonly prescribed phosphate binders available to the nephrology team?

Aluminium hydroxide (AluCap) or sevelamer hydrochloride (Renagel).

Q8. Considering the advantages and disadvantages of each of these agents, which one would you recommend and what would be your suggested starting dose?

Aluminium less likely to be used by nephrologists these days. Concerns over toxicities such as dementia, anaemia and adynamic bone disease, though controversial, mean that many renal units only use it short term, particularly as an additional agent to control severe hyperphosphataemia. However, aluminium binders are cheap and potent – a dose of one AluCap capsule with meals would be an effective starting dose for Mrs A. Sevelamer would be a more likely prescribed drug in many renal units. It has the benefit of being calcium- and aluminium-free but is expensive and has gastrointestinal side-effects to match other binders. Also, it is less potent than aluminium- and probably calcium-based binders so in this case Mrs A would need to start on two or three tablets with meals.

Q9. How can vitamin D therapy cause complications in the management of renal osteodystrophy?

The effectiveness of vitamin D in management of secondary HPT can be limited by its dose-related actions:

- Hypercalcaemia
- Exacerbation of hyperphosphataemia.

Also, overzealous use of vitamin D in CKD patients can lead to excessive suppression of PTH secretion, which increases the risk of inducing low bone turnover forms of renal osteodystrophy (e.g. adynamic bone disease). Target levels for PTH in CKD are not normal range – for example in ESRD usually aim for 3–5 times upper limit of normal range.

Q10. What would you suggest as a vitamin D plan in Mrs A and what are the reasons behind your decision? Stop alfacalcidol? Reduce alfacalcidol dose? Continue alfacalcidol at current dose? Increase alfacalcidol dose?

Using the serum PTH alone, Mrs A needs a dose increase in her alfacalcidol but the elevated calcium and (to a lesser extent) phosphate effectively contraindicate this plan at the moment. However, the hypercalcaemia is only mild so the benefits of continuing alfacalcidol to continue management of HPT probably outweigh the risks of stopping it and seeing PTH rise even higher. Reducing the dose (e.g. to 0.25 µg daily) or even continuing current dose appear to be reasonable options, particularly as you have now switched Mrs A to a calcium-free phosphate binder. In either case, it is very important to check the bone biochemistry more frequently during this period of hypercalcaemia, for example in two weeks time, to review response to changes in the renal bone disease drug regimen.

Q11. What form of renal osteodystrophy is likely to have contributed to Mrs A's fracture and how does it influence bone turnover?

Mrs A's bone disease predominantly appears related to secondary HPT, in view of the raised PTH and alkaline phosphatase. This is known as osteitis fibrosa. The excess PTH is acting on the bone to increase activity of both osteoblasts and especially osteoclasts so it is classed as a high bone turnover form of renal osteodystrophy.

Q12. Why are the doctors concerned about extraskeletal manifestations of an abnormal bone biochemistry profile (i.e. calcification) in Mrs A? At which sites in the body can calcification occur in a CKD patient? How can calcification impact on the morbidity and mortality of CKD patients?

Calcification is increasingly recognised as a significant problem in CKD patients and can be present at various sites, for example:

- Soft tissue and peripheral vasculature (in its most severe form this can progress to calciphylaxis)
- Skin, joints, lungs, cornea, conjunctivae and muscle
- Cardiovascular system (myocardium, coronary arteries, aorta and cardiac valves).

Calciphylaxis is rare but difficult to manage and is associated with a high mortality rate. Cardiovascular calcification is a much greater problem because the most common causes of morbidity and mortality in CKD patients have cardiovascular aetiology. Cardiovascular disease in CKD patients is multifactorial in origin but evidence is accumulating for the importance of the role of calcification and how disturbances of bone biochemistry influence this.

Q13. What are the benefits of prescribing higher doses of calcium-free phosphate binders (sevelamer and/or aluminium hydroxide) for Mrs A in relation to preventing further bone fractures and reducing her calcification risk?

For Mrs A, knowledge of the risks of calcification mean that her abnormal bone biochemistry needs to be managed more aggressively and not simply to protect her bones. Increasing phosphate binder doses will hopefully bring down both serum phosphate and PTH which will have benefits for the bones. More intensive use of calcium-free phosphate binders in Mrs A may also reduce her calcification risk and potentially provide an associated reduction in cardiovascular risk through the following actions:

- Reducing hyperphosphataemia
- Reducing calcium burden by avoiding calcium-based phosphate binders
- Correcting severe HPT with associated fall in serum calcium
- Reducing calcium × phosphate product.

Chapter 7

Q1. What risk factors does he have for CHD?

A TC:HDL-C ratio of 6.9 exceeds the ratio of 6.0 (from the Sheffield table[14]) and indicates a risk of CHD >30% over 10 years. Treatment with a statin and aspirin is indicated. Even without the Sheffield table, diabetes is a risk factor for CHD, as is hypertension and a cholesterol >5 mmol/L. Therefore a statin should be started, at low dose considering his renal impairment.

Q2. What treatment would be suggested with respect to his blood pressure?

He has been hypertensive for some time so drug therapy is indicated. Considering his diabetes an ACE inhibitor would be first choice, with a calcium channel blocker second line. Monitor renal function closely.

Q3. What other advice would be appropriate?

To minimise his CHD risk, he should be advised to stop smoking, given advice on a healthy, low-salt diet, and encouraged to exercise regularly and keep alcohol intake low. He should be referred to a nephrologist and pre-dialysis clinic to minimise his renal disease.

Chapter 8

Q1. At the monthly multidisciplinary meeting, a haemodialysis patient's urea reduction ratio is only 50%. What can be done to improve their adequacy?

Adequacy can be improved by increasing the size of the dialyser, time on dialysis, increasing the blood flow (the patient's access may restrict this). If there are problems with access then the patient should be referred to the vascular surgeon. If possible the patient could be changed to haemodiafiltration.

Q2. Miss RB is an 80-year-old woman recently started on haemodialysis. After about an hour on dialysis she becomes hypotensive. What can be done about it?

The first thing would be to get Miss RB's dry weight assessed. In the acute situation, fluid should be given to the patient and her feet raised above her head. In the longer term, anti-hypertensive medication could be omitted on dialysis days or given post dialysis. If she is not on any blood pressure medication then midodrine (unlicensed) given 1 hour before dialysis or fludrocortisone may be commenced. Sometimes stopping the patient from eating on dialysis can help. In an ideal world, changing to haemofiltration could help, but that is rarely practical. If possible, the patient could be changed to haemodiafiltration, which can improve cardiovascular instability. Again, that is not available in every unit.

Q3. Mr MP has recently started on CAPD and has been having problems with pain on draining in his fluid. What could be the reason for his pain and what dialysis fluid should he use?

The reason for Mr MP's pain could be that the dialysis fluid he is using is too acidic for his peritoneal membrane and that is causing him pain. It could also be that too much fluid is being drained in and he may need the volume reduced initially. Mr MP could also be changed to a more biocompatible fluid with bicarbonate added to it (e.g. Physioneal or Balance). Before these fluids were available sodium bicarbonate or lidocaine were added to the bags, but that sometimes leads to an increased incidence of peritonitis as aseptic technique cannot always be assured.

Q4. Mr BA is a 45 year-old man on peritoneal dialysis. He was admitted with abdominal pain the previous evening. What are the possible causes of his abdominal pain and what should be done?

Possible causes of abdominal pain are constipation or peritonitis. A sample of the peritoneal fluid should be sent off for white cell count and cultures and sensitivities. If the bag is cloudy then peritonitis should be assumed and antibiotics started empirically (e.g. vancomycin and gentamicin) and altered once sensitivities are known (antibiotics may vary between different units). His white cell count came back at 1926 mm^3 with 80% polymorphs. The organism isolated was *Staph. epidermidis*, which is sensitive to vancomycin, so the gentamicin was stopped. An abdominal X-ray should be taken to check for constipation. If constipation is confirmed then treatment with laxatives should be commenced, if there is no success with senna and lactulose then stronger laxatives such as Picolax may be required.

Q5. On checking the notes it appears that Mr BA has had a couple of peritonitis episodes in the past few months and is a known staph carrier. What would you recommend?

He could be started on prophylactic nasal mupirocin for 5 days a month in case that is the reason for his repeated episodes of infection. The peritoneal dialysis team should also check his technique in case he is having problems at home.

Q6. Miss RB did not have good enough veins for a fistula so has a permanent catheter in place. She has come in today and the line is not working. What can be done?

Both urokinase and alteplase can be used to unblock lines. A lock of 5000 IU urokinase or 2 mg alteplase may be tried initially. Both would be left in for an hour. If this did not work then an infusion of urokinase 10 000–250 000 IU over 3–24 hours or alteplase 20–50 mg over 12–20 hours would be done. If all else fails, the line would have to be removed. If it became a chronic problem then she might be started on low-dose aspirin or clopidogrel if she did not tolerate the aspirin.

Q7. Mr MC has only been on haemodialysis a few weeks and it was noticed that his platelet count has fallen quite dramatically. Heparin-induced thrombocytopenia (HIT) has been diagnosed. What can be used as an anticoagulant for his dialysis?

In patients with HIT one of the first things to try would be heparin-free dialysis. If anticoagulation was required then epoprostenol could be used, although it can be quite difficult to get the correct flow rate. Other alternatives would be a bolus dose of danaparoid 2000–3750 units or lepirudin 0.14–0.15 mg/kg pre-dialysis or a bolus dose and continuous infusion of argatroban 2–3 µg/kg/min (started at least 4 hours before dialysis) or as a bolus of 250 µg/kg at the start of dialysis followed by a continuous infusion of 2 µg/kg/min.

Chapter 9

Q1. What recipient factors might have led to JL remaining on the waiting list for over 3 years?

Average waiting times for a kidney transplant are in the order of 2 years. The renal transplant allocation system is complicated and takes into consideration ABO blood group, HLA tissue-type matching, known and declared recipient HLA or ABO antibodies, time on the waiting list and the age and size of both the donor and recipient.

JL has waited longer than average. It is possible that she would have anti-HLA or ABO antibodies from her pregnancies or blood transfusion which might have resulted in a longer wait for a compatible match. It is also possible that she might have been suspended from the transplant waiting list for the periods when she had active peritonitis.

Q2. Which medicines should be stopped at this point and which would normally continue to be prescribed?

The epoetin, B-group vitamins, folic acid, phosphate binder and alfacalcidol can all safely be stopped once a patient is transplanted, even if there is delayed graft function. Alfacalcidol is usually continued only if the recipient has had a parathyroidectomy.

It is usual to stop antihypertensive medications and review if there is a continued need once the kidney is working. Most units will delay starting an ACE inhibitor in the early post-operative period as sudden increases in serum creatinine can be difficult to interpret (rejection, calcineurin inhibitor toxicity or ACE inhibitor induced). However, in the medium term, diabetic kidney transplant recipients will usually receive an ACE inhibitor or angiotensin II receptor blocker, even in the absence of transplant proteinuria.

Aspirin is usually withheld for a few days peri-operatively and reintroduced once the bleeding risk has diminished. There is an enduring indication for a statin. Simvastatin could be continued as tacrolimus is not known to significantly increase the risk of myopathy; however, some units would opt to use a lower dose or an alternative statin.

Subcutaneous insulin would usually be replaced with an intravenous sliding scale peri-operatively.

Q3. What other antirejection strategy might have been considered and could it be justified?

Induction immunosuppression with an IL-2R antibody such as basiliximab is an option which is supported by NICE in combination with a tacrolimus-based triple therapy. In this case the patient has a poorly HLA-matched graft which is a risk factor for acute rejection and so this strategy would be justified.

Q4. Is this tacrolimus level usually considered adequate?

Early tacrolimus levels of between 10 and 15 ng/mL are more normal though some centres opt to use lower doses, particularly where there is a high risk of delayed graft function.

Q5. What might be contributing to this level?

There is great inter-patient variability in the dose of tacrolimus required to achieve target trough levels. This is the main justification for intensive early therapeutic drug monitoring. It is also possible that the carbamazepine required for her diabetic neuropathy has induced higher activity in liver and gut wall cytochrome P450 isoenzymes resulting in greater tacrolimus clearance and lower than expected trough levels.

Q6. What input can the pharmacist make to maximise the chances of medicine regimen adherence?

This patient has a number of potential risk factors for non-adherence in that she is a single person caring for young children, she is blind and has a new and potentially complicated medicine regimen about which she currently knows very little.

The first priority is to simplify JL's regimen into twice daily tablet dosing, the timing of which can be fitted into her life. Medicines can be taken at mealtimes in the same way as she manages with her insulin.

JL needs to be educated about her new medicines. She needs to know the basics of what each medicine is, how she should take it and to develop a strategy for tablet/capsule recognition. This might be best served with a monitored dosage system (MDS) if it is her wish. Care must be taken to ensure that tacrolimus is not taken before clinic visits. In addition JL should be aware of those medicines such as the prophylactic antibiotics which have a fixed duration.

She must then be given as much information as she needs to understand the implications of the medicines. She can pass written information to a family member if desired. If this is satisfactory for her, and she can participate in treatment decisions, her adherence can be as full as is clearly the case with her diabetes care.

Q7. If the transplanted kidney continues to function poorly what could be the possible reasons?

The most likely reasons would be ongoing steroid-resistant rejection, recoverable acute tubular necrosis (ATN) secondary to either an acute rejection or a nephrotoxic level of tacrolimus or lastly a surgical issue such as graft thrombosis.

Q8. What treatment options would be typical?

In such a scenario it is most likely that the graft would be again be re-biopsied to define the problem. Ongoing rejection despite steroid would require treatment with rATG or muromonab-CD3. ATN would require 'watchful waiting'.

Even in light of a known rejection episode a dose adjustment of tacrolimus is necessary for a level of 18 ng/mL. Dose adjustments should be proportional to the desired level; if 12 mg/day results in a level of 18 ng/mL then it is reasonable to assume that 9 mg/day will result in the target range of between 12 and 14 ng/mL

Q9. In addition to co-trimoxazole what other prophylaxis might you expect to see on this recipient's TTA?

Three months of CMV prophylaxis is likely as the donor was CMV positive and the recipient was known to be CMV negative 3 years earlier, making the likelihood of primary infection and disease very high. Most transplant centres will repeat the recipient's CMV IgG status when bloods are taken immediately before the transplant. If this shows that the patient has seroconverted between transplant listing and being called then the choice of whether to continue with prophylaxis is centre-specific. With an improving renal function at the point of discharge it is imperative that the dose of antiviral continues to be correlated with graft function.

Antifungal prophylaxis might also be considered for the early period of transplant immunosuppression.

Chapter 10

Q1. Is the dose of flucloxacillin reasonable for a haemodialysis patient?

The SPC for flucloxacillin states that its use in patients with renal impairment does not usually require a dose reduction. However, it also states that in the presence of severe renal failure (creatinine clearance <10 mL/min) a reduction in dose or extension in dosage interval should be considered. As described in the text previously, patients undergoing intermittent haemodialysis should be considered in the category of CrCl <10 mL/min when choosing drug doses. Although it has stipulated a creatinine clearance for 'severe' renal failure, the SPC does not indicate how to reduce the dose or change the dosage interval. From the SPC we can also see that the usual IV dose for flucloxacillin is 250 mg—1 g four times daily, doubled in severe infection. Following an IV dose, 76.1% is recovered in an active form in the urine and a small proportion of the dose is excreted in the bile. Excretion of flucloxacillin is slowed in the presence of renal failure.

Evidently the excretion of flucloxacillin will be affected by renal failure but as specific dosage instructions are not given in the SPC it is prudent to consult other available texts. The *Renal Drug Handbook* suggests dosing for haemodialysis patients should be the same as those for normal renal function up to a maximum of 4 g per day.[18]

As Mr PT has a sepsis and the source is thought to be the tunnelled line needed for haemodialysis it is important to treat quickly and to get high therapeutic levels. The consequences of undertreating are a deterioration of Mr PT's health due to sepsis and the removal of his haemodialysis line. It would therefore seem appropriate to use the dose of 1 g four times daily.

Q2. Should supplementary doses be given on dialysis days?

Supplementary doses should only be used in haemodialysis if significant drug removal takes place during the haemodialysis and where there is a long delay before the next dose is due. The SPC states 'flucloxacillin is not significantly removed by dialysis and hence no supplementary dosages need to be administered either during or at the end of the dialysis period.' This could also have been predicted from the pharmacokinetic data as flucloxacillin is 95% protein bound and therefore significant removal is unlikely.

Q3. How should Mr PT be monitored?

Mr PT has been prescribed a high dose of flucloxacillin for someone receiving haemodialysis, therefore he should be monitored for signs of toxicity and adverse effects. The SPC can be consulted for the whole list of side-effects but the most important ones are: CNS toxicity including convulsions; hepatitis and cholestatic jaundice (liver function tests should therefore be monitored); and diarrhoea and antibiotic-associated colitis. Any of these would necessitate a change in therapy. It is also important to note that the flucloxacillin injection has a sodium content of 2 mmol/g. This will be important in his fluid assessment and interpretation of blood results.

As important as measuring toxicity Mr PT needs to be monitored for therapeutic efficacy. His temperature and white blood cell count should be regularly monitored as well as the clinical symptoms. If he does not improve a change of antibiotic and/or removal of his haemodialysis line will be required.

The administration of IV iron to Mr PT during his illness should also be reviewed as IV iron may worsen his infection.

Chapter 11

Q1. What are the metabolic abnormalities?

The metabolic abnormalities exhibited by the patient are:

- Acute renal failure
- Hypokalaemia
- Hypomagnesaemia
- Hypocalcaemia.

When all electrolytes are reduced like this, it suggests a renal tubular leak syndrome.

Q2. What has caused these abnormalities?

The cause of these abnormalities is almost certainly cisplatin.

- Cisplatin causes acute renal impairment and a tubular leak syndrome by affecting the S3 segment of the proximal tubule. Thirty per cent of patients are affected. Most recover but up to 20% can be left with a long-term reduction in renal function. Biopsies of these patients show tubular fibrosis. Up to 30% of patients can have long-term magnesium wasting.
- Prednisolone is not nephrotoxic.
- Methotrexate is nephrotoxic, especially in high doses, where it can precipitate in the tubules. It can produce a transient reduction in GFR during infusion but this generally recovers immediately on stopping the drug. It is almost entirely renal excreted and needs dose reduction in renal failure to reduce toxicity.
- Bleomycin is not nephrotoxic but needs dose reduction when the GFR is <25–35 mL/min (i.e. moderate renal impairment).

- In addition, amongst other chemotherapeutic agents, cyclophosphamide can cause haemorrhagic cystitis and lead to bladder malignancy in future. Ifosphamide can give haemorrhagic cystitis but also a Fanconi-like syndrome with metabolic acidosis, hypokalaemia, hypophosphataemia, nephrogenic diabetes insipidus, aminoaciduria and renal impairment.
- Almost all chemotherapy agents can induce a haemolytic uraemic syndrome.
- In cases where the patient has a large tumour mass, you can get a tumour lysis syndrome, where the breakdown products from tumour cell destruction can block the filtering system in the kidneys, causing acute renal failure.

Q3. How can you avoid this complication?

This complication can be avoided in future by:

- Calculating Mr NT's body surface area (BSA) using his ideal body weight rather than his actual body weight. His BSA using his actual weight of 101 kg is 2.09 m². However, calculating his ideal body weight to be 64 kg, his BSA in this instance would be 1.72 m² . This would have a marked impact on the dose of cisplatin he would be given, and dosing according to his ideal body weight BSA would significantly reduce the risk of nephrotoxicity.
- Fluid loading with sodium chloride. Fluid loading increases the renal clearance of these agents by enhancing urine output, but more importantly a high chloride concentration can reduce the toxicity of the platinum drug. Cisplatin is toxic in cells with low chloride concentrations by forming reactive hydroxyl radicals with water. Therefore increasing chloride will reduce toxicity and some suggest giving cisplatin in hypertonic saline (e.g. sodium chloride 1.8%).
- Choosing an alternative chemotherapeutic agent. Carboplatin is said to be less toxic, especially since the dose is based on the area under the curve (AUC) exposure to the drug, and so automatically adjusts for renal impairment, but it may also be less effective with

some tumours. Oxaliplatin may be as effective but less toxic.
- Amifostine is an organic thiophosphate and can donate a thiol group to reduce toxicity. It has only been tested in high-dose platinum therapy in ovary and small cell lung carcinoma, but it reduces nephrotoxicity.

Q4. What has happened now?

Mr NT's pre-existing renal impairment from his previous course of chemotherapy has predisposed him to damage from further renal insults. The subsequent course of cisplatin has now caused the patient to develop cisplatin-induced renal impairment.

By day 4 he already has severe renal impairment (calculated creatinine clearance of 16 mL/min using the Cockcroft and Gault equation) and he will require renal replacement therapy should his renal function deteriorate further.

Q5. Comment on the antibiotic therapy he has been prescribed. Do you need to intervene?

This is not the best choice of antibiotics for neutropenic sepsis and it is probably better to liaise with microbiology for a better combination. However, in the case of this particular combination, several of them are renally excreted, therefore will accumulate in patients with impaired renal function, and cause severe side-effects. Hence, it will be necessary to modify several of the dosage regimens. Note, if a drug is renally excreted and accumulates, the toxicity seen is not necessarily nephrotoxicity, but an exaggeration of whatever the symptoms may be in overdosage of this drug, for example, neurotoxicity, bone marrow suppression, etc.

Q6. What would you recommend?

For the existing prescription, the following points should be taken into account:

- Metronidazole – metabolised by liver, no dosage reduction necessary in renal impairment.
- Ceftazidime – renally excreted, and toxic in overdose (mainly neurotoxicity). Must substantially reduce the dose in renal

impairment. Suggest 1 g three times or twice daily in Mr NT and monitor response.

- Amikacin – exclusively renally excreted, and extremely nephrotoxic and ototoxic. Under no circumstances should the full dose of 7.5 mg/kg twice daily be attempted, as has been prescribed. With Mr NT's current level of renal function, suggest giving a stat dose of 2 mg/kg, waiting 24 hours and doing random trough level, then dosing again as necessary, when the trough is less than 5 mg/L. This dose will need to be reviewed should Mr NT be commenced on renal replacement therapy.

Also note that the patient's renal function is deteriorating rapidly, therefore using the Cockroft and Gault equation to estimate renal function will be unreliable. It will be necessary to reassess the patient's renal function each day, and adjust drug dosages accordingly.

Other possible antibiotics that could be prescribed for neutropenic sepsis include:

- Meropenem – again, this drug is excreted via the renal route, so the dose will need to be reduced in severe renal impairment.
- Tazocin – this drug has dual liver and renal excretion, but the dose should be modified slightly in severe renal impairment.

Chapter 12

Case 1

Q1. What diagnosis is most likely to be made?

The most likely diagnosis is Wegener's granulomatosis. The presence of c-ANCA and granulomatous lesions distinguish it from other types of vasculitis. Haemoptysis is likely to be due to pulmonary haemorrhage which is also more common in Wegener's granulomatosis.

Q2. What initial treatment would you recommend?

Initial treatment should be IV pulsed methylprednisolone 1 g daily for 3 days. Followed by oral prednisolone 1 mg/kg/day. Then IV cyclophosphamide 7.5 mg/kg every two weeks for three doses then monthly for six months. This is the dose adjusted for GFR <10 mL/min. Cyclophosphamide is renally excreted and requires dose adjustment. A further reason for dose reduction would be the patients age as elderly patients are more susceptible to adverse events.

Q3. How would you monitor this therapy?

Cyclophosphamide suppresses the bone marrow so a full blood count including neutrophils is imperative. The nadir for bone marrow suppression is 10 days after administration so this would be the best time to take a blood sample. Cyclophosphamide may also affect liver function so liver enzymes should also be checked. Prednisolone therapy can cause hyperglycaemia, lipid abnormalities and hypertension so these parameters should be checked regularly. A bone density scan may be appropriate if the prednisolone can not be tapered quickly and long-term therapy is required. Success of treatment is measured by a resolution of symptoms, improvement in renal function and a reduction in c-ANCA titre.

Q4. What adjunctive therapies would you consider for this patient?

- Oral mesna for prevention of urothelial toxicity given 2 hours before, 2 hours after and 6 hours after the cyclophosphamide infusion.
- Metoclopramide should be prescribed for nausea. Ondansetron is a suitable alternative if metoclopramide is ineffective.
- Co-trimoxazole for prevention of *Pneumocystis jiroveci* (*P. carinii*) pneumonia. Dapsone may be used in patients allergic or intolerant to co-trimoxazole.
- Proton pump inhibitor such as omeprazole 20 daily to reduce the risk of gastric ulceration while on concomitant prednisolone.
- Osteoprophylaxis with calcium and vitamin D supplements should be considered. Bisphosphonates such as alendronate 70 mg weekly should also be considered though this is unlicensed in patients with a GFR <10 mL/min.

Q5. What advice would you give to the patient regarding their new treatment regimen?

- Patients taking immunosupression are at higher risk of infection and should be advised to seek medical advice at the onset of any signs of infection such as coughs and colds.
- Cyclophosphamide may cause thrombocytopenia so patients should be asked to report any unexplained bruising or bleeding.
- Patients should be asked to carry a steroid card and advised to avoid contact with people with chickenpox.
- The importance of complying with immunosuppressive therapy should be stressed as, in addition to the risk of disease progression, relapses require further immunosuppressive therapy which carries complications.

Case 2

Q1. What drug therapy would you suggest?

First-line therapy for any patient with proteinuria is ACE inhibition. A suitable starting regimen would be ramipril 1.25 mg daily increasing every few days in increments of 1.25–2.5 mg according to blood pressure.

Q2. What is the target blood pressure for this patient?

The target blood pressure in patient with proteinuric renal disease is <125/75 mmHg.

Q3. What is the prognosis for Mr Y?

Mr Y's renal function has deteriorated despite maximal supportive treatment. Hypertension and proteinuria have also persisted which are all poor prognostic markers. Progression of kidney disease is likely to continue if further interventions are not made. It may be appropriate to start an immunosuppressive regimen.

Q4. What further drug therapy would you recommend?

Although evidence for immunosuppression in IgA nephropathy is not definitive, Mr Y's condition is deteriorating quite rapidly so further efforts are required to arrest the decline in renal function as the alternative may be dialysis! An suitable regimen would be oral cyclophosphamide 2 mg/kg/day together with prednisolone 1 mg/kg/day. The prednisolone dose may be tapered gradually provided there is no deterioration in symptoms. There is no consensus on the length of course.

Chapter 13

Q1. How would you determine the baby's GFR?

It is very difficult to determine the GFR accurately. Normal GFR based on age can be determined by Fawer's table = 13 mL/min/1.73 m². However, as the baby's creatinine is measured as 234 µmol/L (normal range 53–97 µmol/L) it can be seen that the baby is in chronic renal failure.

Q2. Describe the therapy that should be initiated and why.

The baby should be started on chronic renal failure medicines. As the phosphate is above 2 mmol/L, calcium carbonate as a phosphate binder should be prescribed. Start with a small dose (125 mg) given with each 4-hourly feed and adjust as necessary. Calcium level is in the normal range but the baby has a very high PTH at 10.0 pmol/L. To ensure strong and healthy bones alfacalcidol should be prescribed, but the serum calcium needs to be monitored.

The haemoglobin is 12 g/dL. Oral iron and folic acid should be prescribed. The kidneys will be unable to produce erythropoietin so epoetin therapy should be initiated at 100 units/kg SC once a week. The ferritin level will need to be measured.

Monitoring of U&Es should continue on a daily basis at this early stage and adjustments to therapy made as necessary.

Blood pressure and fluid balance should be measured daily.

Q3. How would you ensure that the child maintains optimum growth and development?

The baby must be referred to a dietician who will advise on the best feeds whilst encouraging mum to continue to breastfeed. The urea is in the high range of normal so the dietician must improve nutrition to reduce this. The baby must not gain weight in the form of fluid. Regular measurement of weight (daily), length and head circumference must be made and plotted on a growth chart.

Tube feeding may be required if vomiting becomes a problem.

Q4. The parents are told that the baby will need to start dialysis in the very near future, and will ultimately require a transplant. The parents are very keen to donate a kidney as soon as possible. They are aware of the work up required, but what is the earliest age that a transplant could go ahead and why?

Before a transplant can be considered all vaccinations must be up to date. An accelerated immunisation schedule can be carried out but the earliest age at which a child can be transplanted is 19/20 months.

Q5. What is the likely diagnosis and what would you therefore recommend that mum should do?

The baby almost certainly has peritonitis. The baby must be admitted to hospital immediately, and as the baby shows signs of systemic illness IV vancomycin and IV ciprofloxacin should be prescribed. A PDF sample should be sent to microbiology and the peritoneal dialysis regimen should be changed to continuous cycling. Treatment will then be modified according to microbiology results.

Chapter 14

Q1. Assess his renal function, and decide whether it will be necessary to adjust the dosage of his antibiotics and any other medications.

In the acute phase of illness, reviewing clinical findings, particularly urine output, will often give a better guide to renal function than laboratory tests. This is because creatinine and other markers of renal impairment take time to accumulate. Consequently there is a lag time

before results accurately reflect renal function. If you use the serum creatinine results and the Cockcroft and Gault formula you will calculate an estimated creatinine clearance of between 80 and 85 mL/min, but as previously explained this information is likely to be misleading. This is because MF has stopped passing urine, effectively meaning that he is in ARF, and his creatinine clearance is more likely to be less than 10 mL/min.

In the early stage of disease all dosing decisions should therefore be based on a clinical assessment, and creatinine clearance calculations only used once a steady state has been reached. This typically occurs within 3–4 days of admission, depending on the speed of onset and the severity of the renal failure.

The dosage of drugs should be confirmed in standard sources. Additionally, in critically ill patients you need to ensure that therapeutic levels of antibiotics are achieved quickly by using a loading dose. This usually means giving a typical maximum single dose (e.g. cefotaxime 2 g, and 2.4 g benzylpenicillin). Thereafter the dosage should be adjusted to allow for the renal dysfunction (i.e. cefotaxime 1 g four times daily and benzylpenicillin 1.2 g every four hours).

Renal failure should not affect dosage of inotropic agents such as noradrenaline (norepinephrine) and other catecholamines as these have very short half-lives and are not renally cleared. These drugs are always given according to response.

Q2. The standard protocol for sedating patients on the ICU uses a combination of morphine and midazolam. The clinical staff are concerned about drug accumulation with these agents. What are the options to prevent accumulation?

Morphine and midazolam are standard sedative agents in many ICUs but are more likely to cause oversedation in renal failure due to accumulation of active metabolites. There are various options to prevent oversedation. One is to use regular (daily) sedation holds when the sedation is stopped to offset the risk of accumulation. Alternatively non-accumulating agents such as fentanyl or alfentanil for analgesia, and propofol or lorazepam for anaesthesia could be used. These medicines tend to be more expensive but this additional cost maybe cancelled out as delayed recovery from sedation is less likely. The downside is that clinical staff maybe unfamiliar with these agents and therefore use them inefficiently, resulting in poor-quality sedation if too little is given, or accumulation if too much is given. In practice there is no right or wrong drug choice, the key issue is to use the chosen agents carefully.

Q3. The CVVHF system is configured to an ultrafiltration rate of 30 mL/kg/h. Are any dosage modifications required for the drugs mentioned above and for the following additional agents – enoxaparin SC 40 mg once daily, ranitidine IV 50 mg three times daily, and IV insulin infusion to maintain a blood glucose of 5–8 mmol/L?

An ultrafiltration rate of 30 mL/h/kg is equivalent to 30×70 (i.e. 2100 mL/h or 35 mL/min). This is maximum drug clearance that can be achieved by the CVVHF device. As for all other dosage decisions you should always refer to standard sources, but with drugs that are renally cleared you will also need to consider the CVVHF clearance. In this case the following dosages are suitable for a patient with ARF receiving 35 mL/h CVVHF clearance.

- Cefotaxime 2 g four times daily
- Benzylpenicillin 1.8 g every 4 hours
- Sedation, insulin and inotropes – according to response
- Ranitidine 50 mg twice daily
- Enoxaparin 40 mg once daily.

Note: Enoxaparin thromboprophylaxis is usually omitted as the patient will probably be receiving anticoagulation to facilitate the CVVHF. Typical agents used are unfractionated heparin or epoprostenol.

Q4. Are any dosage modifications required for this agent, and are any additional precautions necessary?

Drotrecogin alfa (activated protein C) is cleared systemically so no dosage adjustment is necessary. A more important concern is to stop any additional anticoagulants as this will increase the potential for haemorrhagic side-effects. Drotrecogin alfa will also provide more than adequate anticoagulation for CVVHF.

Q5. What options are available to manage MF's metabolic acidosis?

MF's metabolic acidosis is probably due to a combination of renal impairment and anaerobic metabolism secondary to organ hypoperfusion and sepsis. This anaerobic metabolism is reflected by the raised blood lactate level which is due to excess lactate production and an inability to metabolise this to bicarbonate. The best method to correct this acidosis is to offset the causes (e.g. improve tissue perfusion by use of inotropes and fluid resuscitation) and the use of CVVHF. In this case a bicarbonate-based haemofiltration fluid should be chosen as the replacement fluid as opposed to a lactate-based fluid. The latter will probably aggravate the already raised lactate levels.

Chapter 15

Q1. Comment on this prescription. What interventions might you make?

Prescription for amitriptyline and tramadol MR. Things to consider:

- Tramadol, amitriptyline and fluoxetine can all increase serotonin levels, therefore using all three together gives much increased risk of developing serotonin syndrome. Therefore this combination is best avoided.
- Tramadol, amitriptyline and fluoxetine can all lower the seizure threshold, therefore using all three together increases the risk of this occurring
- Tramadol is 90% excreted in urine and little is removed by dialysis. Use a non-MR (modified release) preparation at 50 mg twice daily in ESRF.
- Tramadol is converted to its active form (M1 metabolite) in the body. It has been proposed that SSRIs block this conversion process, therefore rendering tramadol inactive. This would be another reason for not using these two drugs together.

- In some cases an SSRI and a TCA can be used together. This would usually be in a situation where a patient had neuropathic pain that was responding to a TCA and was also depressed. The first option would be to try and increase the TCA to an antidepressant dose, but often this is not tolerated. Then the next step would be to try an SSRI. If the two classes of drugs were being used together then the dose of amitriptyline would be limited to a maximum of 75 mg once daily. (SSRIs are thought to inhibit the metabolism of TCA by cytochrome P450 CYP2D6 resulting in increased serum concentrations of the TCA.)

Suggestions for treatment:

- Consider using gabapentin at reduced dosage instead of amitriptyline.
- Consider an alternative analgesic to tramadol (e.g. co-codamol 30/500). Would need to discuss what the patient had tried before.

An important point to note is that the patient feels no one believes she has pain, as no physical cause for it has been found. This is quite a common scenario; the majority of chronic pain patients do not have a physical cause for their pain. An important part of the treatment process is to reassure patients that you do believe them and try to help them understand the reasons why their pain is occurring.

Chapter 16

Q1. What might her causes of diabetes be?

Hypertension and/or obesity.

Q2. What might her causes of chronic renal failure be?

Poorly controlled blood glucose and blood pressure.

Q3. Could it have been prevented?

Yes, tight blood glucose and blood pressure has been proven by the DCCT, UKPDS and Kumamoto studies to reduce the risk of developing microvascular complications.

Q4. What might her causes of acute renal failure be?

Sepsis, drug-induced (metformin and or valsartan) or hypovolaemia.

Q5. Explain her drug history and any possible reasons for stopping some of her medication on admission.

Triple OHA therapy, as mentioned in the chapter, may be beneficial for a 2–3 month period as glitazones can take several months to show their full effect, although initiating insulin treatment should not be delayed if there is pancreatic beta cell exhaustion. Metformin, as discussed earlier, is safe to use in chronic renal failure as long as the GFR is above 60 mL/min/1.73 m^2. In this particular case, it is sensible to stop metformin and withhold rosiglitazone and glicazide on admission until investigations are done and DP's blood glucose levels return to above 5 mmol/L and she is able to eat.

ACE inhibitors and angiotension II receptor antagonists have been shown to reduce the rate of progression in both diabetic nephropathy and non-diabetic nephropathy, so it seems sensible for DP to be on valsartan. What is not known is whether this has caused the acute renal episode, so bilateral renal artery stenosis needs to be ruled out, but also DP has presented with extremely low BP. ACE inhibitors/angiotension II receptor antagonists can also cause hyperkalaemia and as DP presented with high potassium the valsartan is stopped.

Beta-blockers should be used with caution in diabetes as they may mask hypoglycaemia, but it is not a contraindication to treatment. NICE have recently published an update for hypertensive treatment and no longer sanction their use unless no other alternative can be found. DP is a long standing patient so it is not unreasonable for this patient to present on this treatment, although it may be an opportunity to trial an alternative agent when her BP begins to normalise.

Flucloxacillin and cefalexin initiated by the GP for cellulitis are known to cause interstitial nephritis, so this may be another cause of acute renal failure, although the likelihood is low. Cephalosporins can also cause diarrhoea, so this may be the culprit for DP's presenting diarrhoea.

Q6. Why would this patient take atorvastatin and aspirin?

The major causes of death in type 2 diabetes are cardiovascular-related illnesses, so all patients with diabetic kidney disease should take a low-dose aspirin and a lipid-lowering agent for vascular protection.

Q7. Why change this patient's diabetic regimen to insulin?

DP has a history of poorly controlled blood glucose levels and a HbA1c result of 9% despite triple OHA therapy. This may be a result of pancreatic beta cell exhaustion. If there is some residual insulin secretion then an option for DP could be a daytime metformin with a nocturnal insulin, although this is probably not an option due to the failure of the triple OHA therapy. The best treatment at this stage for DP is a twice a day insulin regimen, as recommended by the diabetologist with careful monitoring for hypoglycaemia and weight gain.

Q8. Would the regimen differ if the patient had ESRF?

In ESRF the risk of hypoglycaemia is higher as the kidney, with the liver, metabolise circulating insulin, so in kidney impairment or failure this will result in an accumulation of this circulating insulin and thus hypoglycaemia. In ESRF the insulin regimen may require a dose reduction or a switch to a once a day basal human analogue such as glargine or levemir.

Q9. Comment on BP control in diabetes.

As already discussed, ACE inhibitors and angiotensin II receptor antagonists are beneficial in diabetic nephropathy and as there is no renal vascular disease restarting DP on her valsartan is sensible but at a lower dose with a recommendation to titrate the dose to maximise BP control to ≤135/75 mmHg. Beta-blockers, also mentioned before, are not contraindicated in diabetes but this may be an ideal opportunity to recommend an alternate agent. The patient's BP on discharge was below the recommended target so at this stage another antihypertensive agent is not necessary, but a recommendation of a calcium channel blocker could be noted for the follow-up plans.

Q10. What discharge plans should be made for this patient?

The patient has been switched from OHA therapy to injecting insulin therapy, which is a huge change for DP, so she will need education and training for insulin administration and monitoring from a diabetic link nurse. Education on diet and exercise will also be necessary due to the increased side-effect of weight gain with insulin therapy. Awareness of hypoglycaemia needs emphasising to DP again due to the increased incidence with insulin therapy. Follow-up within the community for blood glucose and blood pressure monitoring will also need to be organised as well as regular screening for ESRF.

Chapter 17

Q1. He has been transferred to your ward. As the ward pharmacist, what further information would you like to know?

Drug history – pre-admission, during hospital stay, any allergies.

Q2. At the previous hospital he was given gentamicin, vancomycin and pamidronate? Could any of these contribute to his renal failure?

Gentamicin, vancomycin and pamidronate can all cause ARF.

Q3: What would be your pharmaceutical care plan at this stage?

See ARF pharmaceutical care – avoid nephrotoxic drugs, check fluid status, and consider the need for further therapy of hypercalcaemia and the need for antibiotics.

Q4. Would your pharmaceutical care plan change at this stage? Outline a new pharmaceutical care plan.

- Ensure that the correct doses have been prescribed – any requirement for modification in view of renal impairment?
- Ensure appropriate supportive therapy is prescribed
- Timings of doses relative to dialysis
- Monitor for adverse effects
- Patient counselling.

Q5. After 10 days Mr CB remains haemodialysis-dependent as his renal function has not improved. The renal team would like to treat Mr CB's anaemia and commence an erythropoesis-stimulating agent. What dose would you recommend? Are there any other factors to consider?

Patients with anaemia due to bone marrow infiltration, chemotherapy and kidney disease may require higher doses of chemotherapy. Any of the currently licensed erythropoesis-stimulating agents may be given – see individual summary of product characteristics for detailed dosing advice.

Chapter 18

Q1. What are the possible causes of his pain?

The pain in the left leg could be due to diabetic neuropathy or metastases, and the pain in his shoulder is likely to be due to metastases.

Q2. How would you manage his nausea and vomiting?

Adding in metoclopramide will act as an antiemetic and also help diabetic gastroparesis. Dose reduction in end stage renal disease is recommended, although normal doses are used regularly in practice.

Q3. What might be causing his pain? What other treatment would you consider to relieve his pain?

The pain is likely to be due to restless legs (see Table 18.6).

Q4. What would you discuss at this stage? What medications could you ensure were prescribed for the last few days of life?

Discuss conservative management, including active symptom management, analgesia, antiemetic, sedative and glycopyrronium.

Chapter 19

Q1. What advice would you give him?

For each patient the renal diet is different. It depends on the patient's normal dietary intake, stage of kidney disease, biochemistry and treatment. Dietary restriction may include protein, phosphate, potassium, sodium and fluid. As his biochemistry is within acceptable ranges and his weight is fairly steady, only healthy eating, low salt advice would be given. If Mr Smith is overweight then advice to reduce his weight, leading to a decrease in blood pressure, and some lifestyle advice should be given. This would include advice about increasing exercise and decreasing the amount of salt within his diet by avoiding convenience foods and by cooking with fresh ingredients. If ready-made foods are the only way to ensure that a patient's nutritional status is not compromised then the patient should be advised to look at the food labelling and choose products that contain 0.25 g salt (0.1 g sodium) or less per 100 g.

His biochemistry, weight and appetite should be monitored closely.

Q2. What advice would you give him now?

Advice would be give to limit the dairy foods – milk, cheese, yoghurts, offal meats, nuts, fish with edible bones and shellfish – ensuring that he was meeting his protein and energy requirements to prevent malnutrition.

Q3. What further dietary measures would be needed?

First check for non-dietary causes of hyperkalaemia, such as drugs or blood transfusions. Second, review the diet to check for nonnutritious potassium foods (use of salt substitutes, excessive intake of fruit and fruit juice, vegetables and potatoes that have not been boiled in water). It is essential at this stage to ensure the diet remains nutritionally adequate so a full dietetic assessment is necessary.

Q4. Which supplements would you suggest?

Supplements chosen would depend on the patient's nutritional requirements, biochemistry, other medical history – diabetes, patient likes and dislikes. The basic 1.5 kcal/mL milk-based supplements are Ensure Plus, Fortisip, Fresubin Energy and Resource shake. Other options include fruit juice-based supplements – Enlive, Fortijuice (which are higher in glucose than the milk-based supplements). Supplements not recommended for renal patients are Build-up and Complan. Food fortification is also recommended with fats (fried foods, olive oil, double cream, Calogen) or with sugar (fizzy drinks, glucose-based polymers – Vitajoule, Maxijul).

Always ensure that the patient is referred to a dietician so a detailed nutritional assessment can be carried out and the patient is monitored.

Chapter 20

Case 1

Q1. What are the vaccinations required for travel to these areas?

Check that Ellen's British schedule is up to date. A tetanus booster may be required if her last dose was more than 10 years ago. The Americas are considered polio free, so polio vaccination is not required provided Ellen is fully vaccinated according to the British schedule. Pneumoccocal, influenza, hepatitis A and yellow fever (for Colombia) are normally advised where not medically contraindicated (see below: caution with live vaccines).

Q2. What other considerations need to be taken into account when recommending appropriate vaccinations for Ellen?

Yellow fever is a live vaccine which would not be recommended to an immunocompromised traveller such as Ellen. This should be discussed with travel health experts and the supervising clinician. If she travels unprotected by the vaccine, she should minimise her risk of yellow fever transmission by remaining on the ship in Colombia and taking good insect bite precautions during daylight hours if on deck/land. A yellow fever certificate would be required for onward travel to Barbados (who require certificate of vaccination from all travellers arriving from, or passing through, endemic areas). If Ellen is unable to receive the vaccine, she would require a letter of medical exemption from the vaccination. This may be taken into consideration by port officials but should not be considered an automatic waiver.

Ellen's response to any vaccination may be suboptimal. Food and water hygiene and insect bite precautions should be emphasised.

Q3. What malaria prophylaxis is appropriate?

Ellen is travelling to low-risk areas for malaria and so does not require chemoprophylaxis. Full bite protection measures, however, should be taken. The importance of recognising signs and symptoms of malaria should also be discussed with Ellen. She should be advised to seek rapid medical attention if she develops any flu-like symptoms, fever, or any other unexplained symptoms, 7 days or more after entering a malarial area and for up to one year after exit.

Case 2

Q1. What would be appropriate malaria prophylaxis for travel to these areas?

Dorothy is travelling to Kruger (South Africa), Zambia, and Botswana which are risk areas for falciparum malaria. The Advisory Committee on Malaria Prevention recommends mefloquine, doxycycline, or Malarone.

Q2. Which would be the most appropriate chemoprophylaxis for Dorothy?

Mefloquine would be the most suitable option. Malarone (atovaqone/proguanil) is contraindicated for severe renal failure. Dorothy's calcium-based phosphate binder may interact with doxycycline and reduce its antimalarial effects.

Q3. What advice about malaria prophylaxis should be given to Dorothy?

Dorothy should be advised to ideally start taking the mefloquine three weeks before travel. She should take it at the same time each week, for the duration of her trip and for four weeks after leaving Africa. The importance of taking the medication regularly and for the full duration should be emphasised. She should also be informed about the possible adverse effects of mefloquine, and to seek medical advice should they occur so a suitable alternative can be prescribed.

It is important that Dorothy understands the need for scrupulous mosquito bite precautions in addition to chemoprophylaxis.

Dorothy should also be made aware of the signs and symptoms of malaria. She should be advised to seek rapid medical attention if she develops any flu-like symptoms, fever, or any other unexplained symptoms, 7 days or more after entering a malarial area and for up to one year after exit.

Q4. Which vaccinations are required for travel to these areas?

Check Dorothy's British schedule is up to date and give booster doses of tetanus and polio if her last doses were more than 10 years ago. Pneumococcal, influenza, hepatitis A, hepatitis B and typhoid are normally recommended. Her holiday dialysis unit will also usually require Dorothy's hepatitis B immune status. Rabies vaccine could also be offered, although it is not generally suggested for short trips. Dorothy should be given advice about risk avoidance and the importance of post-exposure treatment for rabies, which is required whether or not pre-exposure vaccine has been received.

Zambia was declared yellow fever free by the World Health Organization in 2002 and Dorothy is not at personal risk of this disease for this itinerary.

Case 3

Q1. What would be appropriate malarial prophylaxis for travel to Punta Cana?

There is a risk of malaria in the Dominican Republic, including recently (2005) to tourist travellers who have only stayed in coastal areas. Chloroquine or proguanil are usually recommended.

Q2. Which agent would be most appropriate for Mary?

Neither drug is ideal for Mary. Proguanil should be avoided due to her previous reaction to the drug. If chloroquine is prescribed there is an increased risk of ciclosporin toxicity, as the plasma concentration of ciclosporin can be increased by chloroquine. Careful monitoring of ciclosporin levels would be required and dose adjustments made accordingly.

Q3. Would any other antimalarial be suitable?

Other agents used for malaria chemoprophylaxis are Malarone, mefloquine and doxycyline. Malarone contains proguanil so is not an option. Mefloquine is contraindicated due to Mary's previous medical history of post-natal depression.

Doxycycline, like chloroquine, may interact with ciclosporin and increase the plasma concentration of ciclosporin. Close monitoring with appropriate ciclosporin dose adjustments would be required to prevent toxicity.

Q4. What advice would you give to Mary?

Mary should consider the option of changing her holiday to a non-malarious destination.

Glossary

Absolute iron deficiency Marked by low serum ferritin.

Accelerated phase hypertension Essential hypertension characterised by acute onset, severe symptoms, rapidly progressive course, and poor prognosis.

Acute tubular necrosis (ATN) The term used to describe the pathology where tubular cells have died and have not yet been replaced by new ones.

Adaptive immune system The cellular aspect of the immune systems of higher life forms which allow recognition and memory of pathogens.

Adynamic bone disease Low turnover bone disease, where bone cell activity is reduced or absent. In contrast to osteomalacia, there is no increase in bones lacking minerals. People with adynamic bone disease have a tendency to develop more fractures and blood vessel calcification.

Allograft A transplanted organ sourced from a non-identical member of the same species.

Amyloidosis Amyloids are insoluble fibrous protein aggregations sharing specific structural traits. Amyloidosis is defined as any extracellular, proteinaceous deposit exhibiting cross-beta structure.

Anaphylactoid Resembling anaphylaxis or anaphylactic shock, i.e. hypersensitivity (as to foreign proteins or drugs) resulting from sensitisation following prior contact with the causative agent.

Antinociception Reduction in the perception of pain (nociception).

Apoptosis One of the main types of programmed cell death. As such, it is a deliberate process of life relinquishment by a cell in a multicellular organism. In contrast to necrosis, which is a form of cell death that results from acute cellular injury, apoptosis is carried out in an ordered process that generally confers advantages during an organism's life cycle.

Atherosclerosis An arteriosclerosis characterised by atheromatous deposits in and fibrosis of the inner layer of the arteries

Anuria Passing less than 50 mL urine per day.

β_2-Microglobulin A component of MHC class I molecules, which are present on almost all cells of the body (red blood cells are a notable exception). In patients on long-term haemodialysis, they can aggregate into amyloid fibres that deposit in joint spaces, a disease known as dialysis-related amyloidosis.

Biocompatible Not having toxic or injurious effects on biological function.

Cachectic A profound and marked state of constitutional disorder; general ill-health and malnutrition

Calciphylaxis An adaptive response that follows systemic sensitisation by a calcifying factor (as a vitamin D) and a challenge (as with a metallic salt) and that involves local inflammation and sclerosis with calcium deposition, leading to necrotic skin lesions.

Cardiogenic shock Shock resulting from failure of the heart to pump an adequate amount of blood as a result of heart disease and especially heart attack.

Carpal tunnel syndrome Swelling within the carpal tunnel causing pain and numbness in one half of the hand.

Chronic allograft nephropathy (CAN) Alternatively termed chronic rejection. The insidious and slow deterioration of transplanted kidney function.

Complex regional pain syndrome A chronic progressive disease characterised by severe pain, swelling and changes in the skin.

C-Reactive protein (CRP) A protein produced by the liver that is normally present in trace amounts in the blood serum but is elevated during episodes of acute inflammation (as those associated with neoplastic disease, chronic infection, or coronary artery disease).

Cryoglobulins Circulating proteins (e.g. IgM) which become insoluble at reduced temperatures – less than 4°C. The reaction is reversible; redissolution occurs at 37°C.

Cryoglobulinaemia The presence in the blood of cryoglobulin, which is precipitated in the microvasculature on exposure to cold.

Cytolytic enzymes Enzymes which cause the death of a cell by bursting, often by osmotic mechanisms that compromise the integrity of the cellular membrane.

Delayed graft function (DGF) The temporary and usually recoverable period where a patient may continue to require dialysis after a transplant.

Darbepoetin An erythropoiesis-stimulating agent made by Amgen.

Dyslipidaemia A condition marked by abnormal concentrations of lipids or lipoproteins in the blood.

Dysplastic kidneys A condition of both kidneys where the tissue is partly normal with some normal glomeruli but laced throughout the kidney is fibrosis (like scar tissue), abnormal cell groups such as little pieces of cartilage, and immature tissue where the kidney did not finish developing.

EBPG European Best Practice Guidelines for renal anaemia.

ElectroCardioGram ECG – a trace of the electrical activity of the heart.

Echocardiography The use of ultrasound to examine and measure the structure and functioning of the heart and to diagnose abnormalities and disease.

Echogenicity Reflecting ultrasound waves.

Ectopic calcification Extraskeletal calcification, i.e. calcium phosphate deposits in soft tissues and blood vessels.

En-bloc transplant Where both kidneys from a single donor are transplanted into a single recipient.

Endothelin Any of several polypeptides consisting of 21-amino-acid residues that are produced in various cells and tissues, which play a role in regulating vasomotor activity, cell proliferation, and the production of hormones, and that have been implicated in the development of vascular disease.

Epoetin Erythropoiesis-stimulating agent made by various companies that is very similar to natural erythropoietin.

Erythrocyte Red blood cell.

Erythropoietin Hormone that stimulates erythropoiesis.

Erythropoiesis The production of red blood cells (as from the bone marrow).

Erythropoiesis stimulating agent ESA – substance that stimulates erythropoiesis (e.g. epoetin or darbepoetin)

Euvolaemia Normal circulatory or blood fluid volume within the body.

Extracorporeal circuit Blood circulation in a circuit occurring or based outside the living body (e.g. blood passing around a haemodialysis circuit).

Fanconi syndrome A disorder in which the proximal tubular function of the kidney is impaired, resulting in decreased reabsorption of electrolytes and nutrients back into the bloodstream. Compounds involved include glucose, amino acids, uric acid, phosphate and bicarbonate. The reduced reabsorption of bicarbonate results in type 2 or proximal renal tubular acidosis,

Fibromyalgia A chronic syndrome characterised by diffuse or specific muscle, joint, or bone pain, fatigue, and a wide range of other symptoms.

Functional iron deficiency Marked by transferrin saturation or % hypochromic cells.

Gastroparesis Also called delayed gastric emptying, a disorder in which the stomach takes too long to empty its contents. Is usually caused by damage to the vagus nerve, especially in diabetic autoneuropathy.

Glomerular filtration The forcing, under high pressure, of small molecules such as water, glucose, amino acids, sodium chloride and urea, from the blood in the renal afferent arteriole across the glomerular basement membrane of the Bowman's capsule and into the nephron.

Glomerulonephritis Nephritis marked by inflammation of the capillaries of the renal glomeruli.

Glycosuria The presence in the urine of abnormal amounts of sugar.

Granulomatous lesions Small nodules that are seen in a variety of diseases such as Crohn's disease, tuberculosis and sarcoidosis, They are composed of a group of epithelioid macrophages surrounded by a lymphocyte cuff.

Haematocrit The percentage of the volume of whole blood that is composed of red blood cells as determined by separation of red blood cells from the plasma usually by centrifugation. A haematocrit ranging from 42% to 52% in males and 35% to 47% in females is typically considered normal – also called packed cell volume.

Haematuria The presence of blood or blood cells in the urine.

Haemodynamic Relating to or functioning in the mechanics of blood circulation.

Haemolytic uraemic syndrome (HUS) An inflammatory reaction leading to acute renal failure (ARF) and disseminated intravascular coagulation (DIC). The fibrin mesh destroys red blood cells and captures thrombocytes, leading to a decrease of both on full blood count. Can be caused by *Escherichia coli* toxin, HIV, lupus, post-partem, malignant hypertension, scleroderma and cancer chemotherapy. There is also familial HUS, an inherited condition.

HbA1c Glycosylated haemoglobin – it is primarily a treatment-tracking test reflecting average blood glucose levels over the preceding 90 days (approximately).

Hepatorenal syndrome Functional kidney failure associated with cirrhosis of the liver and characterised typically by jaundice, ascites, hypoalbuminaemia, hypoprothrombinaemia and encephalopathy

Homeostasis The maintenance of relatively stable internal physiological conditions (as body temperature or the pH of blood) in higher animals under fluctuating environmental conditions.

Hyperacute rejection The almost immediate response to donor antigen where a recipient has preformed antibody.

Hypernatraemia The presence of an abnormally high concentration of sodium in the blood.

Hyperplasia Abnormal increase in the number of normal cells in normal arrangement in an organ or tissue, which increases its volume.

Hyperviscosity syndrome An increase in the viscosity of the blood. This may be caused by an increase in serum proteins and may be associated with bleeding from mucous membranes, retinopathy and especially monoclonal gammopathies such as in multiple myeloma. An increased viscosity secondary to polycythaemia may be associated with organ congestion and decreased capillary perfusion.

Hypoalbuminaemia Hypoproteinaemia marked by reduction in serum albumin.

Hypochromic anaemia An anaemia marked by deficient haemoglobin and usually microcytic red blood cells and associated with lack of available iron.

Hypovolaemia Decrease in the volume of the circulating blood.

Immunomodulation Modification of the immune response or the functioning of the immune system by the action of an immunomodulator.

Induction immunosuppression Drugs used peri-operatively and in the first few weeks after transplant to augment the long-term immunosuppression strategy.

Intimal proliferation Thickening of the walls forming blood vessels or renal tubules.

Left ventricular hypertrophy (LVH) The thickening of the myocardium (muscle) of the left ventricle of the heart. Disease processes that can cause LVH include any disease that increases the afterload that the heart has to contract against (e.g. aortic stenosis, aortic insufficiency and hypertension), and some primary diseases of the muscle of the heart.

Luminal obliteration Shrinkage, leading to disappearance of the lumen of blood vessels or tubules within the kidney.

Maintenance immunosuppression Oral drugs, with different and complimentary mechanisms of action, usually taken in combination for the life of the transplanted organ.

Microalbuminuria The measurement of small amounts of albumin in the urine that cannot be detected by urine dipstick methods, typically the excretion of 30–300 mg of albumin/24 hours.

Microangiopathic Conditions associated with a disease of very fine blood vessels.

Myositis Inflammation of a muscle, especially a voluntary muscle, characterised by pain, tenderness, and sometimes spasm in the affected area.

Nephropathy An abnormal state of the kidney; especially one associated with or secondary to some other pathological process.

Nephrotoxic Poisonous or damaging to the kidney, as in nephrotoxic drugs.

NMDA (N-methyl-D-aspartic acid) An amino acid derivative acting as a specific agonist at the NMDA receptor, mimicking the action of the neurotransmitter glutamate, and associated with learning and memory.

Nocturia Urination at night especially when excessive.

Non-heart beating donor (NHBD) Where the organs originate from a cadaver who does not fall into the typical heart-beating, brain-stem dead donor category.

Nephrosclerosis Hardening of the kidney; *specifically*: a condition that is characterised by sclerosis of the renal arterioles with reduced blood flow and contraction of the kidney that is associated usually with hypertension and that terminates in renal failure and uraemia.

Neuropathic pain Chronic pain resulting from injury to the central or peripheral nervous system.

Oliguria Passing less then 400 mL urine per day.

Osteodystrophy Defective ossification of bone usually associated with disturbed calcium and phosphorus metabolism.

Osteomalacia A disease of adults that is characterised by softening of the bones and is analogous to rickets in the young.

Panel reactive antibodies (PRA) A measure of a patient's level of sensitisation to a standard panel of donor antigens.

Periarticular Relating to, occurring in, or being the tissues surrounding a joint.

Pericarditis Inflammation of the pericardium, the conical sac of serous membrane that encloses the heart and the roots of the great blood vessels.

Peritubular cells Cells found adjacent to or surrounding a renal tubule.

Plasma oncotic pressure In blood plasma, the dissolved compounds have an osmotic pressure. A small portion of the total osmotic pressure is due to the presence of large protein molecules; this is known as the colloidal osmotic pressure, or oncotic pressure.

Plasma exchange A procedure used to separate the plasma from the blood. After plasma separation, the blood cells are returned to the person undergoing treatment, while the plasma, which contains the unwanted antibodies, is discarded and the patient receives replacement donor plasma or saline with added proteins in its place.

Plasmapheresis A procedure used to separate the plasma from the blood. After plasma separation, the blood cells are returned to the person undergoing treatment, while the plasma, which contains the unwanted antibodies, is first treated and then returned to the patient.

Pleural effusion An exudation of fluid from the blood or lymph into a pleural cavity.

Polycystic kidney disease Either of two hereditary diseases characterised by gradually enlarging bilateral cysts of the kidney which lead to reduced renal functioning. (a) A disease that is inherited as an autosomal dominant trait, is usually asymptomatic until middle age, and is marked by side or back pain, haematuria, urinary tract infections, and nephrolithiasis. (b) A disease that is inherited as an autosomal recessive trait, usually affects infants or children, and results in renal failure.

Polyuria Renal disorder characterised by the production of large volumes of pale dilute urine (usually >5 L/24 hours); often associated with diabetes.

Post-herpetic neuralgia A condition resulting after nerve fibres are damaged during a case of herpes zoster, causing chronic pain that may persist or recur for months or years in the area affected.

Postural hypotension Symptoms include dizziness, lightheadedness, headache, blurred vision and fainting, generally occurring after sudden standing. It can be caused by blood pooling in the lower extremities; venous return and cardiac output are further compromised, resulting in further lowering of arterial pressure.

Pure red cell aplasia (PRCA) A type of anaemia affecting the precursors to red blood cells but not to white blood cells. In PRCA, the bone marrow ceases to produce red blood cells. Pure red cell aplasia is regarded as an autoimmune disease.

Purpura The appearance of red or purple discolorations on the skin, caused by bleeding underneath the skin. Small spots are called petechiae, while large spots are called ecchymoses.

Pyelonephritis Inflammation of both the parenchyma of a kidney and the lining of its renal pelvis especially due to bacterial infection.

Renal artery stenosis Narrowing of the major artery that supplies blood to the kidney. Renal artery stenosis can lead to seriously elevated blood pressure. Common causes of renal artery stenosis include atherosclerosis and thickening of the muscular wall (fibromuscular dysplasia) of the renal artery.

Renoprotective Protection against damage to the kidney.

Residual urine output The amount of urine still passed by patients.

Reticulocytes Erythrocyte precursors.

Reticulo-endothelial system A diffuse system of cells of varying lineage that include especially the macrophages and the phagocytic endothelial cells lining blood sinuses and that were originally grouped together because of their supposed phagocytic properties.

Retroperitoneal fibrosis Proliferation of fibrous tissue behind the peritoneum often leading to blockage of the ureters – also called Ormond's disease.

Rhabdomyolysis The destruction or degeneration of skeletal muscle tissue (as from traumatic injury, excessive exertion, or stroke) that is accompanied by the release of muscle cell contents (as myoglobin and potassium) into the bloodstream, resulting in hypovolaemia, hyperkalaemia, and sometimes acute renal failure.

Scleroderma A usually slowly progressive disease marked by the deposition of fibrous connective tissue in the skin and often in internal organs and structures, by hand and foot pain upon exposure to cold, and by tightening and thickening of the skin.

Serum ferritin Protein that reflects iron stored as ferritin in tissues.

Systemic inflammatory response syndrome (SIRS) An inflammatory state of the whole body (the 'system') without a proven source of infection. SIRS can be considered to be a subset of cytokine storm, a general term for cytokine dysregulation.

Thromboxanes Any of several substances that are produced especially by platelets, are formed from endoperoxides, cause constriction of vascular and bronchial smooth muscle, and promote blood clotting.

Transferrin Iron carrier protein, reflects available iron.

UF coefficient A measure of how permeable the dialyser is.

Vasculitis Inflammation of a blood or lymph vessel.

Vasculitides A group of conditions characterised by inflammation of blood or lymph vessels.

Index

Page numbers in *italic* refer to figures, tables and boxes.